American Public Health Association
VITAL AND HEALTH STATISTICS MONOGRAPHS

DIFFERENTIAL MORTALITY IN THE UNITED STATES: A STUDY IN SOCIOECONOMIC EPIDEMIOLOGY

DIFFERENTIAL MORTALITY IN THE UNITED STATES: A STUDY IN SOCIOECONOMIC EPIDEMIOLOGY

EVELYN M. KITAGAWA
and
PHILIP M. HAUSER

1973 / HARVARD UNIVERSITY PRESS
Cambridge, Massachusetts

Library of Congress Catalog Card Number 72-93951
SBN 674-20561-8
Printed in the United States of America

PREFACE

This volume in the monograph series of the American Public Health Association (APHA) brings together the key findings of three research undertakings of the Population Research Center at the University of Chicago. One is the Matched Records Study funded by the National Institutes of Health, which involved matching of death certificates for a sample of persons who died in the United States between May and August 1960 to the 1960 Population Census schedules. The second is the series of investigations of differential mortality in the Chicago area from 1930 to 1960 based on the allocation of deaths to census tract of residence of decedents and using the characteristics of the population in the census tract as socioeconomic controls. The third involved the analysis of special tabulations of 1959-61 deaths from all causes, which were compiled by the National Center for Health Statistics for the APHA monograph series.

The 1960 Matched Records Study was conceived and designed by a combination of University of Chicago and federal government personnel. It was funded by a Research Grant (RG-7134) from the National Institutes of Health to the Population Research Center. Lillian Guralnick of the National Center for Health Statistics and Charles Nam of the Bureau of the Census collaborated with the authors in the design of the study and the collection and processing of the basic data. They had earlier carried out a pretest in Memphis which paved the way for the Matched Records Study. Lillian Guralnick served as a consultant throughout the study with special reference to problems relating to the death records, and Charles Nam served as a consultant in respect to the problems involved in the matching operation at the Bureau of the Census. An informal Advisory Committee was also an important resource in the launching of the investigation. It included Dr. Iwao Moriyama of the National Center for Health Statistics, Dr. Harold Dorn of the National Institutes of Health, and Mr. Mortimer Spiegelman of the Metropolitan Life Insurance Company, who was subsequently the General Editor of the APHA monograph series.

The basic data for the analysis of trends in socioeconomic differentials in the Chicago area were derived from two Ph.D. dissertations and two research projects carried out at the Population Research Center, one of which was funded by a grant from the U.S. Public

Health Service (Research Grant 4397 [R]) to the Population Research Center. The analysis of the 1959-61 tabulations of deaths was subsidized by a Research Grant to the APHA from the Public Health Service (Research Grant CH 00075).

Parts of the materials in this volume have been previously published—some in more condensed form and some in preliminary form, as indicated in the appropriate sections. In coordinated, integrated, and supplemented form they reinforce each other and, it is hoped, have synergistic impact.

The authors are indebted to their colleagues in the Population Research Center for support and counsel, directly and indirectly. Thea Hambright served as Research Assistant on the 1960 Matched Records Project, 1965-66, and supervised most of the computational work carried out during this period. Chen-Tung Chang and Helen Chang, Research Assistants on the project from 1966 to 1969, completed most of the remaining computations for the monograph. Acknowledgment must be made of the supervisory services of Hana Okamoto, Administrative Assistant, and of the editorial and typing services of Wilhelmina Crawford and Adele Kaye. Finally, acknowledgment is gratefully made of the administrative and professional support of Mortimer Spiegelman, who unfortunately did not survive to witness the completion of the volume; and of his successor, Dr. Carl Erhardt, who patiently shepherded the authors into the final tasks of completing this manuscript.

Evelyn M. Kitagawa

Chicago, 1972   Philip M. Hauser

CONTENTS

TABLES

APPENDIX TABLES

FIGURES

FOREWORD

Rapid advances in medical and allied sciences, changing patterns in medical care and public health programs, an increasingly health-conscious public, and the rising concern of voluntary agencies and government at all levels in meeting the health needs of the people necessitate constant evaluation of the country's health status. Such an evaluation, which is required not only for an appraisal of the current situation but also to refine present goals and to gauge our progress toward them, depends largely upon a study of vital and health statistics records.

Opportunity to study mortality in depth emerges when a national census furnishes the requisite population data for the computation of death rates in demographic and geographic detail. Prior to the 1960 census of population there had been no comprehensive analysis of this kind. It therefore seemed appropriate to build up for intensive study a substantial body of death statistics for a three-year period centered around that census year.

A detailed examination of the country's health status must go beyond an examination of mortality statistics. Many conditions such as arthritis, rheumatism, and mental diseases are much more important as causes of morbidity than of mortality. Also, an examination of health status should not be based solely upon current findings, but should take into account trends and whatever pertinent evidence has been assembled through local surveys and from clinical experience.

The proposal for such an evaluation, to consist of a series of monographs, was made to the Statistics Section of the American Public Health Association in October 1958 by Mortimer Spiegelman, and a Committee on Vital and Health Statistics Monographs was authorized, with Mr. Spiegelman as Chairman, a position he held until his death on March 25, 1969. The members of this Committee and of the Editorial Advisory Subcommittee created later are:

Committee on Vital and Health Statistics Monographs

Carl L. Erhardt, D.Sc., Chairman
Paul M. Densen, D.Sc.
Robert D. Grove, Ph.D.
Clyde V. Kiser, Ph.D.
Felix Moore
George Rosen, M.D., Ph.D.

William H. Stewart, M.D.
  (Withdrew June 1964)
Conrad Taeuber, Ph.D.
Paul Webbink
Donald Young, Ph.D.

Editorial Advisory Subcommittee

Carl L. Erhardt, D.Sc., Chairman   Eliot Freidson, Ph.D.
Duncan Clark, M.D.   (Withdrew February 1964)
E. Gurney Clark, M.D.   Brian MacMahon, M.D., Ph.D.
Jack Elinson, Ph.D.   Colin White, Ph.D.

The early history of this undertaking is described in a paper presented at the 1962 Annual Conference of the Milbank Memorial Fund.[1] The Committee on Vital and Health Statistics Monographs selected the topics to be included in the series and also suggested candidates for authorship. The frame of reference was extended by the Committee to include other topics in vital and health statistics than mortality and morbidity, namely fertility, marriage, and divorce. Conferences were held with authors to establish general guidelines for the preparation of the manuscripts.

Support for this undertaking in its preliminary stages was received from the Rockefeller Foundation, the Milbank Memorial Fund, and the Health Information Foundation. Major support for the required tabulations, for writing and editorial work, and for the related research of the monograph authors was provided by the United States Public Health Service (Research Grant CH 00075, formerly GM 08262). Acknowledgment should also be made to the Metropolitan Life Insurance Company for the facilities and time that were made available to Mr. Spiegelman before his retirement in December 1966, after which he devoted his major time to administering the undertaking and to serving as general editor. Without his abiding concern over each monograph in the series and his close work with the authors, the completion of the series might have been in grave doubt. The published volumes will be a fitting memorial to Mr. Spiegelman even though his name does not appear as an author.

The New York City Department of Health allowed Dr. Carl L. Erhardt to allocate part of his time to administrative details for the series from April to December 1969, when he retired to assume a more active role. The National Center for Health Statistics, under the supervision of Dr. Grove and Miss Alice M. Hetzel, undertook the

---

[1] Mortimer Spiegelman, "The Organization of the Vital and Health Statistics Monograph Program," *Emerging Techniques in Population Research* (*Proceedings of the 1962 Annual Conference of the Milbank Memorial Fund*; New York: Milbank Memorial Fund, 1963), p. 230. See also Mortimer Spiegelman, "The Demographic Viewpoint in the Vital and Health Statistics Monographs Project of the American Public Health Association," *Demography*, vol. 3, No. 2 (1966), p. 574.

sizable tasks of planning and carrying out the extensive mortality tabulations for the 1959-1961 period. Dr. Taeuber arranged for the cooperation of the Bureau of the Census at all stages of the project in many ways, principally by furnishing the required population data used in computing death rates and by undertaking a large number of varied special tabulations. As the sponsor of the project, the American Public Health Association furnished assistance through Dr. Thomas R. Hood, its Deputy Executive Director.

Because of the great variety of topics selected for monograph treatment, authors were given an essentially free hand to develop their manuscripts as they desired. Accordingly, the authors of the individual monographs bear the full responsibility for their manuscripts, and their opinions and statements do not necessarily represent the viewpoints of the American Public Health Association or of the agencies with which they may be affiliated.

James R. Kimmey, M.D.
Executive Director
American Public Health Association

NOTES ON TABLES AND FIGURES

1. Symbols used in tables of data:
- - - - Data not available;
   - ... Category not applicable (except Table 4.5, where ...should read ---, and Tables 7.6 and 7.7, which have special definitions);
      - - Quantity zero (*except when* category is used as base of differential or index);
      - 0 Quantity zero (when category is base of differential or index, as in Tables 4.6, 4.8, 6.4, 6.6, 6.9, 7.2, 8.1, 8.3, 8.4, 8.5);
   - 0.0 Quantity more than zero but less than 0.05.
2. Regarding 1959-61 mortality data:
   a. Deaths relate to those occurring in the United States (including Alaska and Hawaii);
   b. Deaths are classified by place of residence (if pertinent);
   c. Fetal deaths are excluded;
   d. Deaths of unknown age, marital status, nativity, or other characteristics have not been distributed into the known categories, but are included in their totals. (This applies to all 1959-61 mortality measures *except* those labelled "corrected" in Chapter 6. The corrections allocate unknown characteristics on the death certificate to categories reported on "matching" census records; see Chapter 6 for details.)
   e. Deaths were classified by cause according to the *Seventh Revision of the International Statistical Classification of Diseases, Injuries, and Causes of Death* (Geneva: World Health Organization, 1957).
3. Geographic classification:[1]
   a. Standard Metroplitan Statistical Areas (SMSA's): except in the New England States, "an SMSA is a county or a group of contiguous counties which contains at least one city of 50,000 inhabitants or more or 'twin cities' with a combined population of at least 50,000 in the 1960 census. In addition, contiguous counties are included in an SMSA if, according to specified criteria, they are (a) essentially metropolitan in character and (b) socially and economically integrated with the central city or cities." In New England, the Division of Vital Statistics of the National Center for Health Statistics uses, instead of the definition just cited, Metropolitan State Economic Areas (MSEA's) established by the Bureau of the Census, which are made up of county units.
   b. Metropolitan and nonmetropolitan: "Counties which are included in SMSA's or, in New England, MSEA's are called metropolitan counties; all other counties are classified as nonmetropolitan."
   c. Metropolitan counties may be separated into those containing at least one central city of 50,000 inhabitants or more or twin cities as specified previously, and into metropolitan counties without a central city.

[1] National Center for Health Statistics, *Vital Statistics of the United States, 1960* (Washington, D.C., 1963), vol. 2, pt. A, sec. 7, p. 8.

DIFFERENTIAL MORTALITY IN THE UNITED STATES: A STUDY IN SOCIOECONOMIC EPIDEMIOLOGY

1 / INTRODUCTION

Increasing attention in recent years to high rates of population growth and the need to control fertility has almost obscured interest in mortality, among both demographers and the general public. Yet, death remains a subject of deep concern to the person, the family, the community, government at all levels, and international agencies. It is becoming widely recognized that decreased mortality increasing the length of human life has been the major factor in the acceleration of rates of population increase. But, by reason of the universal value attached to life, the further reduction of death rates remains a major human goal, and great differentials in mortality continue not only to point toward possibilities of further increases in longevity but, also, to provide motivation to effect such gains.

This analysis of differential mortality in the United States has such a twofold purpose: first, to measure the differences in death rates which persist despite the large general reductions in mortality and, second, to direct attention to the population groupings which have not fully shared in the longevity gains attained. The objects of the study are, of course, both to add to knowledge and to stimulate such programs in public health agencies, in private and social medicine, and through various types of social and economic activities to reduce high death rates. That is, the goal of equal opportunity for all, so deeply ingrained in American ideology, tradition, and law, is still to be implemented in the realm of life itself—the achievement of equal opportunity for survival. No review of the literature on socioeconomic differences in mortality is presented here, because this task has been done by others. Among such summaries are those by Daric (National Center for Health Statistics, 1951), by Stockwell (1961), by Benjamin (1965), and by Antonovsky (1967).

Mortality Trends in the United States

Although the United States, under the Constitution, was among the first nations to provide for national censuses, she was relatively slow to develop a national vital registration system. Massachusetts, however, arranged for the recording of deaths, along with births and marriages, while still a colony as early as 1639, and other colonies followed suit. Only 14 of the 50 states had central death records before 1900. Moreover, despite the growing demand for vital statistics emanating from the public health movement, in the main, the states remained indifferent or opposed to the establishment of central vital statistics systems.

The United States census collected information on deaths in the 12 months prior to the census date from 1850 to 1900, but the data were defective and not worth analyzing. With the establishment of a permanent Bureau of the Census in 1902, provision was made for the annual collection of copies of death certificates from states and cities having satisfactory registration systems. The death registration area, initiated with 10 states and some separate cities, did not cover the entire nation until 1933 with the inclusion of Texas. The United States was, therefore, about a century behind European countries in compiling national mortality data.

The official mortality statistics of the United States, based on the registration system, from 1900 to 1960, have been summarized in two volumes, the first including statistics from 1900 to 1940 (Linder and Grove, 1943, pp. 122-663) and the second covering the period 1940 to 1960 (Grove and Hetzel, 1968, pp. 190-770). Data on mortality prior to 1900 are available in *Historical Statistics of the United States, Colonial Times to 1957* (U.S. Bureau of the Census, Washington, D.C., 1960, pp. 24-30). The data which have been compiled by government, in the censuses and from vital registration systems, permit the rough tracing of mortality trends in the United States from its beginnings as a nation. Systematic mortality information, however, dates only from the beginning of this century and for the entire nation, as has been indicated, only from 1933.

Expectation of life at birth in Philadelphia from 1782 to 1790 approximated 25 years, according to Barton (Dublin, Lotka, and Spiegelman, 1949, p. 36). In Massachusetts and New Hampshire at about the same time, according to Wiggelsworth, the expectation of life was about 35 years. By 1850 expectation of life at birth, according to Meech, had reached 41.8 years for males and 44.9 years for females in Maryland, and for Massachusetts, 38.3 years for males and 40.5 years for females. Glover calculated for Massachusetts in 1890 an expectation of life of 42.5 years for males and 44.5 years for females; and for 1900-1902, 46.1 years for males and 49.4 years for females (Dublin et al., 1949, pp. 39ff). For the nation as a whole, between 1900-1902 and 1959-61 expectation of life at birth for white males rose from 48.2 years to 67.6 years; and for white females from 51.1 years to 74.2 years (Spiegelman, 1966, p. 2). Thus, from the beginning of the nineteenth century to 1960 the reduction in mortality in the United States added some 40 years to expectation of life at birth; and from the beginning of the twentieth century to 1960, expectation of life increased by over 19 years for white males and by 23 years for white females.

During the course of this century death rates also decreased for nonwhites, but nonwhite mortality remained at a relatively high level. In 1919-21 expectation of life at birth for nonwhite males was 47.1 years, or below the level of white males in 1900-02. By 1959-61, expectation of life of nonwhite males had increased by 14.4 years to reach 61.5 years—a level still 6.1 years below that of white males. In 1919-21 expectation of life at birth for nonwhite females was 46.9 years, 4.2 years below white female life expectancy in 1900-1902. Nonwhite female expectation of life increased by 19.6 years between 1919-21 and 1959-61 to reach 66.5 years—a level still 7.7 years below white female life expectancy (Spiegelman, 1966, p. 2). Since 1939-41, however, nonwhite mortality has decreased somewhat more rapidly than white, suggesting possible convergence in the years which lie ahead (Spiegelman, 1966, p. 3).

Declines in mortality from 1900 to 1960 were much greater among infants and the young, in general, than for older persons. Infant mortality for white males in 1959-61, at 25.9 (deaths per 1,000 infants born) was only one-fifth of the level of white male infant mortality in 1900-02, 133.5. Mortality of white males at age 10 in 1959-61 was about one-seventh that in 1900-1902, 0.4 compared with 2.7; at age 20, less than one-third, 1.6 compared with 5.9; at age 45, less than one-half, 5.6 compared with 12.6; and at age 65, only 19 percent below the earlier level, 33.9 compared with 41.7 (Spiegelman, 1966, p. 2). It is evident that the mortality gains diminish as age increases.

The secular decline in mortality in the United States seems to have come to a halt in the early 1950's and remained on a plateau to 1963—that is beyond the period with which this study is concerned (National Center for Health Statistics [NCHS], June 1966, pp. 1-57). Not only did the crude death rate level off but so also did age-specific rates. The age-adjusted death rate of the United States (using the 1940 age distribution of the United States as a standard) was 7.6 in 1954 and 7.6 in 1960, and it remained within the range from 7.3 to 7.8 during the 10-year period from 1954 to 1963. The leveling off of the secular decline in mortality during the fifties was manifest in each sex for both the white and the nonwhite populations (NCHS, June 1966, p. 7). Joan Klebba has attributed the mortality plateau between 1954 and 1963 in large part to the increase in death rates for 12 of the 15 leading causes of deaths, including diseases of the heart, malignant neoplasms, vascular lesions, and accidents, which accounted for 71.4 percent of total deaths in 1963. The 12 causes of death which showed increases during the period accounted for 85 percent of all mortality (NCHS, June 1966, pp. 1-7).

Other economically advanced nations have also experienced a plateau in death rates since the 1950's and some an actual increase in mortality among men over 45 (Bourgeois-Pichat, 1971, p. 50). Bourgeois-Pichat attributes this reversal in trend to two factors: "a) a slowing down of the drop in mortality from infectious and parasitic diseases, b) increase in mortality from degenerative diseases—an increase which had long been masked by the drop in mortality because of infectious diseases." Significantly he states that the explanation for this phenomenon is likely to be found in such factors as social class, nutrition, and illnesses.

The mortality plateau experienced by the United States from 1954 to 1963 does not mean that death rates had reached an irreducible minimum. Among the nations in the world, at least 15 had a longer life expectancy at birth than the United States (Department of Health, Education and Welfare, 1969, p. 6). The fact that many other nations had achieved lower mortality rates than did the United States indicates that this nation can still further reduce her death rates. In view of the fact that the United States is by far the most affluent nation on the globe, her failure to achieve a higher ranking in life expectancy points to the need for a comprehensive investigation into the causes of her relatively high mortality. This study of social and economic differentials in mortality constitutes one element into such an investigation.

The study of socioeconomic mortality differentials constitutes what may be termed "socioeconomic epidemiology" in contrast to biomedical epidemiology. The importance of socioeconomic differentials in mortality is that they point to the possibilities of reducing mortality through the betterment of socioeconomic conditions in the population. Thus, socioeconomic epidemiology is interested in the extent to which differences in socioeconomic status are responsible for differences in mortality and indicates the gains that might be achieved in life expectancy if socioeconomic conditions are improved. This study, then, is an example of socioeconomic epidemiology and its findings have important implications for both the public and the private agencies concerned with the health and longevity of the American people.

The Study of Differential Mortality

The limited information reported on the legal death record in the United States greatly restricts analysis of social and economic differentials in mortality, at least by any direct method wherein deaths tabulated by characteristics reported on death certificates are related to exposed population tabulated by characteristics reported on censuses or surveys. For example, the only measure of socioeconomic status on the death certificate is occupation, but any attempt to utilize this information for analysis of mortality by occupation is limited at the outset by the great discrepancy between the "usual occupation" reported on the death certificate and the "current (or last) occupation" reported in the population census (NCHS, June 1961; Moriyama and Guralnick, 1956). Because children and many women do not have occupations and because occupation is difficult to define meaningfully and consistently (on death and census records) for retired older men who comprise so many of the male decedents, the occupational differentials derived for the United States have typically been limited to men 25-64 years of age. Even in respect to other items on the death certificate, such as age, race, marital status and country of birth, death rates are subject to error because of the lack of correspondence in the information reported for the same person on his death certificate and census schedule (NCHS, June 1968 and May 1969).

Because of these kinds of difficulties, several indirect approaches to the analysis of socioeconomic differentials in mortality have been developed. One that has been used in a number of cities in the United States is based on census tracts, the small, relatively homogeneous geographic subdivisions into which large cities are divided for census purposes and for which population data are published. In this approach, deaths are compiled by census tract of residence of the decedent (using the street address reported on the death certificate) and then deaths and population for each tract are allocated *as a unit* to one of several socioeconomic groups on the basis of a socioeconomic index for the census tract. For example, in Chicago (a city divided into about 900 census tracts in the last four censuses) median rent of dwelling units, median family income, and median years of school completed by adult residents have been used to allocate deaths and population for each tract to one of five socioeconomic groups (see Chapter 4).

In interpreting mortality differentials based on areal indexes of socioeconomic status it should be remembered that they do not represent differences in mortality among subgroups of the population when individual members are used as the basis of classification. That is, the mortality differentials obtained when residents of Chicago are classified according to "median years of school completed by all adults in their census tract of residence" (as in Chapter 4) do not necessarily represent education differentials in mortality when residents of Chicago are individually classified by years of school completed, and they should not be interpreted as "education differentials" per se. In other words, the use of the "census tract" as the unit of aggregating deaths and population, and the allocation of entire tracts to socioeconomic groups on the basis of the median education level of their residents, introduces an "area effect" which is confounded, in the mortality differentials obtained, with education differentials in mortality per se.

The mortality studies using areal indexes of socioeconomic status to define socioeconomic groups have typically been limited to large metropolitan areas because only for such areas have population data been available for the numerous small geographic subdivisions required to allocate persons to socioeconomic groups on the basis of average characteristics of their areas of residence. Although the population living in a particular census tract is never entirely homogeneous, socioeconomic homogeneity is one of the criteria used to delineate tract boundaries, and in very large cities there is great variability among tracts with respect to such variables as median income, median rent, percent of workers in professional occupations, percent of housing units in substandard condition, etc. The validity of this approach is discussed in Chapter 4.

The term "socioeconomic differentials in mortality"—often seen in the literature—is used to refer to differences in mortality among subgroups of the population when ordered in some hierarchy of socioeconomic status, usually without any careful consideration or definition of the concept of socioeconomic status. Sometimes the more general term "social and economic differentials" is used to refer to a broader spectrum of differential mortality including such personal characteristics as marital status, race, ethnic group, education, income, and occupation, as well as such external characteristics as condition of the housing unit of residence. Although many of these characteristics are related to a person's socioeconomic status—however it may be defined—no one of them is directly equated with socioeconomic status in the sense that it is accepted as the sole determinant of such status or that it is a fully satisfactory index of socioeconomic status for all research purposes.

Writers on the subject recognize income, education, and occupation as the three basic aspects of socioeconomic status (Reiss et al., 1961, p. 83). Duncan describes the salient functional connection among them as follows: "Education qualifies the individual for participation in occupational life, and pursuit of an occupation yields him a return in the form of income"; he also documents the importance of occupation as an intervening variable in the translation of educational advantage into income advantage with data from the 1950 census of the United States which show that "differences in income according to level of educational attainment are due, in large measure, to the fact that well-educated persons engage disproportionately in high-income occupations and poorly-educated persons in low-income occupations" (Duncan, 1961, pp. 783-84).

Duncan and others have also argued that there is no such thing as a single index of socioeconomic status suitable for all research purposes and have recommended that objective items such as education, occupation, and income be treated as separate dimensions of social stratification rather than combined into a single index (Reiss et al., 1961, p. 139; Hodge and Siegel, 1968, pp. 319-20). Loose relationship among the several dimensions of socioeconomic status is the compelling reason behind their recommendation. For example, Duncan found that variation between educational levels accounted for only about one-third of the total variation in occupational socioeconomic status and that occupational socioeconomic status accounted for only a minor fraction of the individual variation in income (Reiss et al., 1961, p. 141). Thus they make clear that the various dimensions of socioeconomic status may exhibit quite different relationships to a particular dependent variable—mortality, for example—and that these different relationships themselves may be an important part of the association between the dependent variable and socioeconomic status.

Socioeconomic epidemiology as indicated above is interested in the extent to which differences in socioeconomic status are responsible for differences in mortality. From this perspective, causal paths in the reverse direction can provide distorted socioeconomic patterns. As is made clear in Chapter 2, the income differentials in mortality for men of working age are in all likelihood exaggerated by a reverse causal path in which the approach of death itself is the cause of decreased income during the year prior to death for a substantial number of men of working age. Occupation differentials are also subject to exaggeration for a similar reason, namely, a tendency for men to work at jobs prior to death that are below the level of their long-time or normal occupations. Similarly, reverse causal paths may be involved in the use of areal indexes of socioeconomic status. For example, the very high mortality reported for the lowest socioeconomic group of males in Chicago (Chapter 4) may be inflated by a tendency for men near death to move into the areas with very low socioeconomic indexes, such as skid rows or areas with poor and cheap housing occupied largely by low-income households. Education, then, is the only one of the three basic aspects of socioeconomic status for which data are available that cannot be affected by the approach of death, except of course in the young ages when people are still in process of completing their education. For this reason, when only one variable could be used, education has been relied upon more than the other variables in much of the analysis presented, for example in Chapter 5.

The 1960 Matched Records Study

By reason of the difficulties and limitation of national studies of differential mortality by socioeconomic status from available data, a plan was developed that would permit the analysis of differential mortality by a number of indexes of socioeconomic class. This plan was developed collaboratively by personnel in the National Center for Health Statistics, the Bureau of the Census, and the Population Research Center of the University of Chicago and involved the matching of death certificates to the schedules of the 1960 census of population. The feasibility of the general approach had been pretested in an earlier study by Guralnick and Nam (1959). With funds made available by the National Institutes of Health and with the participation of the National Center for Health Statistics and the Bureau of the Census, some 340,000 of the deaths that occurred during the period May through August 1960 were matched with the 1960 census records in order to obtain social and economic characteristics of decedents as reported in the 1960 census. (See Appendix A for details of the plan and procedures.)

This study provides the first measurements, for a nationwide sample of the United States population, of differential mortality by income, education, and various other characteristics reported on population census schedules but not on death certificates. Although the study does permit separate evaluation of the relationship of mortality to the three basic components of socioeconomic status at a given point in time, there are problems of interpretation arising from the fact that it is a cross-section analysis in which each individual is allocated to socioeconomic level as of 1960. To the extent that the components of socioeconomic status are fixed after age 25, there is no problem of allocating adults to the correct level with respect to each component. But it is also clear that two of the basic components of socioeconomic status—income and occupation—can and often do vary over the lifespan of an individual. This creates problems relating to the concept of socioeconomic status itself. For example, for those individuals who have changed their occupation and income level during the course of their adult lives there is a real problem of how these two components of socioeconomic status should be defined—in terms of an average status, a "normal" status (e.g., longest job held), or perhaps classified in terms of status mobility (upward shifts, downward shifts, etc.). Ideally, one might like to have an occupation and income history for each person which, theoretically at least, might permit some evaluation of status mobility itself on mortality. Unfortunately, such data do not exist.

Outline and Sources

The mortality differentials summarized in this monograph were derived primarily from three studies: (1) the 1960 Matched Records Study, described briefly in the preceding section and in more detail in Appendix A, which provided the national statistics on education, income, and occupation differentials for persons 25 and over discussed in Chapters 2, 3, and 5, and also the data for differential mortality by parity of married women in Chapter 6; (2) the series of Chicago studies utilizing the indirect approach based on areal indexes of the type described earlier, which provided the materials for the analysis of socioeconomic differentials in a metropolis during the 30-year period 1930-1960 which are discussed in Chapters 4 and 5; (3) the special tabulations of 1959-61 deaths for the entire nation compiled by the National Center for Health Statistics especially for this series of monographs, which provided age-adjusted death rates for the geographic differentials in Chapter 7 and also for the differentials in mortality by race, nativity, country of origin, and marital status in Chapter 6. The accuracy of the analysis by race, nativity, country of origin, and marital status—factors known to be subject to response error because of discrepant reporting on the death certificate and census schedule—was increased by the availability of tabulations from the Matched Records Study which compared responses to these questions on the census and death records for a sample of the deaths matched with census records in the 1960 study. Chapter 8 summarizes the findings on differential mortality and discusses their implications in terms of the "excess mortality" experienced by various subgroups of the population.

2 / EDUCATION AND INCOME DIFFERENTIALS

It has never been possible to compute death rates by education or income level directly from official tabulations of deaths for the United States because neither item is reported on the legal death record. The first direct assessment of education and income differentials for a representative sample of the nation's adult population was derived from the 1960 Matched Records Study,[1] which provided the basic data for the education and income differentials presented in this chapter. Some preliminary findings have been published elsewhere (Kitagawa, 1971; Kitagawa and Hauser, 1971); others are reported here for the first time. The design and methodology of the study are described in Appendix A. Problems in respect of the limitations and interpretations of the data are discussed at the end of this chapter.

Education Differentials Among Adults

Among adults (persons 25 or older) in the United States, mortality varied inversely with level of educational attainment.[2] The range of the education differentials was much larger among persons 25-64 years of age than among older persons, and greater among women than men. Although smaller numbers and poorer quality of data limited the analysis for nonwhites to two or three broad levels of education, whites and nonwhites exhibited similar patterns of mortality by education level. After age 65, a marked inverse association between mortality and education persisted only among white families.

White Population

The three general patterns of education differentials described above—an inverse relationship to mortality that is stronger for women than men, and stronger below age 65 than above age 65—are documented for the white population in Table 2.1. For example, among white males 25-64 years of age mortality ratios by education decreased consistently from a high of 1.15 for men with less than 5 years of school to a low of 0.70 for men with at least 4 years of college, a differential of 64 percent.[3] That is, the age-adjusted mortality ratio for men 25-64 years of age who completed less than 5 years of school was 64 percent higher than the comparable ratio for men the same age who completed at least 4 years of college. In contrast to this, the education differential in mortality for white males 65 and over was only 4 percent, ranging from a mortality ratio of 1.02 for persons with less than 5 years of school to a ratio of 0.98 for persons with at least one year of college.[4] Among white females 25-64 years old the mortality ratio of 1.60 for women with less than 5 years of school was 105 percent higher than the ratio of 0.78 for women with at least 4 years of college, as compared with the comparable differential of 64 percent for men. It should be noted, however, that this larger education differential for women is due entirely to the very high mortality—relatively speaking—of women in the lowest education group, that is, those who completed less than 5

Table 2.1. Mortality ratios by years of school completed for the white population 25 years of age and over, by sex and family status: United States, May-August, 1960

Family status and years of school completed	Mortality ratios[a]						Population (percent distribution)			
	White males			White females			White males		White females	
	25 & over	25-64 years	65 & over	25 & over	25-64 years	65 & over	25-64 years	65 & over	25-64 years	65 & over
All persons..........	1.00	1.00	1.00	1.00	1.00	1.00	100.0	100.0	100.0	100.0
0-4 years.............	1.02	1.15	1.02	1.27	1.60	1.17	5.0	20.7	3.9	15.6
5-7 years.............	1.04	1.14	1.00	1.08	1.18	1.04	12.0	23.1	10.1	20.4
8 years...............	1.02	1.07	1.00	1.05	1.08	1.03	16.7	27.5	15.4	28.8
High school, 1-3 years....	1.01	1.03	} .99	.87	.91	} .94	20.4	10.8	21.0	13.3
High school, 4 years......	.98	.91		.92	.87		24.7	8.2	32.8	12.2
College, 1-3 years........	.98	.85	} .98	.73	.82	} .70	9.8	5.2	10.2	6.4
College, 4 years or more..	.80	.70		.71	.78		11.4	4.5	6.6	3.4
0-7 years..............	1.03	1.14	1.01	1.16	1.31	1.10	17.0	43.8	14.0	36.0
College, 1 year or more...	.89	.77	.98	.72	.80	.70	21.1	9.7	16.8	9.7
0-8 years..............	1.02	1.11	1.01	1.11	1.19	1.06	33.7	71.3	29.4	64.8
High school or college....	.96	.91	.98	.85	.87	.88	66.3	28.7	70.6	35.2
Family members..........	1.00	1.00	1.00	1.00	1.00	1.00	100.0	100.0	100.0	100.0
0-7 years..............	1.03	1.13	1.02	1.17	1.26	1.10	16.4	13.6	13.6	38.1
8 years...............	1.00	1.06	.98	1.04	1.06	1.01	16.7	27.8	15.3	29.5
High school, 1-3 years....	1.02	1.04	} .99	.88	.93	} .91	20.6	11.0	21.3	12.7
High school, 4 years......	.99	.92		.87	.88		25.3	8.2	33.6	11.4
College, 1 year or more...	.90	.81	.98	.75	.85	.70#	21.0	9.9	16.1	8.3
0-8 years..............	1.02	1.09	1.00	1.11	1.16	1.06	33.1	70.9	28.9	67.6
High school or college....	.97	.92	.99	.85	.89	.86	66.9	29.1	71.1	32.4
Unrelated individuals...	1.00	1.00	1.00	1.00	1.00	1.00	100.0	100.0	100.0	100.0
0-8 years.............	.98	1.10	.99	1.07	1.28	1.05	37.5	72.9	32.6	58.5
High school, 1-4 years....	} 1.04	.99	} 1.02	.84 } .91		} .93	37.0	18.0	41.3	28.6
College, 1 year or more...		.72#			.77#		25.5	9.1	26.1	13.0
Inmates of institutions.	1.00	1.00	1.00	1.00	1.00	1.00	100.0	100.0	100.0	100.0
0-8 years..............	1.04	1.09#	1.04	1.08	1.10#	1.07	59.1	73.6	59.4	63.8
High school or college....	.90#	.85#	.88#	.86	.84#	.87	40.9	26.4	40.6	36.2

Source: Population Research Center, University of Chicago, study based on matching death certificates with 1960 Census records (see Appendix A).

Does not meet reliability requirement that the Special Sample Survey of May-August deaths (which provided data for estimating characteristics of deaths not matched with census records) include at least 10 unmatched decedents whose survey questionnaires allocate them to this subgroup of the population.

[a] The mortality ratios in this table measure the range of education differentials in mortality within each color-sex-age-family status subgroup of the population. They were derived from the ratios of actual to expected deaths described in Appendix A, Section 3, by setting the ratio for each subgroup total equal to 1.00.

years of school. Above this level of schooling the differentials are quite similar for men and women 25-64 years of age. The most striking contrast between the education differentials for men and women lies in the persistence of a marked inverse association between mortality and education level among women after age 65. The mortality ratios for white females 65 and older decreased from 1.17 for those who completed less than 5 years of school to 0.70 for those who completed at least one year of college, a differential of 67 percent as compared with the differential of 4 percent already cited for white males 65 and over.

Table 2.1 also reports education differentials in mortality within three family status subgroups of the white population: family members, unrelated individuals, and inmates of institutions. The percentage of the white population in each family status subgroup is summarized below, to indicate the relative importance of the three subgroups in different sex-age groups of the population. It is clear from these distributions that the age group 25-64 years is composed almost entirely of family members (92 percent of both males and females). Consequently, the more detailed education differentials shown for all persons 25-64 years of age in Table 2.1 should apply with very little modification to family members 25-64 years of age. Among those 65 and over, 4 out of 5 men, and 2 out of 3 women were family members.

	Total	Family Members	Unrelated Individuals	Inmates
White males 25 and over	100.0	90.1	8.4	1.6
25-64 years	100.0	91.8	7.0	1.2
65 years and over	100.0	80.8	15.8	3.4
White females 25 and over	100.0	87.4	11.3	1.3
25-64 years	100.0	91.9	7.5	0.6
65 years and over	100.0	66.8	28.9	4.3

Education differentials appeared to be very similar among family members, unrelated individuals, and inmates, although the limited number of education levels for the last two groups do not permit a detailed verification of this conclusion. However, examination of the education differentials for family members in the same broad categories as reported for unrelated individuals and inmates reveals similar patterns.

Nonwhite Population

There was a strong inverse relationship between mortality and level of educational attainment in the nonwhite population of the United States in 1960 (Table 2.2). Although, as mentioned earlier, relatively small numbers made it necessary to limit the education classification for nonwhites to three broad levels and to combine any amount of high school or college education as a single interval, the differentials are substantial, especially among nonwhites 25-64 years of age. In this age group males with less than 5 years of school had a mortality ratio (1.14) that was 31 percent higher than the ratio (0.87) for males with at least one year of high school. Females 25-64 years old with less than 5 years of school had a mortality ratio (1.26) that was 70 percent higher than the ratio (0.74) for females the same age who had at least one year of high school.

By Region

Although there were some differences in the size of education differentials within the two broad regions of the United States for which mortality ratios could be calculated separately—the South and a combined North and West region—in general the pattern of the education differentials in the two regions were similar (Table 2.3).

Table 2.2. Mortality ratios by years of school completed for the non-white population 25 years of age and over, by sex: United States, May-August, 1960

Sex and years of school completed	Mortality ratios[a]			Population (percent distribution)		
	25 & over	25-64 years	65 & over	25 & over	25-64 years	65 & over
Nonwhite males......	1.00	1.00	1.00	100.0	100.0	100.0
0-4 years.............	1.01	1.14	1.04#	27.7	23.4	57.0
5-8 years.............	.98	.97	.93#	35.2	35.8	31.3
High school or college.	1.00	.87	.97#	37.1	40.8	11.7
Nonwhite females....	1.00	1.00	1.00	100.0	100.0	100.0
0-4 years.............	1.04	1.26	1.05	19.6	15.4	48.7
5-8 years.............	1.01	1.06	.93	36.9	36.9	37.2
High school or college.	.89	.74	1.01#	43.5	47.7	14.1

Source: Same as Table 2.1.

Does not meet reliability requirement specified in Table 2.1.

[a] See note a, Table 2.1, for definition of ratios.

Table 2.3. Mortality ratios by years of school completed, by color, sex, and region: United States, May-August, 1960

Color, sex and years of school completed	Mortality ratios for persons aged:[a]					
	25 and over		25-64 years		65 and over	
	North & West	South	North & West	South	North & West	South
White males..........	1.00	1.00	1.00	1.00	1.00	1.00
0-7 years...............	1.05	.99	1.19	1.06	1.02	.98
8 years.................	1.00	1.08	1.07	1.09	.97	1.09
High school, 1-4 years...	1.00	.99	.97	.99	1.00	.93
College, 1 year or more..	.87	.94	.75	.82	.97	1.04
White females.........	1.00	1.00	1.00	1.00	1.00	1.00
0-7 years...............	1.17	1.15	1.36	1.25	1.10	1.09
8 years.................	1.04	1.07	1.08	1.05	1.01	1.06
High school, 1-4 years...	.91	.86	.90	.85	.95	.91
College, 1 year or more..	.72	.74	.78	.88	.70	.71
Nonwhite males........	--*	--*	1.00	1.00	--*	--*
0-8 years...............	--*	--*	1.04	1.03	--*	--*
High school or college...	--*	--*	.93	.87#	--*	--*
Nonwhite females......	--*	--*	1.00	1.00	--*	--*
0-8 years...............	--*	--*	1.21	1.07	--*	--*
High school or college...	--*	--*	.72#	.80	--*	--*

Source: Same as Table 2.1.

Does not meet reliability requirement specified in Table 2.1.

[a] See note a, Table 2.1, for definition of ratios.

--* Ratio not computed because Special Sample Survey had too few unmatched decedents 65 and over from each region to derive estimates for even two levels of education.

Small frequencies prevented more detailed geographical comparisons. Among white males 25-64 years old, education differentials were substantially larger in the North and West than in the South. In the North and West, mortality ratios ranged from 1.19 for those with less than 8 years of school to 0.75 for those with one year or more of college, a differential of 59 percent; in the South comparable ratios ranged from 1.06 to 0.82, a differential of 29 percent. A similar regional pattern obtained among white females 25-64 years old, for whom comparable ratios ranged from 1.36 to 0.78 in the North and West, a differential of 74 percent; and from 1.25 to 0.88 in the South, a differential of 42 percent. Among white persons 65 and over, education differentials were similar in both regions; that is, there was no consistent pattern among white males and a marked inverse association between mortality and education level among white females. In fact, the differentials for white females 65 and over in both regions were comparable to those observed for white males 25-64 years of age.

Among nonwhites 25-64 years of age, the only age group for which nonwhite mortality ratios could be calculated separately by region, education differentials were very similar by region for males, but were smaller in the South than in the North and West for females.

Education and Length of Life

Differences in mortality by level of educational attainment—or any other factor—can be quantified and summarized in more than one way. It has been demonstrated that various alternative indexes of mortality can, and often do, appreciably affect the results obtained (Kitagawa, 1964 and 1966). The analysis thus far has been based on the age-standardized ratios of actual to expected deaths defined in note a, Table 2.1 (a form of indirect standardization). The same basic data for all white males and females have also been summarized in terms of life expectancies and probabilities of dying between certain ages; these measures are presented in Table 2.4.[5]

The life expectancies indicate, for example, that a cohort of women exposed, from age 25 on, to the age-specific schedule of mortality experienced by white females with one year or more of college could expect to live 56.4 years after age 25. This is almost 10 years longer, on the average, than a cohort exposed to the schedule of mortality experienced by white females with less than 5 years of school. Although the education differential for white females did decrease with age, at age 65 it was still large—6.0 years more of life for the college-educated women. Among white males, the differences in life expectancy were much smaller: at age 25, only 3.2 years longer life on the average for college-educated men than for men with less than 5 years of school; at age 45, only 2.2 years longer for the college-educated men; and by age 65, there was no significant difference in the life expectancy by education.

The relative size of the education differentials in mortality is considerably less when measured in terms of life expectancies (Table 2.4) than by age-adjusted mortality ratios (Table 2.1). For example, among white females 25 and older the mortality ratio was 78 percent higher for those having less than 5 years of school than for those having completed 4 years of college (1.27 as compared with 0.71). However, the same data yield a life expectancy at age 25 that is only

Table 2.4. Selected life table functions for the white population, by sex and years of school completed: United States, 1960

Sex and years of school completed	Probability of dying[a] between ages:			$(\mathring{e}_x)$ average years of life remaining at age:		
	25 & 45	45 & 65	65 & 75	25	45	65
White males						
0-4 years..............	.0680#	.3086	.4156	43.9	26.2	12.7
5-7 years..............	.0878	.2944	.4051	43.6	26.7	12.9
8 years................	.0634	.2863	.3997	44.8	27.1	13.0
High school, 1-3 years.	.0562	.2777	.3757#	45.6	27.6	13.5
High school, 4 years...	.0431	.2637	.3919	46.0	27.5	12.9
College, 1 year or more	.0345	.2284	.3803	47.1	28.4	13.1
White females						
0-4 years..............	.0838#	.2123#	.3004	46.8	30.0	14.8
5-7 years..............	.0407#	.1667	.2660	50.5	32.1	16.0
8 years................	.0332#	.1569	.2599	51.1	32.4	16.2
High school, 1-3 years.	.0323	.1247	.2319#	53.4	34.8	18.0
High school, 4 years...	.0239	.1297	.2435	52.2	33.2	16.3
College, 1 year or more	.0289#	.1099	.1833#	56.4	37.7	20.8

Source: Same as Table 2.1.

Does not meet reliability requirement specified in Table 2.1.

a Computed from ℓ_x column of abridged life table.

21 percent higher for women having completed 4 years of college than for those having less than 5 years of school (56.4 years as compared with 46.8 years). These results illustrate the point made at the beginning of this section, that different indexes of mortality may produce different quantitative evaluations of mortality differentials with respect to a given socioeconomic characteristic. Each of the evaluations, however, adds to available knowledge and helps to clarify the socioeconomic epidemiological problems involved, the need for policies and programs to effect further mortality reductions, and the impact of the gains to be achieved.

Income Differentials Among Adults

The relationship between income and mortality in the United States in 1960 was similar in many respects to the relationship between education and mortality. For example, income also was inversely related to mortality and the range of income differentials also was much larger and the pattern more consistent among persons 25-64 years of age than among older persons. However, there were a few striking differences between the education and income differentials, and the income data have special limitations—especially for white males 25-64 years of age—which should be taken into account in interpreting the data. These problems are discussed later in the section on "evaluation of education and income differentials."

Table 2.5 summarizes income differentials in mortality separately for (1) white family members, using total family income in 1959 as the basis of the income classification; and (2) white unrelated individuals, using personal income of each individual in 1959 as the basis of the income classification. The use of family income for family members was preferred because it was judged to be a better index of the socioeconomic status of individual family members, especially for women and retired family members. Income data for inmates were not available in the 1960 census, and in any case the

Table 2.5. Mortality ratios by income level, for white family members and unrelated individuals, by sex and age: United States, May-August, 1960

Family status and income in 1959	Mortality ratios[a]			Population (percent distribution)		
	25 & over	25-64 years	65 & over	25 & over	25-64 years	65 & over
Family members by family income						
White male family members..............	1.00	1.00	1.00	100.0	100.0	100.0
Under $2,000......................	1.14	1.51	1.10	9.3	6.3	27.6
$2,000-3,999.....................	1.03	1.20	.99	14.8	12.8	27.0
$4,000-5,999.....................	.97	.99	} .92	22.8	23.9	16.3
$6,000-7,999.....................	.91	.88		21.0	22.6	10.9
$8,000-9,999.....................	1.00	.93	} .96#	13.2	14.2	6.6
$10,000 or more...................	.89	.84		19.0	20.2	11.6
Under $4,000.....................	1.09	1.32	1.05	24.1	19.1	54.6
$8,000 or more...................	.93	.88	.96#	32.2	34.4	18.2
White female family members...........	1.00	1.00	1.00	100.0	100.0	100.0
Under $2,000......................	1.05	1.20	.96	10.8	8.5	25.7
$2,000-3,999.....................	1.02	1.12	.96	15.4	14.1	24.2
$4,000-5,999.....................	1.00	1.00	} 1.05	22.2	23.0	17.1
$6,000-7,999.....................	1.01	.98		20.3	21.5	12.2
$8,000-9,999.....................	.95	.92#	} 1.01	12.9	13.7	7.8
$10,000 or more...................	.92	.86		18.4	19.3	13.0
Under $4,000.....................	1.04	1.15	.96	26.2	22.6	49.9
$8,000 or more...................	.93	.88	1.01	31.3	33.0	20.8
Unrelated individuals by personal income						
White male unrelated individuals.........	1.00	1.00	1.00	100.0	100.0	100.0
Under $2,000......................	.97	1.26	1.00	40.5	28.7	68.8
$2,000-3,999.....................	} 1.05	1.02#	} 1.01	23.4	25.5	18.4
$4,000 or more....................		.77		36.1	45.8	12.8
White female unrelated individuals.......	1.00	1.00	1.00	100.0	100.0	100.0
Under $2,000......................	1.06	1.27	1.05	59.3	42.8	79.0
$2,000-3,999.....................	} .80	.73#	} .80#	22.0	29.2	13.3
$4,000 or more....................		.79#		18.8	28.1	7.6

Source: Same as Table 2.1.

Does not meet reliability requirement specified in Table 2.1.

[a] See note a, Table 2.1, for definition of ratios.

census definition of income has only limited applicability to inmates of institutions.

Among white family members 25-64 years of age, the inverse relationship between family income and mortality was very marked, especially for males. For example, among males of this age the mortality ratio of 1.51 for those from families with less than $2,000 income in 1959 was 80 percent higher than the ratio of 0.84 for those from families with income of $10,000 or more. Comparable indexes for white females in the 25-64 age group ranged from 1.20 for those from families with less than $2,000 income to 0.86 for those from families with more than $10,000 income, a differential of 40 percent. After age 65, however, the mortality ratio for men from families with less than $2,000 income was only 15 percent higher than that for men from families with income of $8,000 or more. Among women 65 and older, there was no consistent pattern of declining mortality with increasing family income.

Among white unrelated individuals 25-64 years of age, there also was a strong inverse association between mortality and income. In fact, given the broad income intervals necessitated by small numbers of unrelated individuals and the need for some adjustment to effect comparability of family income and personal income, the decreases in mortality level as income increased appear to be more marked among unrelated individuals than among family members. For example, if it is assumed that a given amount of personal income (for an unrelated individual) is roughly comparable to twice as much family income (for a family member), then differentials in mortality ratios by personal income intervals ranging from "under $2,000" to "$4,000 or more," for unrelated individuals would be roughly comparable—in terms of implied socioeconomic level—to differentials in mortality ratios by family income intervals ranging from "under $4,000" to "$8,000 or more" for family members. When this comparison is made for white males 25-64 years of age, the income differential of 64 percent for unrelated individuals (the proportionate difference between the mortality ratio of 1.26 for those with under $2,000 income and the ratio of 0.77 for those with $4,000 or more income) is larger than the income differential of 50 percent for family members (the proportionate difference between mortality ratios of 1.32 and 0.88 for those with under $4,000 and $8,000 or more family income respectively).[6] Among white females 25-64 years of age, the income differential of 61 percent for unrelated individuals (based on ratios ranging from 1.27 to 0.79) was almost twice as large as the differential of 31 percent for family members (based on ratios ranging from 1.15 to 0.88).

Among white unrelated individuals over 65 years of age, there was no indication of an inverse association between mortality and income for men, although women did maintain a differential of 31 percent. This pattern is in direct contrast to that described above for family members over 65 years of age, among whom an inverse association was found for men but not for women.

The fact that the income differentials appear to be more marked among unrelated individuals than among family members under age 65 is not surprising if account is taken of the limitations of income as an index of socioeconomic status in the study of mortality. As pointed out in Chapter 1, the basic presupposition in studies of socioeconomic differentials in mortality is that socioeconomic status has an effect on mortality; that is, the direction of the relationship is presumed to be that differences in socioeconomic status are responsible for differences in mortality. In the case of the income differentials, however, this causal path is complicated by a reverse path because the approach of death itself is often the cause of decreased income during the year preceding death, and also because income as measured in the census excludes savings and other forms of capital which are important economic assets and criteria of socioeconomic status.[7] The reverse causal path is especially important between ages 25 and 64, ages when illness prior to death removes from the work force persons who otherwise would be working,[8] and it is also likely to have a more pronounced effect on the personal income of an unrelated individual prior to death than on the family income of a family member (on the assumption that other family members contribute to family income). Thus, it is quite likely that the excessively high mortality of white males 25-64 years of age (both family members and unrelated individuals) in the low income groups in 1959 reflects, in part at least, the fact that large numbers of male decedents 25-64 years of age must have been reported in the low income groups in 1959 not because they normally belonged there but because they were unable to work at their normal level during the year preceding their death. Among white females under age 65 the very large income differential for unrelated individuals may have a similar explanation—assuming that their personal income would normally be derived primarily from their own work—while the smaller income differential for family members may be explained by the fact that family income is much less dependent on the income of

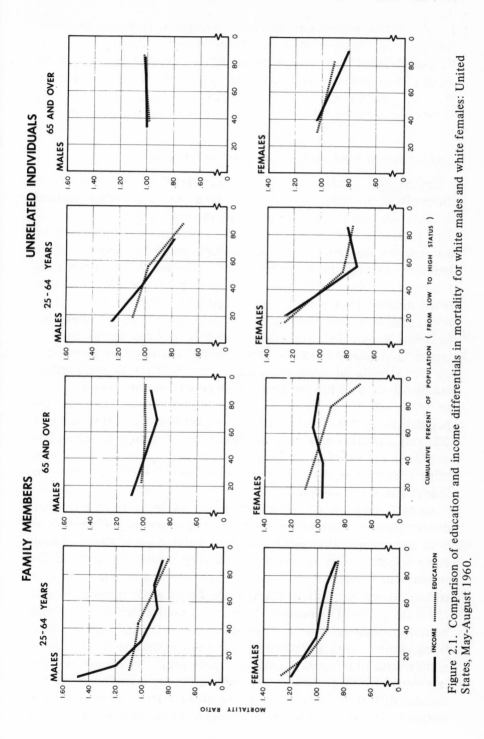

Figure 2.1. Comparison of education and income differentials in mortality for white males and white females: United States, May-August 1960.

female than of male family members. Bolstering these conclusions is the fact that among white female family members 25-64 years of age the education differentials in mortality are at least as large as the income differentials, whereas among white male family members of the same age the education differentials are much smaller than the income differentials. This point is elaborated in the next section.

Comparison of Education and Income Differentials

Among white females in the United States in 1960, education differentials in mortality were as large or larger than income differentials, while the opposite was the case among white males. This pattern is evident in Figure 2.1, where income and education differentials are drawn on the same graph for each sex-age subpopulation by plotting the mortality ratios on the vertical axis against the midpoints of the cumulative percent distribution of the population when ordered from low to high education (or income) level on the horizontal axis, and connecting successive points on the education (income) graph. This procedure not only enables the plotting of income and education on the same axis of each graph but also makes an approximate adjustment for differences between the proportionate distribution of the population into education and income groups. In other words, in Figure 2.1 the percent distributions of the population by education and income level found in Tables 2.1 and 2.5, respectively, are viewed as allocations of family members and unrelated individuals into groups ranked from low to high status, using education as the index of status in Table 2.1 and income as the index of status in Table 2.5.

Among women who were members of families in 1960, education differentials in mortality were larger than income differentials in both age groups, although below age 65 the slope of the education curve appears to be only very slightly steeper than the slope of the income curve. After age 65, however, the inverse association between education and mortality remains quite strong while income shows if anything a slight tendency toward a positive relationship with mortality. Among women classified as unrelated individuals—those living alone or with unrelated persons—education and income differentials were quite marked and also quite similar below age 65, and less marked and not quite so similar after age 65. Above age 65, income differentials appeared to be slightly larger than education differentials. Among men, on the other hand, income differentials in mortality were consistently larger than education differentials, with the single exception among unrelated individuals 65 and over, for whom there were virtually no differences in mortality between the two categories of education and income.

These comparisons do not necessarily justify the conclusion that income is a more important factor in mortality among men than women, nor even that income is more important than education as a factor in male mortality. As was pointed out in the preceding section, the income differentials may be quite misleading because the very high mortality of the low-income groups—especially for persons under age 65—no doubt reflects in part a reverse causal path in which the approach of death causes "lower than normal income" during the year preceding death.

Mortality and Socioeconomic Status

The discussion in Chapter 1 reviewed some of the problems involved in defining and measuring socioeconomic status. Education, occupation, and income were recognized as three basic components of socioeconomic status, with the admonition that they be treated as separate dimensions of socioeconomic status rather than being combined into a single index, primarily because they are not highly intercorrelated and are capable of quite different relationships with a dependent variable. The latter expectation is realized in the important differences between the education and income differentials in mortality summarized in the preceding sections of this chapter.

Despite these considerations, however, some judgments concerning the comparative worth of these education and income differentials as indicators of differential mortality by socioeconomic status do appear to be warranted. *In our judgment, the education differentials probably provide more reliable indicators of socioeconomic differentials in mortality in the United States in 1960 than do the income differentials.* The income differentials are subject to criticism for two reasons. First, the reverse causal path tends to inflate income differentials for subgroups of the population heavily represented in the work force, especially males 25-64 years of age and female unrelated individuals of the same age. Second, education as an index of socioeconomic status has the advantage of being fixed after young adulthood; income, on the other hand, is subject to variation over time and for many persons income during a given year, especially as reported in a census enumeration, may be a poor indicator of the "wealth" component of socioeconomic status.

This judgment is made not to imply that there is a single pattern of socioeconomic differentials in mortality which the education differentials are more likely to approximate, but rather to emphasize the deficiencies of the census definition of income as a measure of the wealth component of socioeconomic status, especially for mortality studies. Nor does the judgment imply that differences in the impact of education and wealth on mortality may not be in the directions indicated. For example, wealth may in fact have a greater impact than education on male mortality, and a greater impact on male than on female mortality. The point made here is simply that such conclusions are not warranted from the data available for the United States in 1960 because the income differentials, especially for males,

Table 2.6. Mortality ratios by years of school completed (standardized for age and income level), for white family members 25-64 years of age, by sex: United States, May-August, 1960

Years of school completed	Ratios standardized for age only[a]		Ratios standardized for age and income level[b]	
	White males	White females	White males	White females
Family members 25-64 years..	1.00	1.00	1.00	1.00
0-7 years................	1.13	1.27	1.05	1.21
8 years..................	1.06	1.07	1.04	1.05
High school, 1-3 years....	1.04	.93	1.05	.93
High school, 4 years......	.91	.87	.95	.90
College, 1 year or more...	.81	.84	.87	.89

Source: Same as Table 2.1.

[a] Minor differences between the age-standardized mortality ratios in this table and comparable ratios in Table 2.1 are the result of different "standard rates" used to compute expected deaths. In this table expected deaths for white males were computed by multiplying age-specific death rates for all white male family members during the period May-August, 1960 (instead of age-specific rates for the total population during the year, 1960), by the 1960 age composition of white male family members in each education subgroup; expected deaths for white females were similarly computed by multiplying age-specific death rates for all white female family members during the period May-August, 1960, by the 1960 age composition of white female family members in each education subgroup.

[b] Ratios standardized for both age and family income level were computed in the same manner as those standardized for age only, except that expected deaths were computed by multiplying age-income-specific death rates for white male and white female family members for the period May-August, 1960, by the 1960 age composition of white male and white female family members in each education subgroup of the population. Ten-year age intervals were used to standardize for age, and the income intervals reported in Table 2.7 were used to standardize for family income.

are no doubt exaggerated by a reverse causal path and the extent of this inflation unfortunately is impossible to estimate.

Independent Influence of Education and Income

Although the relationship between education and mortality and between income and mortality in the United States in 1960 were not entirely independent of each other, substantial inverse associations remained between education and mortality when income was controlled, as well as between income and mortality when education was controlled. These conclusions are documented for white family

Table 2.7. Mortality ratios by level of family income (standardized for age and education level), for white family members 25-64 years of age, by sex: United States, May-August, 1960

Family income, 1959	Ratios standardized for age only[a]		Ratios standardized for age and education[b]	
	White males	White females	White males	White females
Family members 25-64 years..	1.00	1.00	1.00	1.00
Under $2,000..............	1.49	1.21	1.40	1.11
$2,000-3,999..............	1.20	1.12	1.13	1.06
$4,000-5,999..............	.99	1.00	.96	.98
$6,000-7,999..............	.88	.97	.89	.99
$8,000-9,999..............	.93	.92#	.96	.96#
$10,000 or more...........	.84	.86	.90	.93

Source: Same as Table 2.1.

Does not meet reliability requirement specified in Table 2.1.

[a] Minor differences between the age-standardized mortality ratios in this table and comparable ratios in Table 2.5 are the result of different "standard rates" used to compute expected deaths. In this table expected deaths for white males were computed by multiplying age-specific death rates for all white males (instead of age-specific rates for the total population) for the year, 1960, by the 1960 age composition of white male family members in each income subgroup; expected deaths for white females were similarly computed by multiplying age-specific death rates for all white females in 1960 by the 1960 age composition of white female family members in each income subgroup.

[b] Ratios standardized for both age and education were computed in the same manner as those standardized for age only, except that expected deaths were computed by multiplying estimated annual age-education-specific death rates for all white males and all white females in 1960 (see Appendix A, Section 4, for procedures used to estimate these annual rates) by the 1960 age composition of white male and white female family members in each income subgroup. Ten-year age intervals were used to standardize for age, and the education levels reported in Table 2.6 were used to standardize for education.

members 25-64 years of age in Table 2.6, which reports education differentials standardized for income as well as age, and in Table 2.7, which reports income differentials standardized for education as well as age.

The education differential of 40 percent for white males (the proportionate difference between the age-standardized mortality ratio of 1.13 for those with less than 8 years of school and the ratio of 0.81 for those with at least one year of college) was reduced to a differential of 21 percent (the proportionate difference between ratios of 1.05 and 0.87) when income was also controlled (Table 2.6). Among white females, the education differential of 51 percent (ratios ranging from 1.27 to 0.84) was reduced to 36 percent (ratios ranging from 1.21 to 0.89) when income was also controlled.

Similarly, the income differential of 77 percent for white males (ratios from 1.49 to 0.84) was reduced to a differential of 56 percent (ratios from 1.40 to 0.90) when education was controlled (Table 2.7). Among white females the income differential of 41 percent (ratios from 1.21 to 0.86) was reduced to a differential of 19 percent (ratios ranging from 1.11 to 0.93).

These findings are not surprising given the low intercorrelations between education and income in the United States in 1960 which were cited in Chapter 1. They imply, of course, that persons with both high education and high income have lower mortality, on the average, than persons high on education but low on income or than persons high on income but low on education. Clearly both education and income have important *independent* associations with mortality.

Education Differentials by Age

The preceding analysis has shown that the range of socioeconomic differentials in mortality—as measured by both education and income—was much larger among persons 25-64 years of age than among persons 65 and over. Differentials by age within these broad age groups were not explored, in large part because the very small numbers of deaths below age 45 preclude any detailed analysis by socioeconomic level within 10-year, or even 20-year, age intervals. However, it was possible, by condensing the detail of socioeconomic level, to obtain reasonably stable socioeconomic differentials for the white population within 10-year and 20-year age groups, based on 5 levels of educational attainment without controls for other variables (Table 2.8).

As might be expected—from the patterns described earlier for the two broad age groups—the relative size of socioeconomic differentials in mortaltiy decreased with increasing age, especially among white males. Thus, the range of differentials was from 2.67 to 1.00 from the lowest (less than 8 years of school) to the highest education level (1 year or more of college) for white males 25-34, and then decreased sharply as age increased to a range of only 1.10 to 1.00 in the age group 65-74. Above age 74, the mortality of college-educated males was slightly higher than that for men with less education.

Among white females, there were less marked socioeconomic

Table 2.8. Estimated annual death rates (per 1,000 population) by years of school completed for the white population 25 years and over, by sex and age: United States, 1960

Sex and age	Deaths per 1,000 population					Index of death rate (college 1 year or more as base)				
	Less than 8 years	8 years	High school		College 1 year or more	Less than 8 years	8 years	High school		College 1 year or more
			1-3 years	4 years				1-3 years	4 years	
AGE-SPECIFIC RATES										
Males										
25-34 years.........	3.2	2.3#	1.8#	1.4#	1.2	2.67	1.90#	1.47#	1.18#	1.00
35-44 years.........	5.4	4.3	4.0	3.0	2.4	2.23	1.77	1.67	1.24	1.00
45-54 years.........	11.4	9.7	9.6	8.4	7.4	1.54	1.32	1.31	1.14	1.00
55-64 years.........	23.6	23.5	22.4	21.8	18.2	1.29	1.29	1.23	1.19	1.00
65-74 years.........	50.7	49.1	46.5		46.1	1.10	1.06	1.01		1.00
75 years & over......	123.7	122.4	123.0		128.6	.96	.95	.96		1.00
Females										
25-34 years.........	1.7	1.3#	1.1#	0.8#	1.0#	1.78	1.31#	1.11#	.80#	1.00#
35-44 years.........	3.6	2.1#	2.2#	1.6	1.9#	1.84	1.07#	1.13#	.84	1.00#
45-54 years.........	5.7	5.3	4.2#	4.2	3.7#	1.54	1.42	1.12#	1.14	1.00#
55-64 years.........	13.9	11.7	9.1	9.6	7.9#	1.77	1.48	1.16	1.22	1.00#
65-74 years.........	32.1	29.4	26.5		19.9#	1.61	1.48	1.33		1.00#
75 years & over......	106.0	100.8	94.3		69.9#	1.52	1.44	1.35		1.00#
AGE-ADJUSTED RATES[a]										
Males										
25 years & over......	16.6	15.5	14.7	14.6	13.5	1.23	1.15	1.09	1.08	1.00
25-64 years.........	9.0	8.0	7.6	6.8	5.7	1.57	1.40	1.32	1.18	1.00
25-44 years.........	4.2	3.2	2.8	2.1	1.8	2.38	1.81	1.58	1.21	1.00
45-64 years.........	16.3	15.3	14.8	13.8	11.8	1.39	1.30	1.26	1.18	1.00
65 years & over......	72.1	70.5	68.9		70.4	1.02	1.00	.98		1.00
Females										
25 years & over......	11.0	9.7	8.2	8.8	6.8	1.62	1.42	1.21	1.29	1.00
25-64 years.........	5.2	4.1	3.4	3.2	3.0	1.72	1.37	1.13	1.08	1.00
25-44 years.........	2.6	1.7#	1.6	1.2	1.4#	1.81	1.16#	1.12	.81	1.00#
45-64 years.........	9.1	7.9	6.2	6.4	5.4	1.68	1.46	1.14	1.19	1.00
65 years & over......	53.7	50.4	46.4		34.6	1.55	1.46	1.34		1.00

Source: Population Research Center, University of Chicago, 1960 Matched Records Study. Estimated annual death rates by 10-year age intervals for each education subgroup were calculated following the procedures described in Appendix A, section 5, steps 1-4.

\# Does not meet reliability requirement specified in Table 2.1.

[a] Age-adjusted death rates were calculated from the age-specific death rates, using the total 1940 U.S. population as standard.

differentials between ages 25 and 45—as compared with males—and much less contraction of socioeconomic differentials with increasing age. For example, the mortality index for the lowest education level varied only between 1.78 and 1.52 by 10-year age intervals, with no consistent pattern by age. In addition, there were some inconsistencies in the inverse pattern between the third and fourth education levels (1-3 and 4 years of high school), which may, however, be the result of small numbers of deaths. Moreover, even above age 75, the death rate for women with less than 8 years of school was over 50 percent higher than that for women with 1 year or more of college.

Infant Mortality Rates

Infant mortality rates in the United States, 1964-66, were inversely related to family income and to the level of educational attainment of both parents (Table 2.9). For example, there were 34.8 infant

Table 2.9. Infant mortality rates by education of parents, color, and family income: United States, 1964-66

Subject	Total	Years of school completed				
		None or elementary	High school		College	
			1-3 years	4 years	1-3 years	4 years or more
Infant mortality rate						
by education of mother....	22.8	34.8	27.4	19.2	15.7	19.7
by education of father....	22.8	32.7	27.1	18.8	20.4	17.1
Index of infant mortality						
by education of mother....	1.00	1.53	1.20	.84	.69	.86
by education of father....	1.00	1.43	1.19	.82	.89	.75

Subject	Total	Family income				
		Under $3,000	$3,000-4,999	$5,000-6,999	$7,000-9,999	$10,000 or more
Infant mortality rate, total.	22.8	31.8	24.9	17.9	19.6	19.6
White...................	20.5	---	---	---	---	---
Nonwhite...............	37.1	---	---	---	---	---
Index of infant mortality,						
total...................	1.00	1.39	1.09	.79	.86	.86

Source: National Center for Health Statistics, The Health of Children—1970 (Washington: Government Printing Office, 1970). The infant mortality rate is the number of deaths that occurred to infants under 1 year of age during the 3-year period, per 1,000 live births that occurred during the same period.

deaths per 1,000 live births to mothers having no more than an elementary school education, as compared with only 19.7 infant deaths per 1,000 live births to women with 4 years or more of college. Thus, the infant mortality rate was 77 percent higher for mothers who had only an elementary school education than for mothers who graduated from college. Differentials in infant mortality were very similar by level of educational attainment of father, and only slightly less marked by family income.

These data were compiled from the National Sample Surveys of Natality and Mortality conducted by the National Center for Health Statistics. More details on education and income differentials by color and sex, as well as for cross classifications of the socioeconomic indicators, were discussed in a recent paper (MacMahon, 1970). It is expected that these materials will be published in the NCHS series of published reports.

Limitations of Data

The mortality differentials by education and income obtained from the Matched Records Study are subject to various sources of error, of which the most important are sampling error and a potential seasonal bias. The design of the study and the procedures by which estimates of education and income differentials were derived are described in Appendix A. Sampling errors for the mortality ratios were not estimated for several reasons. First, because the study was limited to deaths occurring during a four-month period (May through August), the possibility of a seasonal bias raised questions concerning the applicability of random sampling theory. Second, the adjustments made for discrepancies in the response to the same questions on the 1960 census schedules and the NCHS Special Survey questionnaires, although they provided improved estimates of mortality differentials, raised similar questions with respect to the applicability of random sampling theory. Third, age-adjusted mortality ratios of the kind used here would undoubtedly have exceedingly complex sampling variance formulas—if they could be evaluated at all from present knowledge on the subject. In any case, the simplifying assumptions utilized by Keyfitz to estimate sampling errors of standardized death rates (Keyfitz, 1968, chapter 15) are not applicable to the ratios cited here, given the definitions of the ratios and the numerous steps in the estimation procedures, especially those for estimating census characteristics of unmatched decedents and the adjustments made for discrepancies in response to the same characteristics on death certificates and census records (see Appendix A).

Although data from the Matched Records Study did not permit direct measurement of seasonal bias, it was possible to determine that there was very little *seasonal selection by cause of death* during the May-August period, and that what selection did exist had virtually no effect on the size and pattern of education differentials for all causes of death combined. Indexes of seasonal selection (the percentage of all 1960 deaths covered in the "total Stage II Census") for some 20 different causes of death among the white population are reported in Appendix Table A.14, column 7. With the exception

Table 2.10 Mortality ratios by years of school completed (adjusted for seasonal selection by cause of death) for the white population 25 years and over, by sex: United States, May-August, 1960

Age and years of school completed	White males		White females	
	Unadjusted[a] (May-August)	Adjusted for seasonal selection[b]	Unadjusted[a] (May-August)	Adjusted for seasonal selection[b]
Total 25 & over.......	1.00	1.00	1.00	1.00
0-7 years..............	1.03	1.05	1.16	1.17
8 years................	1.02	1.02	1.05	1.06
High school, 1-4 years..	1.00	.97	.90	.88
College, 1 year or more.	.89	.88	.72	.71
25-64 years..........	1.00	1.00	1.00	1.00
0-7 years..............	1.14	1.15	1.31	1.31
8 years................	1.07	1.06	1.08	1.08
High school, 1-4 years..	.97	.97	.89	.89
College, 1 year or more.	.77	.77	.80	.81
65 & over............	1.00	1.00	1.00	1.00
0-7 years..............	1.01	1.01	1.10	1.09
8 years................	1.00	.99	1.03	1.03
High school, 1-4 years..	.99	.98	.94	.94
College, 1 year or more.	.98	.99	.70	.70

Source: Same as Table 2.1.

[a] See note a, Table 2.1, for definition of ratios.

[b] The seasonal adjustment was made by (1) inflating estimates of "actual deaths for May through August" for each of nine major causes of death, to total 1960 deaths from that cause, with controls by sex and age; and (2) summing these annual estimates for the nine causes of death to obtain an annual estimate of actual deaths from all causes of death. The nine causes selected for this purpose are those numbered 1 to 9 in Table A-15, Appendix A. The seasonal index, or the percent of total 1960 deaths included in the estimated actual deaths for May through August, is reported for each cause of death in column 7 of Table A-15.

of influenza and pneumonia, almost all of the seasonal indexes fall between 6.5 and 8.5, a relatively narrow range around the indexes of 7.3 and 7.2 for all causes of death for white males and females 25 and over.[9] The indexes for influenza and pneumonia were considerably lower (between 4.2 and 5.0 percent for the different sex-age subgroups), indicating relatively fewer deaths from these causes during the summer months. That these variations in seasonal indexes by cause of death had virtually no effect on the education differentials in mortality from all causes of death combined is evident from the adjusted and unadjusted indexes reported in Table 2.10. The unadjusted indexes are comparable to those reported in Tables 2.1 to 2.7 of this chapter; the adjusted indexes incorporate a correction for reweighting the nine major causes of death (causes 1, 2, 3, 4, 5, 6, 7, 8, and 9 in Appendix Table A.14) by the proportions they comprised of total 1960 deaths for each sex-age subgroup of the white population. Therefore, to the extent that seasonal variations in education (and probably other socioeconomic) differentials in mortality are the result of seasonal selection by cause of death, there is reason to believe that the education differentials for the May through August period are not distorted by seasonal bias. This does, of course, still leave one with the assumption that education (and other socioeconomic) differentials observed for each cause of death during the May through August period are representative of the pattern of differentials for all deaths from that cause during the year. It should not be forgotten, however, that the bias of any time period is "relative" in the sense that any time period selected for a study of mortality is subject to distortion by particular circumstances during the period. Thus, even deaths for an entire year are subject to a "period" bias, a reason often cited for combining deaths for several years.

The 1960 education differentials summarized in this chapter are compared with similar differentials derived from age-adjusted death rates for three broad education levels in 1962-63 in Table 2.11. Although it may be tempting to interpret some of the differences between the two sets of data in terms of a possible seasonal bias in the differentials for May-August 1960, such an interpretation does not appear to be justified. The small sample frequencies in the 1962-63 study (which was based on a mail survey of 10,822 deaths occurring during the two-year period), the fact that no corrections were made for discrepancies in response to the same questions in the 1962-63 death survey questionnaire and the current population

Table 2.11. Mortality ratios by years of school completed, by sex, age and color: United States, 1962-63 and May-August, 1960

Age and highest grade of school completed	1962-63 (2-year total)[a]				May-August, 1960[b]			
					White		Nonwhite	
	All males	All females	All white	All non-white	Males	Females	Males	Females
25-64 years....	1.00	1.00	1.00	1.00	1.00	1.00	1.00	1.00
Elementary school	1.25	1.26	1.22	1.13	1.11	1.19	1.05	1.13
High school......	.91	.86	.91	.79	.97	.89	} .87	.74
College..........	.70	.85	.80	.91	.77	.80		
65 years & over	1.00	1.00	1.00	1.00	1.00	1.00	1.00	1.00
Elementary school	1.07	1.05	1.07	1.06	1.01	1.06	1.00	1.00
High school......	.84	.90	.87	.53	.99	.94	} .97	1.01
College..........	.86	.90	.88	.91	.98	.70		

Source: Ratios for May-August, 1960 from same source cited in Table 2.1. Ratios for 1962-63 calculated from age-specific death rates (for age intervals 25-44, 45-54, 55-64, 65 and over) reported in National Center for Health Statistics, Series 22, Number 9 (February, 1969), Socioeconomic Characteristics of Deceased Persons, United States, 1962-63 Deaths, Table 3. The age-specific death rates for 1962-63 were based on (1) estimates of deaths derived from a mail survey covering a sample of 10,822 decedents drawn by systematic selection of one in 330 death records from the microfilm copies of all death certificates for 1962-63; and (2) estimates of population derived from the Current Population Survey for March, 1962.

[a] The 1962-63 mortality ratios for ages 25-64 were calculated from age-adjusted death rates standardized by the direct method, using the total 1960 U.S. population as standard; ratios for ages 65 and over were computed from the death rate for persons 65 and over.

[b] The 1960 mortality ratios are defined in note a, Table 2.1; they are equivalent to ratios based on age-adjusted death rates indirectly standardized for 10-year age intervals (up to ages 75 and over) within the two broad age intervals reported here.

survey schedule, and the fact that no corrections apparently were made for nonrespondents in the 1962-63 death survey (8 percent of the questionnaires mailed out were not returned), make it virtually impossible to use the 1962-63 study as a base for evaluating a possible seasonal bias in the 1960 education differentials.

The main differences between the two sets of differentials in Table 2.11 are a larger education differential for males in both age groups in the 1962-63 study and a smaller differential for females 65 and over in the 1962-63 study. The differentials for females 25-64 are quite similar in the two studies. In the 1962-63 study, the education differentials for males 25-64 years of age are larger than the differentials for females 25-64 years of age, and an inverse association persists for males after age 65.

It may also be noted that most of the mortality differentials reported from the 1960 Matched Records Study were based on ratios of actual to expected deaths standardized for age by the indirect method (see note 3, this chapter, and Appendix A); the only exceptions are in Tables 2.4 and 2.8. That the indirect and direct methods of standardization give virtually identical education differentials for the white population in 1960 is evident in Table 2.12, which compares the relative size of education differentials calculated by the two methods.

Table 2.12. Comparison of socioeconomic differentials in mortality based on directly and indirectly standardized measures of mortality: United States, 1960

Sex and years of school completed	Index of mortality (college-educated as base)					
	Directly standardized for age[a]			Indirectly standardized for age[b]		
	25-44 years	45-64 years	65 & over	25-44 years	45-64 years	65 & over
White males						
Less than 8 years......	2.38	1.39	1.02	2.34	1.37	1.03
8 years...............	1.81	1.30	1.00	1.79	1.30	1.01
High school, 1-3 years.	1.58	1.26 ⎫ .98		1.60	1.26 ⎫ 1.00	
High school, 4 years...	1.21	1.18 ⎭		1.22	1.17 ⎭	
College, 1 year or more	1.00	1.00	1.00	1.00	1.00	1.00
White females						
Less than 8 years......	1.81	1.68	1.55	1.83	1.69	1.57
8 years...............	1.16#	1.46	1.46	1.13#	1.45	1.48
High school, 1-3 years.	1.12	1.14 ⎫ 1.34		1.12	1.14 ⎫ 1.35	
High school, 4 years...	.81	1.19 ⎭		.83	1.19 ⎭	
College, 1 year or more	1.00#	1.00	1.00	1.00#	1.00	1.00

Does not meet reliability requirements specified in Table 2.1.

[a] Differentials calculated from age-specific death rates reported in Table 2.8 (calculations based on rates to 3 decimal places, which may differ slightly from results using rates to 1 decimal as reported in Table 2.8).

[b] Differentials calculated from same ratios of actual to expected deaths which provided the mortality ratios reported in Table 2.1 (see Appendix A for detailed definition).

3 / OCCUPATION DIFFERENTIALS

Differences in mortality by occupation have been among the major interests in studies in differential mortality. One reason for this, a pragmatic one as indicated in Chapter 1, is that occupation has been one of the few, and in many places including the United States the only, item on the death certificate that could be used as an index of the decedent's socioeconomic status. To be sure, knowledge of a person's occupation provides a significant insight into his physical environment, his social milieu, his educational background, his income, and his life style. Moreover, since there is great variability among occupations in hazards and risks to health and life there have been many investigations focused on differential mortality as induced by occupation. There are, however, a number of difficulties which impair the use of occupation as an index of socioeconomic status in general and, also, specifically, in the study of differential mortality.

First, it is to be emphasized that despite the interrelationships of occupation, income, and education, each of these items considered as an independent variable may differ in its relationship to any given dependent variable. In this study, the latter point is clearly demonstrated in the differences between income, education, and occupational differentials in mortality. In addition, occupational data have a number of specific limitations in the study of mortality differentials. Since an occupational death rate requires the relating of occupational returns on death certificates with occupational returns on census schedules, any differences in the reporting of occupation on these respective documents obviously distort the rates. It has been assumed in the past that the use of the broad major groupings of occupations as socioeconomic indicators would help to control the discrepancy between the occupational return in the death certificate which affects the numerator of the death rate, and that in the census which affects the denominator of the rate. For example, such a practice was followed in the Registrar General's Decennial Supplements for England and Wales for 1921, 1931, and 1951. The same practice was followed in the United States in 1950 (Moriyama and Guralnick, 1956). However, this procedure has by no means eliminated the problems of comparability and interpretation of the data. A comparison of the occupational returns on death certificates in the United States and in the 1950 census based on matching of these records for a sample of males 45-64 years of age revealed significant differences in the reporting of occupation in the two sets of records (NCHS, June 1961). A similar study in England, although it indicated that discrepant reporting may have been somewhat less than in the United States, gave comparable results (General Register Office, 1958, pp. 41-45 and 50-56, cited in NCHS [June 1961], p. 17).

The data available also greatly restrict conclusions about differential occupational mortality risk. The occupation of a decedent at the time of death may be quite different from that at which he spent most of his working life. Moreover, even if this question does not arise, the risk of death for any person includes not only his occupational exposure but also the other exposures of his total life space, including his neighborhood, his housing, his level of living, his personal habits, his nutrition, and all the diverse elements that make up his style of life. In consequence, mortality studies have tended to use occupational data more as indicators of general socioeconomic level than as a measurement of differential occupational mortality risks.

The use of occupational returns as a general socioeconomic indicator, despite distortions, does provide a picture of differential mortality with reasonable validity. This conclusion is bolstered by various studies in which the mortality of wife classified by occupation of husband shows patterns of differentials which match those of their husbands (Benjamin, 1965, p. 33). Additional difficulties are found in efforts to obtain occupational differences in mortality for females. Since a relatively small proportion of women are in the labor force and the proportion has increased over time, and since women have a much higher in and out of the labor force mobility, occupational death rates for women are much more difficult both to compile and to interpret. When, however, what is desired is an analysis of differential female mortality by socioeconomic level the occupation of the husband can be used, as indicated above. By reason of the unavailability of data, however, such studies have not been possible heretofore, for the United States.

In the 1960 Matched Records Study for the United States, the problems of discrepant reporting of occupation in the census and on the death certificate were, of course, resolved by matching the two records. It is doubtful if the cost of the matching could be justified if the purpose had been merely to control differences in the occupational returns. Such a doubt has, indeed, been expressed by Benjamin (Benjamin, 1965, p. 32). The other problems of interpreting the occupational data were, of course, not obviated by the matching procedure.

In this chapter analysis of differential mortality by occupation in the United States in 1960 is given for white males 25 to 74 years of age with age subgroupings and, by reason of smaller numbers, for nonwhites 25 to 64 years old. Males "employed" during the census week, the last week in March 1960, for whom "current" occupation was reported were combined with males who had worked at any time since 1949, for whom "last" occupation was reported. This practice was followed because, of the males 25 to 74 years of age who died between May and August in 1960, a large proportion were not reported in the census as employed because of incapacitation or illness. This, in effect, provides information for all males in 1960 in the age groups with work experience since 1950.

The proportion of matched records varied by occupational grouping and by age of the male decedent. The general procedure for adjusting the data for the unmatched records in the 1960 Matched Records Study was followed. Further detail on the procedures followed in the analyses of mortality by occupation is contained in Appendix A, Section 3.

Previous Findings

Occupation has been the major item used in earlier efforts to study class differentials in mortality based on the characteristics of the person. Much of the earlier literature on differential occupational mortality has been effectively summarized by a number of scholars. Reviews of the literature on occupational mortality are contained in the works of Daric (National Center for Health Statistics [NCHS], 1951), Stockwell (1961), Benjamin (1965), and Antonovsky (1967). Benjamin has placed mortality studies by occupation in the context of general studies on social and economic factors affecting mortality (1965). Moriyama and Guralnick (1956) have analyzed occupational differences in mortality for the United States in 1950, and, in the context of social class differences, in comparison with mortality in England and Wales. The largest time series of occupational mortality rates are those for England and Wales initiated by William Farr in 1851 and made available for every census year since, except for 1941, when World War II greatly restricted statistical output. In the United States official differential occupation mortality data were tabulated in 1890 and in each census year since except for 1940. But the data were published only for 1890, 1900, 1930, and 1950. In 1950 five "Special Reports" were devoted to mortality by occupation, by occupation and industry, by occupation and cause of death, by industry and cause of death, and by occupational level and cause of death (NCHS, *Vital Statistics—Special Reports*, vol. 53, nos. 1, 2, 3, 4, and 5, 1961). The Actuarial Society of America using life insurance data has also tabulated and published occupational mortality statistics since 1915, with special interest in occupational hazards to life.

It has been known for some time that some categories of occupations are associated with low and others with high death rates. Farr in 1851, for example, found that in England and Wales farmers enjoyed relatively low death rates, whereas miners, bakers, butchers, and innkeepers had relatively high death rates (Farr, 1885, p. 397). In the study of occupational mortality in England and Wales in 1949-53 great differences in mortality by occupation were still in evidence. "Farmers and farm managers," 20 to 64 years of age, for example, experienced mortality 30 percent below all workers the same age, whereas "tunnel miners" had a mortality rate more than twice that of the average—a Standard Mortality Ratio of 225 (Benjamin, 1965, pp. 33, 34). Other occupations with well below average mortality included "civil service higher officers"; "heads or managers of office departments"; "bankers, bank managers and inspectors"; "teachers (not music)"; and "costing and accounting clerks." Occupations with higher than average mortality included "makers of glass and glassware," "labourers and other unskilled workers," "sand blasters," "workers in chemical and allied trades," and "in coal mines."

These differentials in mortality reflect in part socioeconomic differences and in part variations in occupational hazards and risks. Examples of occupations with high mortality which in large measure is attributable to hazards and risks in the employment include sand blasters, glass blowers, and machine minders. The fact that mortality in these occupations is above levels that can be attributed to socioeconomic status is indicated by the much lower relative mortality of their wives. Whereas sand blasters 20-64 years of age experienced mortality 73 percent above average their wives had mortality 4 percent below average. Glass blowers' wives had mortality 33 percent above average for workers' wives; but their husbands, working as glass blowers, experienced mortality 89 percent above average. Machine tenders' wives had mortality levels 23 percent above average whereas the mortality of the machine tenders was 60 percent above average.

Most occupations in relation to mortality serve more as indicators of socioeconomic status than as sources of special hazards to life. This conclusion is based on the similarity in mortality differentials of husbands in such occupations and of their wives. For example, "clergymen of the Church of England" experienced mortality 19 percent below average and their wives 20 percent below; "teachers" 34 percent below average and wives 23 percent below; "bankers, etc." 22 percent below average and their wives 18 percent below average.

Moriyama and Guralnick (1956) used broad occupational groups as an indicator of socioeconomic status in their comparison of differential mortality in the United States and in England and Wales using the data from the 1950 census in the United States and 1951 census in England. They found for men 20 to 64 years of age, that death rates (per 100,000 population) varied significantly by five "occupational levels." The occupational levels together with the distribution of males by level for the United States follows:

Occupational Level	Percent
I. Professional Workers	4
II. Technical, Administrative, and Managerial Workers	9
III. Proprietors, Clerical, Sales, and Skilled Workers	37
IV. Semiskilled Workers	25
V. Laborers, except Farm and Mine	10
Agricultural Workers	13

Their standardized mortality ratio, "the age-adjusted rate as a ratio to the average death rate for all men 20-64," varied from 84 for the highest level, the professionals, to 165 for the lowest level, laborers. Although, in general, there was a pattern of increase in death rates with lower occupational levels, there tended to be relatively small differences among the first four occupational levels and a wide difference between them and the fifth level—laborers. The standardized mortality ratio for agricultural workers was almost identical with occupational level II (technical, administrative, and managerial workers). A similar "clustering" was evident in the age-specific rates for the first four occupational levels, with considerable overlapping for men aged 45 to 64. (See Table 3.1.)

Although conclusions about differences are difficult because of possible differences in discrepant reporting and other differences

Table 3.1. Ratios of death rates by occupation level to total death rates, by age, for men 20 to 64 years old: United States and England and Wales, 1950

Occupation level	20-24 years	25-34 years	35-44 years	45-54 years	55-59 years	60-64 years
United States, all males......	100	100	100	100	100	100
England and Wales, all males..	100	100	100	100	100	100
Occupation level I:						
United States...............	49	53	66	87	94	97
England and Wales..........	102	90	83	98	99	100
Occupation levels II, III, IV:						
United States...............	80	84	91	96	99	101
England and Wales..........	94	95	96	97	99	101
Occupation level V:						
United States...............	190	232	219	178	146	128
England and Wales..........	122	138	143	129	115	106
Agricultural workers:						
United States...............	132	125	92	84	84	85
England and Wales..........	139	104	87	75	75	72

Source: I.M. Moriyama and L. Guralnick, "Occupational and Social Class Differences in Mortality," in Milbank Memorial Fund, Trends and Differentials in Mortality (Papers presented at the 1955 Conference of the Milbank Memorial Fund, New York, 1956), p. 69.

between the censuses in England and the United States, the general patterns revealed by the data are similar. The occupational mortality differences for England and Wales tended to be smaller than those for the United States at all ages. In both countries the differences decreased with increasing age, with the greatest variations occurring for ages 25 to 34. A highly significant finding in 1950 was that at the highest occupational level, professional workers, the United States had lower relative mortality than in England and Wales, whereas at the lowest level, laborers, the United States had higher relative mortality. Among agricultural workers mortality in the United States was also relatively higher than in England and Wales at all ages except males 20 to 24 years of age.

Antonovsky has summarized changes in patterns of differences in mortality by social class over time. Using the occupational data for England and Wales from 1910-12, 1921-23, 1930-32, and 1949-53 (1967, p. 63), he shows that mortality differentials between the middle classes and the highest class have narrowed or disappeared but that the lowest class remains very much worse off than the other classes. Also manifest, over time, is the fact that the greatest differences in mortality by occupational class are found in the younger and middle ages.

In summary, the studies of differentials in mortality by occupation have revealed with great consistency an inverse relationship between the chances of dying and socioeconomic level. Earlier studies have also revealed that some occupations are much more hazardous to life than others; but mortality studies by occupation have, in the main, used occupational groupings as indicators of social class. Previous studies have also shown that class differences in mortality, with class measured by occupation, have narrowed over time. But despite the narrowing of mortality differences there appears, as yet, always a lower class that experiences relatively high mortality. That is, most of the diminution in class differences in mortality is confined to the social classes above the lowest. Also evident in earlier studies is the fact that class differences in mortality are greatest in the younger and middle years of life and that they tend to blur, disappear, and even to become inverted at the older ages. The general patterns of differential mortality by occupation revealed by earlier studies, with

Table 3.2. Mortality ratios by occupation, for males 25-74 years of age, by color and age: United States, May-August, 1960

	Mortality ratios				Percent distribution of males				
	Nonwhite	White			Nonwhite	White			
Major occupation group	25-64 years	25-74 years	25-64 years	65-74 years	25-64 years	25-74 years	25-64 years	65-74 years	75 & over
Total males........................	1.07	1.07	1.04	1.10	100.0	100.0	100.0	100.0	100.0
Did not work 1950 or later.................	1.90#	1.64	2.04	1.57	7.2	5.9	4.3	18.4	52.5
Worked 1950 or later[a].....................	1.00	1.00	1.00	1.00	100.0	100.0	100.0	100.0	100.0
1 Professional, technical, & kindred workers.....	--[b]	.88	.80	1.04#	3.8	10.6	11.1	6.2	6.6
2 Managers, officials, & proprietors, except farm	--[b]	.91	.91	.92	2.4	12.2	12.3	12.0	11.1
3 Clerical & sales workers....................	--[b]	1.02	1.02	1.02	6.0	13.2	13.2	13.0	12.6
4 Craftsmen, foremen & kindred workers...........	--[b]	.98	.97	.97	10.9	22.1	22.3	20.7	17.2
5 Operatives & kindred workers...................	--[b]	1.08	1.07	1.08	24.1	19.2	19.7	14.7	10.5
6 Service workers (incl. private h.h.)...........	--[b]	1.16	1.37	.97#	5.4	4.9	9.6	10.8	
7 Laborers, except farm and mine.................	--[b]	1.16	1.19	1.13	20.8	5.5	5.4	6.9	7.2
8 Agricultural workers...........................	--[b]	.82	.76	.90	9.9	7.7	7.1	13.3	19.4
9 Occupation not reported.......................	1.56	1.22	1.25	1.19	8.6	4.0	4.0	3.5	4.7
COMBINATIONS OF GROUPS									
Worked 1950 or later[a]......................	1.00	1.00	1.00	1.00	100.0	100.0	100.0	100.0	100.0
White collar workers (Groups 1, 2, 3)...........	.93	.94	.92	.98	12.2	36.0	36.6	31.2	30.3
Blue collar workers (Groups 4 to 8).............	.95	1.06	1.07	1.02	79.2	59.9	59.4	65.2	65.1
Craftsmen & operatives (Groups 4, 5)..........	.91	1.02	1.01	1.02	35.0	41.3	42.0	35.4	27.7
Service workers & laborers (Groups 6, 7).......	.98	1.16	1.28	1.04	34.3	10.9	10.3	16.5	18.0
Agricultural workers (Group 8).................		.82	.76	.90	9.9	7.7	7.1	13.3	19.4
Occupation not reported (Group 9)..............	1.56	1.22	1.25	1.19	8.6	4.0	4.0	3.5	4.7

Source: Population Research Center, University of Chicago, study based on matching death certificates with 1960 Census records.

Does not meet reliability requirement that the Special Sample Survey of May-August deaths (which provided data for estimating characteristics of deaths not matched with census records) include at least 10 unmatched decedents whose survey questionnaires allocate them to this subgroup of the male population.

[a] Includes decedents for whom "year last worked" was not reported (following procedures used in 1960 Census of Population). Persons not employed at time of 1960 Census are classified by last occupation.

[b] Mortality index not computed because of small numbers of deaths.

occupational grouping used as an indicator of social class, are supported by the findings in this study, as reported below.

Findings in the 1960 Matched Records Study

Occupational differences in mortality in the United States in 1960 are shown for males with work experience by color and by age group in such detail as the data permit in Table 3.2. About 96 percent of white males 25 to 64 years old and 82 percent of those 65 to 74 had worked at some time since 1950 and could therefore be classified by occupation. Of the nonwhite males 25 to 64 years old 93 percent had worked at some time since 1950 and were tabulated by occupation. The numbers of nonwhites above age 65 were too small to permit analysis. About 4 percent of the whites and 9 percent of the nonwhites with work experience since 1950 fell into the "occupation not reported" category. Mortality ratios were not computed for males 75 and over because less than half of this age group had worked since 1950 and could be classified by occupation.

The broad general findings may be briefly summarized. Mortality ratios for those with no work experience since 1950 are substantially higher than those with work experience. This is not unexpected, because the former group includes persons not employable for health reasons.

The mortality ratios for males 25-64 tend to decrease as "level of occupation" increases, although there are some deviations from this pattern, at least if it is assumed that the major occupations are ranked by level in Table 3.2. Among the white males, clerical and sales workers had higher mortality than craftsmen, and service workers had higher mortality than laborers. Among the nonwhite males, craftsmen had lower mortality than white-collar workers. Among both white and nonwhite males, agricultural workers had mortality ratios markedly lower than those of any other major occupation group.

White Male Mortality

White males over the entire age range considered, those 25 to 74 years old, who had not worked since 1950 experienced mortality 64 percent above the level of those who had a work record since that date. The disparity in mortality was much greater for the younger men, 25 to 64, who had not worked since 1950 than for those 65 to

74. White males, 25 to 64, with a mortality ratio of 2.04, experienced mortality more than twice as great as that of those with work experience. The older males, 65 to 74, had a mortality ratio, 1.57, that was 57 percent above that of their age counterparts with work experience. Clearly the higher mortality of the men without work experience since 1950 suggests that they were men who were unable to work because of incapacitation or illness which adversely affected their longevity, especially if they were under 65 years of age at the time of the census. It is to be observed that the proportion of white men without such work experience averaged 5.9 percent for all between 25 and 74 years of age; only 4.3 percent for those 25 to 64; and 18.4 percent for those 65 to 74.

White males for whom occupation was not reported experienced relatively high mortality, with mortality ratios 22 percent above average for the total 25 to 74 years of age, 25 percent above for workers 25 to 64, and 19 percent above for those 65 to 74. These data suggest that such persons may have had marginal health which increased their movements into and out of the labor force, so that an occupational return was relatively difficult to obtain.

Among all the white males 25 to 74 years of age there was considerable variation in mortality by occupation. The group with the highest mortality ratio, 1.22, comprised those for whom occupation was not reported (4.0 percent of the total with work experience). Among those for whom occupation was reported white males employed as service workers and laborers (except farm and mine) experienced the highest mortality, a level 16 percent above that for all white males 25 to 74. The other major occupational group with above average mortality was "operatives," 8 percent above. "Clerical and sales" personnel, with a mortality ratio 2 percent above average, experienced about average mortality. The group with the lowest mortality was that in agricultural occupations ("farmers and farm managers" and "farm laborers and foremen") with a mortality ratio of 0.82, 18 percent below the average. The other occupational groups with below average mortality were "professional and technical," 12 percent below average; "managers, officials, proprietors," 9 percent below. "Craftsmen and foremen," experienced about average mortality, with a mortality ratio only 2 percent below. The occupational groupings with the lowest mortality, apart from the agricultural occupations, were white-collar occupations with relatively high income and prestige. Contrariwise, the groupings with the highest mortality were the manual occupations with relatively low income and prestige. The white-collar occupations with relatively low income and prestige, "clerical and sales," and the manual occupations with relatively high income and high prestige, "craftsmen and foremen," experienced about average mortality. These findings show the complexity involved in using occupation as a sole indicator of socioeconomic level.

The range of mortality differences by occupation is much greater among the younger white males, those 25 to 64, than among the older group, 65 to 74. This is to be expected because it is in the younger ages, as the data on education and income reveal, that socioeconomic differences have the greater impact on mortality. At the older ages socioeconomic differences in death rates are dampened by reason of the fact that those who have survived to older age, and especially those in the lower socioeconomic groupings, possess relatively hardy organisms less subject to exogenous influences in the play of forces making for mortality. Among the younger white males with work experience, those 25 to 64 years old, mortality ratios range from a high of 1.37 for "service workers" to a low of 0.76 for those in the agricultural occupations, a range of 61 points. In contrast, among the comparable older white males, those 65 to 74, the mortality ratios range from a high of 1.13 for "laborers" to a low of 0.90 for the agricultural occupations, a range of only 23 points or little more than one-third of the range among the younger males. Expressed in another way the highest mortality ratio by occupation in the younger category was 80 percent above the lowest. In contrast, among the older men the highest mortality ratio was but 26 percent above the lowest.

Among white males 25 to 64 years of age the occupational categories with above average mortality included "service workers," 37 percent above; "laborers (except farm and mine)," 19 percent above; and "operatives," 7 percent above. White males 25 to 64 in "clerical and sales" occupations experienced about average mortality. The occupations with below average mortality were the "agricultural," 24 percent below; "professional and technical," 20 percent below; and "managers, officials and proprietors," 9 percent below. "Craftsmen and foremen" experienced about average mortality.

Among the white males 65 to 74 years old the occupational groupings with above average mortality were "laborers," 13 percent above; and "operatives," 8 percent above. The occupational groups with below average mortality were the "agricultural," 10 percent below; and "managers, officials, and proprietors," 8 percent below.

Among these older workers, also, the white-collar occupations with relatively low income and prestige and the manual occupations with relatively high income and prestige experienced about average mortality. The numbers of "professional, technical and kindred" and "service workers" for the older workers were too small to permit analysis.

In Table 3.3, earnings and years of school completed are shown by occupational groups for males 25 to 64 years of age in the experienced civilian labor force in 1960 with earnings in 1959. These data throw light on the role of occupational groupings as an indicator of socioeconomic level. The order in which the occupational groups are presented is the usual order of socioeconomic status, from high to low, based on the Edwards' scale, with the exception of the agricultural occupations (Edwards, 1943). The latter are kept separate as a group because of their special implications for mortality differentials—indicating as they do a rural, as compared with an urban, way of life. The 1959 earnings data in Table 3.3 corroborate the rank ordering of the major occupation groups by the Edwards' scale. Earnings in 1959 are relatively high for "occupation not reported," but this is a mixed category which is difficult to interpret. Fortunately, it is relatively small.

When the proportion of persons with 4 or more years of schooling is taken as a basis for ordering socioeconomic status a number of inversions occur. "Clerical and sales" workers have about the same level of education, by this index, as "managers, officials, and proprietors," but they experience appreciably higher mortality. "Service workers" have more education than "operatives" but experience higher mortality. These inversions are probably attributable to the heterogeneous character of each of these occupational groupings which include occupations with a great range in educational requirements. But the inversions in order may point to the differences, despite their overlap, between education, income, and occupation in relation to mortality. In Chapter 2 the specific effects of income and education when the other is controlled were considered. Unfortunately, sample size precludes such an assessment among occupation, income, and education.

Nonwhite Male Mortality

Because of small numbers, mortality data for nonwhites are restricted to the single age group 25 to 64 years of age. As for white

Table 3.3. Earnings and level of education of males 25-64 years old in the experienced civilian labor force, by color and major occupation group: United States, 1960

Major occupation	Number worked 1950 or later (1,000's)	Number with earnings in 1959 (1,000's)	Percent with 1959 earnings	Mean earnings 1959 Each group	Mean earnings 1959 Combined groups	Percent who completed High School
White males 25-64 years...............	35,017	32,758	93.5	$6,112	$6,112	47.1
Professional, technical & kindred workers..	3,887	3,748	96.4	8,881		91.5
Managers, officials, & prop., exc. farm....	4,292	4,083	95.1	9,478		66.2
Clerical workers...........................	} 4,626	2,179 }	94.8	5,458 }	6,256	63.1
Sales workers..............................		2,207 }		7,043 }		67.3
Craftsmen, foremen & kindred workers.......	7,799	7,394	94.8	5,678		36.9
Operatives & kindred workers..............	6,903	6,493	94.1	4,866		26.5
Service workers (incl. pvt. hh.)...........	1,728	1,568	90.7	4,279		33.1
Laborers, except farm & mine..............	1,876	1,658	88.4	3,895		18.6
Farmers & farm managers...................	1,911	1,693	88.6	3,576 }	3,278	31.9
Farm laborers & foremen...................	586	485	82.8	2,237 }		14.2
Occupation not reported...................	1,408	1,248	88.6	5,856		45.1
Nonwhite males 25-64 years............	3,797	3,350	88.2	3,260	3,260	22.9
Professional, technical & kindred workers..	145	136	93.8	5,519 }		89.0
Managers, officials, & prop., exc. farm....	89	81	91.0	4,823 }	4,761	44.4
Clerical workers...........................	} 229	171 }	92.1	4,282 }		56.7
Sales workers..............................		40 }		4,105 }		50.0
Craftsmen, foremen & kindred workers.......	415	377	90.8	3,757 }	3,526	23.9
Operatives & kindred workers..............	916	829	90.5	3,421 }		17.2
Service workers (incl. pvt. hh.)...........	512	453	88.5	2,922 }	2,850	21.9
Laborers, except farm & mine..............	789	681	86.3	2,802 }		10.0
Farmers & farm managers...................	154	124	80.5	1,551 }	1,392	6.5
Farm laborers & foremen...................	221	183	82.8	1,285 }		2.7
Occupation not reported...................	327	271	82.9	3,560		25.5

Source: Bureau of the Census, 1960 Census of Population, Subject Report PC(2)-7B, Table 1, except third column from special tabulation of 5 percent sample of 1960 Census compiled for Population Research Center, University of Chicago.

males, nonwhite males 25 to 64 years of age who had not worked since 1950 experienced higher mortality than those with work experience since that date. Their mortality ratio of 190 was almost twice that of nonwhite males in the experienced civilian work force in 1960 and, undoubtedly, is high for the same reason as for whites. They were probably unable to work since 1950 because of incapacity or bad health, which was reflected in their higher mortality. Non-whites without work experience since 1950 made up 7.2 percent of all nonwhite males of the same age. Also, as for white males, the nonwhite males with "occupation not reported" had a relatively high mortality ratio—56 percent above that of all nonwhite experienced workers.

Since it was not possible to analyze occupational differences for nonwhite males in the same detail as for whites, mortality ratios are shown for combinations of the broad occupational groups. Four categories are given in Table 3.2, namely, white collar and blue collar, with blue collar subdivided into "craftsmen and operatives" and all other groupings including agricultural workers. For purposes of comparability the same combinations are shown for white workers.

Occupational class made much less difference in the mortality of nonwhites than of whites except among workers for whom occupation was not reported. The mortality ratio for nonwhite white-collar workers was 0.93, almost the same as that for nonwhite blue-collar workers, 0.95. The ratio for craftsmen and operatives was 7 percent below that for other blue-collar workers.

The relative insensitivity of mortality ratio by occupation class for nonwhites may be the result of the necessary broader grouping, because of sample size, of occupational classes. The broader groupings are more heterogeneous than more detailed categories and, therefore, obscure possible differences in the factors affecting mortality. Particularly unfortunate in this respect was the need to combine service workers, laborers, and all agricultural workers into one group for nonwhites, because of small numbers and discrepant reporting of occupation on their death certificates and census returns. Among white males, for example, a similar grouping would have combined occupations experiencing the highest mortality (service workers and laborers) with those experiencing the lowest mortality (agricultural workers).

4 / SOCIOECONOMIC DIFFERENTIALS IN A METROPOLIS

Prior to the 1960 Matched Records Study, which provided the data on nationwide differentials in mortality by education, income, and occupation summarized in Chapters 2 and 3, most studies of socioeconomic differentials in mortality in the United States were based on an indirect form of analysis in which indexes of socioeconomic status for small geographic areas were used to classify residents of these areas by socioeconomic level. For example, analyses were made for a number of large cities or metropolitan areas, utilizing census tracts, the small relatively homogeneous geographic subdivisions into which large cities are subdivided for census purposes, or other combinations of areal units within political units (e.g., Hauser, 1938; Sheps and Watkins, 1947; Mayer and Marks, 1954; Yeracaris, 1955; Stockwell, 1962; Seidman, Garfinkle, and Craig, 1962). The studies cover a considerable span of time and, for some areas, permit analysis of trends in socioeconomic differentials. The most comprehensive time series of socioeconomic differentials in mortality in a metropolis pertain to the Chicago metropolitan area, and these materials are analyzed in the present chapter.

In these studies, deaths are typically compiled by census tract of residence of the decedent (using the street address reported on the death certificate), and then deaths and population for each tract are allocated *as a unit* to one of several groups on the basis of a socioeconomic index for the census tract. In general, despite the limitation of this approach, which attributes to each individual residing in a given census tract the average characteristics for the tract as a whole, it has demonstrated that there are wide variations in mortality by socioeconomic status within metropolitan areas. These studies, as those based on individual characteristics, reveal an inverse relationship between mortality and socioeconomic status. Moreover, a methodological analysis comparing socioeconomic differentials in fertility based on census tract indexes with differentials for the same population based on individual characteristics supported the general validity of findings of studies in differential fertility in which areal indexes provided the only measure of socioeconomic status (Duncan, 1964, p. 89). Presumably Duncan's conclusion can be extended to the analysis of socioeconomic differentials in mortality.

Four previous studies of mortality in Chicago, together with new materials generated for this monograph, provided the basic data for the areal socioeconomic differentials discussed in this chapter (Hauser, 1938; Dollar, 1942; Mayer, 1950; Kitagawa and Hauser, 1964). The Chicago studies cover the period from 1920 to 1960, but problems of comparability between 1920 and later dates, as well as inadequate age detail in the 1920 materials, led to the elimination of the 1920 data. Mortality differentials among five socioeconomic groups *within the city of Chicago* for the period 1930 through 1950 were analyzed in a 1964 report (Kitagawa and Hauser, 1964). New materials added for the present chapter include: (1) comparable mortality measures for socioeconomic groups in the city of Chicago in 1960; and (2) comparable mortality measures for the entire Chicago Standard Metropolitan Statistical Area (SMSA)[1] and the ring of the SMSA in 1950 and 1960, the only years for which the basic death statistics for these areas are available.

Data and Method

The population figures needed as bases for mortality rates were obtained from published reports of the United States Censuses of Population for 1930 through 1960. The death statistics were based on the allocation of deaths to the census tract of residence of the deceased.[2] The number of deaths covered in the studies are compared below with the nationally compiled totals for Chicago in 1940, 1950, and 1960, as published in official reports, *Vital Statistics of the United States*, for these years (no such report was compiled for 1930):

Source	1960	1950	1940
SMSA total, official report	62,194	54,452	—
SMSA total, Chicago study	62,066	54,363	—
City total, official report	42,879	40,920	37,582
City total, Chicago study	42,550	40,688	37,184
Sum of 5 SE Groups, Chicago study	42,304	39,269	37,184

The five socioeconomic groups within the city of Chicago were obtained by assigning residents of each of the census tracts in Chicago to a socioeconomic group on the basis of median rent (1930 and 1940) or median family income (1950 and 1960) of the tract. The underlying rationale was to allocate the white and nonwhite population of Chicago to socioeconomic groups in approximately the same proportionate distribution on each date. In 1930, census tracts were classified as being in one of five socioeconomic groups according to 1930 median rent as follows: under $30; $30-$44; $45-$59; $60-$74; and $75 or more. In 1940, tracts were classified according to 1940 median rent as follows: under $20; $20-$29; $30-$39; $40-$49; $50 or more. (In both 1930 and 1940, median rent included the equivalent monthly rental value of owner-occupied dwelling units.) In 1950 and 1960, tracts were classified in five socioeconomic groups according to median family income. However, the heavy in-migration of low-income Negroes to Chicago during the decade 1940-50 resulted in a disproportionate weighting of Negroes in the low-income groups and made it impossible to use the same income intervals to define socioeconomic groups of whites and nonwhites without grossly violating the condition that their proportionate distributions by socioeconomic group should be approximately the same in 1940 and 1950.[3] For this reason, different income intervals were used to define white and nonwhite socioeconomic groups in 1950 and 1960, as specified below:

| | Median Family Income of Tract | |
Socioeconomic Group	1950	1960
White, total city		
SE 1 (low)	Under $3,600	Under $6,100
SE 2	$3,600-3,999	$6,100-6,799
SE 3	$4,000-4,499	$6,800-7,799
SE 4	$4,500-5,099	$7,800-8,499
SE 5 (high)	$5,100 or more	$8,500 or more
Nonwhite, total city		
SE 1 (low)	Under $2,400	Under $4,200
SE 2	$2,400-2,999	$4,200-5,499
SE 3 (high)	$3,000 or more	$5,500 or more

As a result, the socioeconomic groups of whites and nonwhites in 1950 and 1960 are not comparable and, therefore, do not provide a basis for measuring white-nonwhite differences in mortality at the same socioeconomic level on each date. This limitation does not apply to the rates for 1930 and 1940, however, since white and nonwhite socioeconomic groups are defined on the same basis in these years.

The proportionate allocation of the city's white and nonwhite population into socioeconomic groups is given in Table 4.1, in the

Table 4.1. Percent distribution of population by color and socioeconomic group: Chicago Standard Metropolitan Statistical Area (SMSA) and City of Chicago, 1930-1960

Color and socioeconomic group[a]	1960	1950	1940	1930
Chicago SMSA, total population.........	100	100	100	100
City of Chicago.....................	57	70	74	76
Ring (outside City).................	43	30	26	24
Chicago SMSA, white population.........	100	100	100	100[b]
City of Chicago.....................	51	67	73	75
SE 1 (low).......................	9	12	13	---
SE 2.............................	11	14	17	---
SE 3.............................	16	21	21	---
SE 4.............................	10	12	16	---
SE 5 (high)......................	6	8	7	---
Ring (outside City).................	49	33	27	25
Chicago SMSA, nonwhite population......	100	100	100	100[b]
City of Chicago.....................	91	92	92	92
SE 1 (low).......................	27	28	20	---
SE 2.............................	42	43	42	---
SE 3 (high)......................	23	21	30	---
Ring (outside City).................	9	8	8	8
City of Chicago, white population......	100	100	100	100[c]
SE 1 (low).......................	17	17	17	17
SE 2.............................	21	21	23	23
SE 3.............................	31	32	28	25
SE 4.............................	20	17	22	25
SE 5 (high)......................	11	12	10	10
City of Chicago, nonwhite population...	100	100	100	100[d]
SE 1 (low).......................	29	30	22	22
SE 2.............................	46	47	45	38
SE 3 (high)......................	25	23	33	40
Percent of population nonwhite				
Chicago SMSA..........................	15	11	7	6[b]
City of Chicago......................	24	14	8	7[b]
Ring of SMSA.........................	3	3	2	2[b]

Source: Published reports for Decennial Censuses, 1940 to 1960, and census tract summary cards for 1950; E. W. Burgess and Charles Newcomb, Census Data of the City of Chicago, 1930 (Chicago: University of Chicago Press, 1933). Percents not adjusted to sum to 100.

[a] See text for definition of socioeconomic groups.

[b] Figures for whites and nonwhites adjusted to conform to definitions in later censuses by reclassifying, as "white," persons of Mexican ancestry classified as "nonwhite other than Negro" in 1930 census. Adjusted figures not available for socioeconomic groups.

[c] The white population allocated to socioeconomic groups excludes 19,362 persons of Mexican ancestry (0.6 percent of the "adjusted" total).

[d] Refers to Negroes only (see note b).

fourth and fifth panels of percentage distributions. These distributions document the stability of the proportionate distribution of the city's white population throughout the 30-year period, with 17 percent in the lowest socioeconomic group on all four census dates and 10-12 percent in the highest socioeconomic group. The nonwhite population had somewhat higher proportions in the lowest group in 1950 and 1960 (29 and 30 percent) than in 1930 and 1940 (22 percent), and also had lower proportions in the high group in 1950 and 1960 than in 1930 and 1940. Over the 30-year period the proportion of nonwhites in the city increased from 7 to 24 percent; in the ring of the SMSA, from 2 to 3 percent; and in the SMSA as a whole, from 6 to 15 percent (sixth panel of the table).

The percent distributions in the first three panels of Table 4.1 show the proportionate allocation of the Chicago SMSA's population into two major components of the city and the ring, with the city's component further subdivided into five socioeconomic groups. The

Table 4.2. Percent change in population, by color: United States, Chicago Standard Metropolitan Statistical Area (SMSA) and City of Chicago, 1930-1960

Area and color	Percent change in population				Population	
	1930-60	1950-60	1940-50	1930-40	1960	1930[a]
United States[b]..	45	18	14	7	178,464,236	122,775,046
White........	44	17	14	7	158,454,956	110,286,740
Nonwhite.....	60	27	17	8	20,009,280	12,488,306
Chicago SMSA....	40	20	13	3	6,220,913	4,449,646
White........	27	15	8	2	5,300,912	4,189,053
Nonwhite.....	253	66	80	18	920,001	260,593
City of Chicago.	5	-2	7	1	3,550,404	3,376,438
White........	-13	-13	0	-1	2,712,748	3,137,093
Nonwhite.....	250	64	80	18	837,656	239,345
Ring of SMSA....	149	72	33	9	2,670,509	1,073,208
White........	146	71	32	9	2,588,164	1,051,960
Nonwhite.....	288	83	78	19	82,345	21,248

Source: Data for United States from Bureau of Census, 1960 Census of Population, Vol. I, Tables 42 and 44. Data for Chicago SMSA, City and Ring compiled from published census reports as summarized in E.M. Kitagawa and K.E. Taeuber, Local Community Fact Book, Chicago Metropolitan Area, 1960 (Chicago Community Inventory, University of Chicago, 1963).

[a] Figures for whites and nonwhites have been adjusted to conform to definitions used in later censuses (see note b, Table 4.1).

[b] Coterminous United States (excludes Alaska and Hawaii).

important change in these distributions during the 30-year period is the increasing proportion of the SMSA's population living in the ring; this proportion increased from 25 percent in 1930 to 49 percent in 1960.

The population for the nation, Chicago SMSA, the city, and the ring are shown for 1930 and 1960, together with changes for the period and for each decade, in Table 4.2. Between 1930 and 1960, while the population of the nation increased by 45 percent, that of the SMSA increased by 40 percent, that of the city by only 5 percent, and that of the ring by 149 percent. While white population in the nation grew by 44 percent, that in the SMSA increased by only 27 percent, that in the city decreased by 13 percent, and that in the ring increased by 146 percent. In contrast, while nonwhite population in the nation experienced an increment of 60 percent, that in the SMSA increased by 253 percent, that in the city by 250 percent, and that in the ring by 288 percent.

In consequence, by 1960, whites in the city had decreased from 3.1 million in 1930 to 2.7 million; while nonwhites in the city had increased from 239,000 to 838,000. In contrast, in the ring, whites increased from 1.1 million in 1930 to 2.6 million in 1960 while nonwhites increased from about 21,000 to about 82,000. The exodus of whites from the city has undoubtedly had the effect of decreasing the relative socioeconomic status of whites who remained, and since the nonwhites who increased in number and proportion were, as in-migrants, of lower socioeconomic status, it may be inferred that the socioeconomic status of the inhabitants of the city was lowered, relatively, over the 30-year period. The inclusion of data for the SMSA and the ring for 1950 and 1960 helps to provide a reasonably comparable picture of the range of variations in mortality over the period. Data, as has been indicated, were not available for the SMSA and the ring prior to 1950. But the relatively slow growth of the ring prior to 1950 makes the absence of the data for the earlier period less likely to result in distortions of the range of mortality differences prior to 1950 and over the entire period.

Mortality in Chicago Area and in the United States

Trends

Over the 30-year period from 1930 to 1960 the age-adjusted death rate in the United States has taken but one direction, downward, for

Table 4.3. Age-adjusted death rates by color, sex and socioeconomic group: Chicago Standard Metropolitan Statistical Area (SMSA) and City of Chicago, 1930-1960

Color, sex, age and socioeconomic group[a]	Age-adjusted death rate				Index (U.S. as base)			
	1960	1950	1940	1929-1931[b]	1960	1950	1940	1929-1931[b]
White males, all ages								
United States............	9.2	9.6	11.6	12.8	1.00	1.00	1.00	1.00
Chicago SMSA............	9.9	10.6	---	---	1.08	1.10	---	---
City of Chicago......	11.0	11.4	12.6	14.4	1.20	1.19	1.09	1.12
SE 1 (low)........	16.0	14.6	16.6	18.8	1.74	1.52	1.43	1.47
SE 2..............	11.3	11.6	13.4	15.4	1.23	1.21	1.16	1.20
SE 3..............	10.1	9.7	11.5	13.6	1.10	1.01	.99	1.06
SE 4..............	9.2	9.4	10.8	12.4	1.00	.98	.93	.97
SE 5 (high).......	9.6	8.7	11.0	11.6	1.04	.91	.95	.91
Ring (outside City)..	8.4	9.1	---	---	.91	.95	---	---
White males, under 65								
United States............	4.7	5.2	6.6	7.9	1.00	1.00	1.00	1.00
Chicago SMSA............	5.0	5.8	---	---	1.06	1.12	---	---
City of Chicago......	5.8	6.2	7.1	9.1	1.23	1.19	1.08	1.15
SE 1 (low)........	8.6	8.6	10.4	13.2	1.83	1.65	1.58	1.67
SE 2..............	6.0	6.4	7.8	9.9	1.28	1.23	1.18	1.25
SE 3..............	5.2	5.1	6.3	8.4	1.11	.98	.95	1.06
SE 4..............	4.5	4.9	5.6	7.2	.96	.94	.85	.91
SE 5 (high).......	4.7	4.2	5.8	6.6	1.00	.81	.88	.84
Ring (outside City)..	4.0	4.7	---	---	.85	.90	---	---
White males, 65 & over								
United States............	69.1	69.9	79.2	78.7	1.00	1.00	1.00	1.00
Chicago SMSA............	76.6	77.4	---	---	1.11	1.11	---	---
City of Chicago......	82.2	81.0	87.2	86.3	1.19	1.16	1.10	1.10
SE 1 (low)........	116.2	95.9	101.6	94.3	1.68	1.37	1.28	1.20
SE 2..............	83.7	82.6	89.5	89.3	1.21	1.18	1.13	1.13
SE 3..............	76.9	72.0	83.4	85.4	1.11	1.03	1.05	1.09
SE 4..............	73.0	71.2	81.5	82.8	1.06	1.02	1.03	1.05
SE 5 (high).......	76.6	69.8	81.0	79.6	1.11	1.00	1.02	1.01
Ring (outside City)..	66.9	69.4	---	---	.97	.99	---	---
White Females, all ages								
United States............	5.6	6.5	8.8	10.6	1.00	1.00	1.00	1.00
Chicago SMSA............	6.1	7.1	---	---	1.09	1.09	---	---
City of Chicago......	6.7	7.5	9.4	11.6	1.20	1.15	1.07	1.09
SE 1 (low)........	9.0	9.1	12.2	14.5	1.61	1.40	1.39	1.37
SE 2..............	7.0	7.8	10.1	12.5	1.25	1.20	1.15	1.18
SE 3..............	6.2	7.0	9.1	11.3	1.11	1.08	1.03	1.07
SE 4..............	5.8	6.6	8.3	10.5	1.04	1.02	.94	.99
SE 5 (high).......	5.9	6.0	7.6	9.0	1.05	.92	.86	.85
Ring (outside City)..	5.5	6.4	---	---	.98	.98	---	---

(continued)

Table 4.3. Age-adjusted death rates by color, sex and socioeconomic group: Chicago Standard Metropolitan Statistical Area (SMSA) and City of Chicago, 1930-1960--(continued)

Color, sex, age and socioeconomic group[a]	Age-adjusted death rate				Index (U.S. as base)			
	1960	1950	1940	1929-1931[b]	1960	1950	1940	1929-1931[b]
White females, under 65								
United States...........	2.5	3.1	4.6	6.3	1.00	1.00	1.00	1.00
Chicago SMSA...........	2.8	3.4	---	---	1.12	1.10	---	---
City of Chicago.....	3.1	3.6	4.9	7.0	1.24	1.16	1.07	1.11
SE 1 (low).......	4.7	4.9	7.1	9.9	1.88	1.58	1.54	1.57
SE 2.............	3.4	3.8	5.4	7.8	1.36	1.23	1.17	1.24
SE 3.............	2.9	3.3	4.6	6.6	1.16	1.06	1.00	1.05
SE 4.............	2.4	3.0	4.0	5.9	.96	.97	.87	.94
SE 5 (high)......	2.5	2.7	3.6	4.8	1.00	.87	.78	.76
Ring (outside City).	2.3	2.9	---	---	.92	.94	---	---
White females, 65 & over								
United States...........	47.0	52.3	65.3	68.8	1.00	1.00	1.00	1.00
Chicago SMSA...........	52.0	58.2	---	---	1.11	1.11	---	---
City of Chicago.....	54.6	60.3	70.4	74.2	1.16	1.15	1.08	1.08
SE 1 (low).......	68.0	66.6	82.8	77.5	1.45	1.27	1.27	1.13
SE 2.............	55.5	61.9	74.5	77.1	1.18	1.18	1.14	1.12
SE 3.............	50.9	58.5	69.9	75.0	1.08	1.12	1.07	1.09
SE 4.............	51.2	55.6	66.1	73.3	1.09	1.06	1.01	1.07
SE 5 (high)......	51.8	51.2	62.8	66.7	1.10	.98	.96	.97
Ring (outside City).	48.0	53.8	---	---	1.02	1.03	---	---
Nonwhite males, all ages								
United States...........	12.1	13.6	17.6	21.0	1.00	1.00	1.00	1.00
Chicago SMSA...........	12.7	14.9	---	---	1.05	1.10	---	---
City of Chicago.....	13.1	15.4	20.7	26.1	1.08	1.13	1.18	1.24
SE 1 (low).......	16.7	17.7	25.9	30.6	1.38	1.30	1.47	1.46
SE 2.............	13.5	14.7	19.9	27.9	1.12	1.08	1.13	1.33
SE 3 (high)......	9.8	12.5	18.5	21.7	.81	.92	1.05	1.03
Ring (outside City).	9.8	--*	---	---	.81	--*	---	---
Nonwhite males, under 65								
United States...........	8.0	9.4	13.1	16.2	1.00	1.00	1.00	1.00
Chicago SMSA...........	8.1	10.0	---	---	1.01	1.06	---	---
City of Chicago.....	8.3	10.3	15.3	20.2	1.04	1.10	1.17	1.25
SE 1 (low).......	10.9	12.4	19.7	24.7	1.36	1.32	1.50	1.52
SE 2.............	8.5	9.9	15.6	21.9	1.06	1.05	1.19	1.35
SE 3 (high)......	5.7	7.5	12.3	16.0	.71	.80	.94	.99
Ring (outside City).	5.8	--*	---	---	.72	--*	---	---
Nonwhite males, 65 & over								
United States...........	68.1	70.2	80.0	86.5	1.00	1.00	1.00	1.00
Chicago SMSA...........	76.4	81.6	---	---	1.12	1.16	---	---
City of Chicago.....	77.7	85.3	93.7	105.8	1.14	1.22	1.17	1.22
SE 1 (low).......	95.0	89.9	109.9	110.9	1.40	1.28	1.37	1.28
SE 2.............	81.0	79.9	78.5	110.1	1.19	1.14	.98	1.27
SE 3 (high)......	65.4	80.6	103.2	98.4	.96	1.15	1.29	1.14
Ring (outside City).	63.9	--*	---	---	.94	--*	---	---

(Continued)

Table 4.3. Age-adjusted death rates by color, sex and socioeconomic group: Chicago Standard Metropolitan Statistical Area (SMSA) and City of Chicago, 1930-1960--(continued)

Color, sex, age and socioeconomic group[a]	Age-adjusted death rate				Index (U.S. as base)			
	1960	1950	1940	1929-1931[b]	1960	1950	1940	1929-1931[b]
Nonwhite females, all ages								
United States.............	8.9	10.9	15.0	19.2	1.00	1.00	1.00	1.00
Chicago SMSA.............	9.3	11.1	---	---	1.04	1.02	---	---
City of Chicago.......	9.5	11.3	15.5	21.3	1.07	1.04	1.03	1.11
SE 1 (low).........	11.5	13.1	18.5	25.1	1.29	1.20	1.23	1.31
SE 2...............	9.8	11.1	15.5	23.1	1.10	1.02	1.03	1.20
SE 3 (high)........	8.1	9.3	13.8	17.7	.91	.85	.92	.92
Ring (outside City)...	6.8	--*	---	---	.76	--*	---	---
Nonwhite females, under 65								
United States.............	5.9	7.6	11.4	15.3	1.00	1.00	1.00	1.00
Chicago SMSA.............	6.1	8.0	---	---	1.03	1.05	---	---
City of Chicago.......	6.3	8.1	12.1	17.1	1.07	1.07	1.06	1.12
SE 1 (low).........	8.1	9.7	14.6	21.2	1.37	1.28	1.28	1.39
SE 2...............	6.3	7.8	12.3	18.2	1.07	1.03	1.08	1.19
SE 3 (high)........	4.8	6.4	10.4	14.0	.81	.84	.91	.92
Ring (outside City)...	4.4	--*	---	---	.75	--*	---	---
Nonwhite females, 65 & over								
United States.............	50.3	55.8	64.7	73.1	1.00	1.00	1.00	1.00
Chicago SMSA.............	52.6	54.0	---	---	1.05	.97	---	---
City of Chicago.......	53.7	55.8	61.9	78.0	1.07	1.00	.96	1.07
SE 1 (low).........	57.7	59.0	71.8	78.4	1.15	1.06	1.11	1.07
SE 2...............	56.8	56.9	58.5	89.5	1.13	1.02	.90	1.22
SE 3 (high)........	53.7	49.5	59.6	67.9	1.07	.89	.92	.93
Ring (outside city)...	38.2	--*	---	---	.76	--*	---	---

Source: United States age-adjusted rates for all ages from <u>Vital Statistics of United States, 1960</u>, Vol. II, Table 1-B; age-adjusted rates for two broad age groups calculated from age-specific rates in sources cited in headnote of same table. Age-adjusted rates for Chicago SMSA, City and Ring calculated at Population Research Center, University of Chicago (see text for sources of data). All rates standardized by direct method using 1940 total U.S. population as standard.

--* Age-adjusted rate not computed because more than half of the age-specific deaths based on less than 20 deaths.

[a] See text for definition of socioeconomic groups.

[b] United States rates are for the year 1930 and refer to 47 states and the District of Columbia, which comprised the death registration area in 1930. Rates reported for nonwhites in the City of Chicago and the socioeconomic groups refer to Negroes; however, in 1930 Negroes comprised 98 percent of the nonwhite population of Chicago.

each color, sex, and age group shown in Table 4.3. Only one inversion occurs in the pattern of decreasing mortality, that for white males 65 and over, between 1930 and 1940. For both the Chicago SMSA and the city of Chicago, the same pattern of decreasing mortality is evident; and decreasing mortality is the pattern also, without exception, for the years for which the data are available for the metropolitan ring.

Over the entire 30 years, with only one exception, that for nonwhite females 65 and over in 1940 and 1950, the age-adjusted death rate for each color, sex, and age group for the city of Chicago was higher than that for the nation. The Chicago SMSA, in 1950 and 1960, also had a higher age-adjusted death rate than the nation had for each color-sex-age group, except for nonwhite females 65 and over in 1950. In contrast, with no exception, mortality in the ring in 1950 and 1960 was below that of the nation for every group.

Socioeconomic Patterns

For each white sex and age group, mortality in the two lowest socioeconomic groupings is consistently above that of the nation, the SMSA, and the city. For nonwhites the pattern is more variable. Nonwhite mortality in the two lower socioeconomic groups is with two exceptions higher than nonwhite mortality in the nation. The exceptions are found among both males and females 65 and over in 1940. Although nonwhite mortality in the lowest socioeconomic group was consistently above that for nonwhites in the SMSA and the city, that in the intermediate socioeconomic grouping (SE 2) was sometimes above and sometimes below nonwhite mortality for the SMSA and the city.

Although whites in the intermediate socioeconomic class (SE 3), had lower death rates than those which obtained among whites in the SMSA and the city, they were consistently above white mortality for the nation except for white males under 65 in 1940 and 1950, and white females under 65 in 1940. Among white males and females under 65, mortality in the two highest socioeconomic groups (SE 4 and 5) was, with only two exceptions, below national as well as consistently below SMSA and city mortality. The two exceptions were males and females under 65 in 1960 in the highest class, in which year their mortality just matched national mortality. For white males 65 and over, age-adjusted death rates in the two highest socioeconomic groupings were consistently above those for the nation although below those for the SMSA and the city. White females 65 and over in the highest socioeconomic class (SE 5), had lower mortality than their counterparts in the nation, except in 1960; whereas their mortality in the second highest class (SE 4) was above the comparable national level over the entire period.

Both nonwhite males and females under 65 in the highest socioeconomic class (SE 3) had lower mortality than the comparable national level over the entire period. Nonwhite males 65 and over in the highest class had higher than national mortality except in 1960. Nonwhite females 65 and over in the highest class, in contrast, had lower than national mortality except in 1960. Unfortunately, the patterns of differences for nonwhites are subject to relatively large errors as a result of misreporting of age and census underenumeration, as elaborated in Chapter 7. Consequently, it is difficult to ascertain whether some of the nonwhite patterns indicate real differences in the direction and degree indicated in Table 4.3.

Over the 30-year period, the ratio of city to national mortality increased for whites but decreased for nonwhites. For the two periods, 1950 and 1960, for which data for the SMSA are available the ratio of local to national mortality decreased, except for white females. The relative increase in white mortality in the city and the decrease in the ring undoubtedly reflect in part at least the out-migration of more affluent whites from the city to suburbia. The relative decrease in nonwhite mortality is attributable to the rising socioeconomic position of nonwhites in the city and the SMSA. Even though nonwhites are still in a disadvantaged position relative to whites, their improving status in the Chicago area has had an impact on their previously very high levels of mortality.

Range of Differences

The degree of difference in age-adjusted death rates is also presented (Table 4.3). Among white males the highest relative level of mortality over the 30 years is found among males under 65 in the lowest socioeconomic group (SE 1) in 1960, when the age-adjusted death rate was 83 percent above that of the comparable group in the nation (index 1.83). The lowest relative mortality for white males is found among those under 65 in the highest socioeconomic group in 1950, when their age-adjusted death rate was 19 percent below that for comparable males in the nation (index 0.81). Among white females the greatest relative mortality is found among those under 65 in the lowest socioeconomic class, also in 1960, when their age-adjusted death rate was 88 percent above the comparable figure for the nation (index 1.88). For white females the lowest relative mortality is found among those under 65 in the highest socioeconomic class in 1960, when their age-adjusted death rate was 24 percent below the comparable national figure (index 0.76).

Among nonwhite males the highest relative mortality occurred among those under 65 in the lowest socioeconomic group in 1930, when their age-adjusted death rate was 52 percent above the national level (index 1.52). Their lowest relative mortality is found among those under 65 in the highest socioeconomic class in 1960, when their age-adjusted death rate was 29 percent below the national level (index 0.71). For nonwhite females relative mortality was highest among those under 65 in the lowest class in 1930, when their age-adjusted death rate was 39 percent above the national level (index 1.39); and lowest among those under 65 in the highest class in 1960, with a death rate 19 percent below the national level (index 0.81).

For both whites and nonwhites 65 and over, as was to be expected from the preceding chapters, the range of mortality differences was smaller than for those under 65. The relatively high mortality of nonwhites at the beginning of the 30-year period and their relatively low mortality at the end of the period in 1960 were to be expected with the improved status of nonwhites over the years. Unexpected, however, is the pattern evident for whites. The fact that the highest relative mortality for whites occurs at the end of the period under study, 1960, indicates that socioeconomic differences are, over time, more adversely affecting mortality in Chicago even as mortality for the nation and for the city have declined, that is, socioeconomic differences produced greater variations in mortality among whites at the end of the period than at the beginning. More light will be thrown on this phenomenon as the mortality changes over time are considered.

Percentage Change by Decade

Between 1930 and 1960 age-adjusted death rates in the United States for white males decreased by 28 percent (Table 4.4). For the

Table 4.4. Percent change in age-adjusted death rates by color, sex and
socioeconomic group: Chicago Standard Metropolitan Statistical
Area (SMSA) and City of Chicago, 1930-1960

Color, age and socioeconomic group[a]	Percent change in age-adjusted death rate							
	Males				Females			
	1930-60	1950-60	1940-50	1930-40	1930-60	1950-60	1940-50	1930-40
White, all ages								
United States..........	-28	-4	-17	-9	-47	-14	-26	-17
Chicago SMSA..........	---	-7	---	---	---	-14	---	---
City of Chicago....	-24	-4	-10	-12	-42	-11	-20	-19
SE 1 (low)......	-15	10	-12	-12	-38	-1	-25	-16
SE 2............	-27	-3	-13	-13	-44	-10	-23	-19
SE 3............	-26	4	-16	-15	-45	-11	-23	-19
SE 4............	-26	-2	-13	-13	-45	-12	-20	-21
SE 5 (high).....	-17	10	-21	-5	-34	-2	-21	-16
Ring (outside City)	---	-8	---	---	---	-14	---	---
White, under 65								
United States..........	-41	-10	-21	-16	-60	-19	-33	-27
Chicago SMSA..........	---	-14	---	---	---	-18	---	---
City of Chicago....	-36	-6	-13	-22	-56	-14	-27	-30
SE 1 (low)......	-35	0	-17	-21	-53	-4	-31	-28
SE 2............	-39	-6	-18	-21	-56	-11	-30	-31
SE 3............	-38	2	-19	-25	-56	-12	-28	-30
SE 4............	-38	-8	-12	-22	-59	-20	-25	-32
SE 5 (high).....	-29	12	-28	-12	-48	-7	-25	-25
Ring (outside City)	---	-15	---	---	---	-21	---	---
White, 65 & over								
United States..........	-12	-1	-12	1	-32	-10	-20	-5
Chicago SMSA..........	---	-1	---	---	---	-11	---	---
City of Chicago....	-5	1	-7	1	-26	-9	-14	-5
SE 1 (low)......	23	21	-6	8	-12	2	-20	7
SE 2............	-6	1	-8	0	-28	-10	-17	-3
SE 3............	-10	7	-14	-2	-32	-13	-16	-7
SE 4............	-12	3	-13	-2	-30	-8	-16	-10
SE 5 (high).....	-4	10	-14	2	-22	1	-18	-6
Ring (outside City)	---	-4	---	---	---	-11	---	---
Nonwhite, all ages								
United States..........	-42	-11	-23	-16	-54	-18	-27	-22
Chicago SMSA..........	---	-15	---	---	---	-16	---	---
City of Chicago....	-50	-15	-26	-21	-55	-16	-27	-27
SE 1 (low)......	-45	-6	-32	-15	-54	-12	-29	-26
SE 2............	-52	-8	-26	-29	-58	-12	-28	-33
SE 3 (high).....	-55	-22	-32	-15	-54	-13	-33	-22
Ring (outside City)	---	--*	---	---	---	--*	---	---

(continued)

Table 4.4. Percent change in age-adjusted death rates by color, sex and socioeconomic group: Chicago Standard Metropolitan Statistical Area (SMSA) and City of Chicago, 1930-1960--(continued)

Color, age and socioeconomic group[a]	Percent change in age-adjusted death rate							
	Males				Females			
	1930-60	1950-60	1940-50	1930-40	1930-60	1950-60	1940-50	1930-40
Nonwhite, under 65								
United States..........	-51	-15	-28	-19	-61	-22	-33	-26
Chicago SMSA..........	---	-19	---	---	---	-24	---	---
City of Chicago....	-59	-19	-33	-24	-63	-22	-33	-29
SE 1 (low)......	-56	-12	-37	-20	-62	-17	-34	-31
SE 2............	-61	-14	-37	-29	-65	-19	-37	-32
SE 3 (high).....	-64	-24	-39	-23	-66	-25	-38	-26
Ring (outside City)	---	--*	---	---	---	--*	---	---
Nonwhite, 65 & over								
United States..........	-21	-3	-12	-8	-31	-10	-14	-12
Chicago SMSA..........	---	-6	---	---	---	-3	---	---
City of Chicago....	-27	-9	-9	-11	-31	-4	-10	-21
SE 1 (low)......	-14	6	-18	-1	-26	-2	-18	-8
SE 2............	-26	1	2	-29	-37	0	-3	-35
SE 3 (high).....	-34	-19	-22	5	-21	8	-17	-12
Ring (outside City)	---	--*	---	---	---	--*	---	---

Source: Table 4.3. See Table 4.3 for notes a and --*.

city of Chicago the comparable decline was smaller, 24 percent. For females the mortality decline in the nation was greater than for males, 47 percent. Similarly, death rates for females in the city decreased more rapidly than for males, 42 percent.

During the fifties, the only decade for which data were available for the SMSA and the ring, white male mortality declined more sharply in the SMSA, 7 percent, and in the ring, 8 percent, than in the nation, 4 percent. During the same decade, the decrease in white male mortality in the city matched that for the nation; white female mortality declined by the same percentage for the nation, the SMSA, and the ring, 14 percent, and by a smaller percentage in the city, 11 percent.

As was to be expected, the decrease in age-adjusted death rates was greater for both white men and women under 65 than for those 65 and over. The same pattern of differences obtained, however, between the city and the nation. The mortality of white males under 65 decreased over the 30 years by 41 percent in the nation and by 36 percent in the city; for white males 65 and over the comparable declines were 12 and 5 percent, respectively. For white females under 65 mortality declined by 60 percent in the nation and 56 percent in the city. Corresponding percentages for females 65 and over were 32 percent and 26 percent, respectively—substantially larger than the declines in male mortality. Mortality declines were consistently greater during the forties than in either of the other two decades for both men and women in each of the age groups.

For nonwhites the patterns of change in mortality differed in significant respects from those of whites. For the nation the decrease in age-adjusted death rates of nonwhite males of both age groups was greater than for comparable whites. For nonwhite females in both age groups, however, the mortality decrease in the nation was almost the same as for comparable whites. For the city the decline in nonwhite mortality exceeded that in white for each sex and age group.

The greatest decrease in age-adjusted death rates for nonwhites over the 30-year period occurred among females under 65, a 61 percent decline in the nation and 63 percent in the city. The mortality of nonwhite males under 65 decreased by 51 percent in the nation and 59 percent in the city. For nonwhites 65 and over mortality decreased by 21 percent in the nation and by 27 percent in the city for males. Comparable changes for females were 31 percent both in the nation and in the city.

Infant Mortality

Among whites, infant mortality in the city of Chicago for both males and females was below that of the nation prior to 1960, but above that of the nation in 1960 (Table 4.5). Both male and female infant mortality in Chicago were relatively lowest in 1940, when the city rate for males was 38 percent below (index 0.62) and for females 35 percent below (index 0.65) the national level. In 1960, however, the city infant mortality for males was 3 percent above, and for females one percent above, the national level. In both 1950 and 1960, the only periods for which SMSA data are available, infant mortality for both males and females was below the national and city levels in the ring.

Among nonwhites, infant mortality, although much higher than that of whites, was lower in the city than in the nation for every period shown. As for whites, the lowest relative infant mortality rates occurred in 1940, when nonwhite male infant mortality was 42 percent below (index 0.58) and female, 51 percent (index 0.49), below the national level. By 1960, in contrast with 1940, nonwhite male infant mortality was only 11 percent below the national level and female, only 6 percent below.

Over the 30 years infant mortality decreased in the nation slightly more than in the city for each sex and color group; white infant mortality for each sex declined slightly more than nonwhite in both the nation and the city; and white female infant mortality in both the nation and the city decreased slightly more than male. Nonwhite female infant mortality decreased more rapidly than male in the nation but not in the city. However, there were marked differences—between the city and the nation—in the timing of the decline in infant mortality during the 30-year period. In the city of Chicago the greatest improvement in infant mortality during a single decade occurred during the depression years, 1930-40, when infant death rates were at least cut by one-half among both whites and nonwhites; the largest decrease (59 percent) occurred among nonwhite females. Infant mortality rates for the nation decreased much less (24 to 29 percent) during the same decade. It was during the next decade, 1940-50, that the nation experienced its sharpest decreases in infant mortality, 37 to 40 percent in the four sex and color groups, as compared with comparable decreases of 13 to 20 percent in the city. During the decade 1950-60, infant mortality rates actually increased in the city, by a small 1 to 3 percent for white males and females and nonwhite males, and by a very substantial 32 percent for nonwhite females. Nevertheless, it is significant that at the end of the period infant mortality among nonwhites in the city was still 6 to 11 percent below that of the nation, while white infant mortality was 1 to 3 percent higher than in the nation. Clearly, the city's position relative to that of the nation has been better for infant mortality than for mortality over all ages (see Table 4.3). Moreover, the changes in infant mortality rates in Table 4.5 reveal the extent to which the large cities (or at least one large city) led the nation in the reduction of infant mortality. For example, the rates achieved in the city of Chicago by 1940 were still prevailing in the nation in 1950 (for example, 30.0 and 48.0 for white and nonwhite males in the city in 1940, as compared with 30.2 and 48.9 for comparable groups in the nation in 1950).

Socioeconomic Differentials in the Chicago Area

Among both whites and nonwhites of each sex and age group there is evident an inverse relationship between socioeconomic status and

Table 4.5. Infant mortality rates (deaths to infants under one year of age, per 1,000 live births) by color, sex and socioeconomic group: Chicago Standard Metropolitan Statistical Area (SMSA) and City of Chicago, 1930-1960

Color, sex and socioeconomic group[a]	Infant mortality rate				Index (U.S. as base)				Percent change in rate				
	1960	1950	1940	1929- 1931[b]	1960	1950	1940	1929- 1931[b]	1930- 1960	1940- 1960	1950- 1960	1940- 1950	1930- 1940
White males													
United States..........	26.0	30.2	48.3	66.6	1.00	1.00	1.00	1.00	-61.0	-46.2	-13.9	-37.5	-27.5
Chicago SMSA..........	25.1	26.0	---	---	.97	.86	---	---	---	---	-3.5	---	---
City of Chicago....	26.8	26.3	30.0	61.0	1.03	.87	.62	.92	-56.1	-10.7	1.9	-12.3	-50.8
SE 1 (low)......	33.0	...	34.8	83.9	1.27	...	.72	1.26	-60.7	-5.2	...	...	-58.5
SE 2............	28.7	...	31.1	68.9	1.10	...	.64	1.03	-58.4	-7.7	...	...	-54.9
SE 3............	23.6	...	28.8	52.6	.91	...	.60	.79	-55.1	-18.1	...	...	-45.3
SE 4............	23.1	...	27.5	49.2	.89	...	.57	.74	-53.1	-16.0	...	...	-44.1
SE 5 (high).....	25.1	...	26.5	36.7	.97	...	.55	.55	-31.6	-5.3	...	...	-27.8
Ring (outside City)	23.5	25.5	---	---	.90	.84	---	---	---	---	-7.9	---	---
White females													
United States..........	19.6	23.1	37.8	53.2	1.00	1.00	1.00	1.00	-63.2	-48.2	-15.2	-38.9	-29.0
Chicago SMSA..........	17.9	19.2	---	---	.91	.83	---	---	---	---	-6.8	---	---
City of Chicago....	19.7	19.7	24.4	48.0	1.01	.85	.65	.90	-59.0	-19.3	0.0	-19.3	-49.2
SE 1 (low)......	23.5	...	27.9	68.0	1.20	...	.74	1.28	-65.5	-15.8	...	...	-59.0
SE 2............	20.5	...	26.8	52.8	1.05	...	.71	.99	-61.2	-23.5	...	...	-49.3
SE 3............	17.7	...	22.6	43.4	.90	...	.60	.82	-59.2	-21.7	...	...	-47.9
SE 4............	17.1	...	20.6	36.5	.87	...	.54	.69	-53.2	-17.0	...	...	-43.6
SE 5 (high).....	19.2	...	25.4	29.0	.98	...	.67	.55	-33.8	-24.4	...	...	-12.4
Ring (outside City)	16.2	18.1	---	---	.83	.78	---	---	---	---	-10.5	---	---
Nonwhite males													
United States..........	47.9	48.9	82.2	108.7	1.00	1.00	1.00	1.00	-55.9	-41.7	-2.1	-40.5	-24.4
Chicago SMSA..........	42.5	41.4	---	---	.89	.85	---	---	---	---	2.7	---	---
City of Chicago....	42.6	41.3	48.0	94.7	.89	.84	.58	.87	-55.0	-11.3	3.1	-14.0	-49.3
SE 1 (low)......	44.0	...	41.6	104.1	.92	...	.51	.96	-57.7	5.8	...	...	-60.0
SE 2............	43.3	...	55.5	102.4	.90	...	.68	.94	-57.7	-22.0	...	...	-45.8
SE 3 (high).....	38.8	...	41.2	78.3	.81	...	.50	.72	-50.5	-5.8	...	...	-47.4
Ring (outside City)	--*	--*	---	---	--*	--*	---	---	---	---	--*	---	---
Nonwhite females													
United States..........	38.5	39.9	65.2	90.9	1.00	1.00	1.00	1.00	-57.7	-41.0	-3.5	38.8	-28.3
Chicago SMSA..........	35.7	28.4	---	---	.93	.71	---	---	---	---	25.7	---	---
City of Chicago....	36.3	27.9	31.7	77.1	.94	.70	.49	.85	-52.9	14.5	30.1	-12.0	-58.9
SE 1 (low)......	35.7	...	31.5	80.1	.93	...	.48	.88	-55.4	13.3	...	...	-60.7
SE 2............	37.9	...	31.4	80.7	.98	...	.48	.89	-53.0	20.7	...	...	-61.1
SE 3 (high).....	33.2	...	32.3	70.1	.86	...	.50	.77	-52.6	2.8	...	...	-53.9
Ring (outside City)	--*	--*	---	---	--*	--*	---	---	---	---	--*	---	---

Source: Rates for United States from National Center for Health Statistics, Vital Statistics of the United States: 1950, Vol. I, Table 8.49, and 1960, Vol. II, Part A, Table 3-B. Birth and death statistics for Chicago SMSA, City and Ring from sources cited for deaths in Table 4.3. Rates for SE groups in 1950 are not reported because 1950 births were not tabulated by sex for SE groups within the City.

See Table 4.3 for notes a, b and --*.

mortality. This is shown in Table 4.3, which was previously examined largely to relate mortality in the Chicago area to national mortality. Few exceptions to an inverse pattern are to be found in the death rates by socioeconomic class.

In the analysis of socioeconomic differentials, the statistics for the ring supplement the range of socioeconomic groups within the city, and also raise the question of assigning a socioeconomic level to the ring. Between 1950 and 1960, the proportion of the white population living in the ring increased from one-third to almost one-half. On both dates, the median income of families living in the ring ($4,550 in 1950 and $8,095 in 1960)[4] was within the range of median income levels for census tracts included in SE group 4 of the white population and below the minimum income level of tracts in the highest socioeconomic group within the city. Thus, using median family income of the ring as an index of the average socioeconomic level of the ring, it would appear as a whole to fall within the range of SE group 4 in the city.

With this perspective, it is interesting to note that the 1950 death rates for whites in Table 4.3 show a consistent inverse pattern of declining mortality with increasing socioeconomic level, since the death rates for whites are in general higher in the ring than in SE group 5 in the city. However, by 1960 the white death rate in the ring was below that for SE group 5 in the city, although its average family income still remained below that for the highest group in the city. This shift in pattern between 1950 and 1960 suggests that the known out-migration of affluent whites from the city to the suburbs during the decade may have been selective of persons subject to lower mortality, or that the total life style and environment in the suburbs in 1960 *independent of socioeconomic level* was conducive to lower mortality. Some support for the former hypothesis is suggested by the fact that the death rate was lower in SE group 4 than in SE group 5 in 1960, among both males and females. In any case, this shift in pattern between 1950 and 1960 resulted in a shift in the base for measuring the relative size of socioeconomic differentials during the 30-year period. Table 4.6 reports the trends in the size of differentials in terms of the percentage by which the death rate for each socioeconomic group exceeds that of SE group 5 for the years 1930 to 1950, and the percentage by which it exceeds that of the ring in 1960.

In quick overview, the following generalizations emerge from an analysis of these data. First, socioeconomic differentials were much greater among persons under 65 than among persons 65 and over throughout the 30-year period. Second, the relative differences between the death rates of the lowest and highest socioeconomic groups were larger in 1960 than in 1930 except for white females under 65 and nonwhite females 65 and over. During the decade 1930 to 1940, however, there was some convergence between rates for the lowest and highest socioeconomic groups of white males and females under 65, which was offset by a divergence in rates between 1940 and 1960. Patterns for intermediate socioeconomic groups varied. White males experienced increases in the relative differential for all socioeconomic groups in 1960 as compared with 1930 except for those under 65 in SE group 2. White females under 65 in SE groups 2 and above showed some convergence of differentials during the

Table 4.6. Relative size of socioeconomic differentials in age-adjusted death rates, by color and sex: Chicago Standard Metropolitan Statistical Area (SMSA) and City of Chicago, 1930-1960

Color, age and socioeconomic group[a]	Socioeconomic differentials[b]							
	Males				Females			
	1960	1950	1940	1929-31	1960	1950	1940	1929-31
White, all ages								
City of Chicago, SE 1 (low)	90	68	52	62	64	51	60	61
SE 2	35	34	22	33	27	29	32	39
SE 3	20	12	5	18	13	17	19	26
SE 4	10	8	-2	7	5	10	8	16
SE 5 (high)	14	0	0	0	7	0	0	0
Ring (outside City)	0	5	---	---	0	7	---	---
White, under 65 years								
City of Chicago, SE 1 (low)	115	105	79	101	104	79	96	108
SE 2	50	52	35	51	48	41	49	63
SE 3	30	22	8	27	26	20	30	39
SE 4	13	16	-4	10	4	12	11	23
SE 5 (high)	18	0	0	0	9	0	0	0
Ring (outside City)	0	12	---	---	0	7	---	---
White, 65 & over								
City of Chicago, SE 1 (low)	74	37	25	19	42	30	32	16
SE 2	25	18	10	12	16	21	19	16
SE 3	15	3	3	7	6	14	11	12
SE 4	9	2	1	4	7	9	5	10
SE 5 (high)	14	0	0	0	8	0	0	0
Ring (outside City)	0	-1	---	---	0	5	---	---
Nonwhite, all ages								
City of Chicago, SE 1 (low)	70	42	40	41	41	40	34	42
SE 2	37	18	7	29	20	19	12	30
SE 3 (high)	0	0	0	0	0	0	0	0
Ring (outside City)	0.0	--*	---	---	-16	--*	---	---
Nonwhite, under 65 years								
City of Chicago, SE 1 (low)	92	66	60	54	69	52	40	51
SE 2	49	33	27	36	32	22	18	30
SE 3 (high)	0	0	0	0	0	0	0	0
Ring (outside City)	2	--*	---	---	-8	--*	---	---
Nonwhite, 65 & over								
City of Chicago, SE 1 (low)	45	12	7	13	7	19	21	15
SE 2	24	-1	-24	12	6	15	-2	32
SE 3 (high)	0	0	0	0	0	0	0	0
Ring (outside City)	-2	--*	---	---	-29	--*	---	---

Source: Table 4.3. See Table 4.3 for notes a and --*.

[b] Differentials indicate the percent by which the age-adjusted rate for each SE group and the Ring exceeds (or is less than, if negative) the rate for persons of the same sex and color in SE group 5 except for whites in 1960, when the Ring of the SMSA was used as the base.

30-year period, but white females 65 and over did not. For nonwhite males in SE group 2, the socioeconomic differential at both age levels was larger in 1960 than in 1930. Among nonwhite females in SE group 2, the differential was about the same in 1960 as in 1930 for those under 65, but there was some convergence for those 65 and over.

Infant Mortality

Socioeconomic differentials in infant mortality in the Chicago area during the 30 years from 1930 to 1960 are summarized in Table 4.5, which has already been analyzed from the perspective of comparing the area's rates with those of the nation. The data reveal a marked inverse association between infant mortality and socioeconomic level in 1930. Among white males the rate declined sharply, from 83.9 infant deaths per 1,000 live births in the lowest socioeconomic group to 36.7 in the highest group; rates for females showed a comparable decline from 68.0 to 29.0 from the lowest to highest socioeconomic groups. Nonwhites also showed a consistent, though less marked, pattern of infant mortality. However, by 1940 the inverse association was much weaker among whites and had disappeared among non-whites. For example, among white males the infant mortality rate declined from 34.8 for SE 1 to 26.5 for SE 5, and among white females the rate declined from 27.9 for SE 1 to 20.6 for SE 4 and then increased to 25.4 in SE 5. In 1960, there was a similar exception to the inverse pattern among whites in the 3 upper socioeconomic groups (SE 4, 5 and the ring), and a weak and inconsistent pattern among nonwhites.

This marked convergence of socioeconomic differentials in infant mortality in the Chicago area between 1930 and 1960 is in sharp contrast to the lack of convergence of socioeconomic differentials in age-adjusted death rates over all ages (see Table 4.6 and the analysis above). The relatively small differentials in infant mortality in Chicago in 1960 are also markedly different from the very large socioeconomic differentials in infant mortality in the nation during 1964-66. For example, infant mortality rates in the United States, 1964-66, decreased sharply from 32.7 for infants whose fathers had only an elementary education to 17.1 for infants whose fathers had completed four years or more of college (see Table 2.9). These comparisons suggest that biomedical knowledge and other factors responsible for the reduction of infant mortality were in 1960 much more equally available at all socioeconomic levels within the Chicago area than within the nation as a whole. It also indicates that socioeconomic differentials in infant mortality may converge in the absence of any convergence of differential mortality at the older ages.

The indexes of excess mortality analyzed in Chapter 8 (Tables 8.4 and 8.5) provide summary measures over all socioeconomic groups combined of the relative impact of socioeconomic differentials in mortality in the Chicago area during the 30-year period.

Percent Change for SE Groups

Among whites in the city over the 30-year period, no consistent pattern of change in mortality is discernible by socioeconomic status and the range of changes by class is relatively narrow (Table 4.4). Among males under 65 the greatest decline is found in the second lowest group (SE 2), 39 percent, and the smallest in the highest socioeconomic class (SE 5), 29 percent. Among white females under 65 the largest decline is found in the second highest class (SE 4), 59 percent, and the lowest decline in the highest socioeconomic class (SE 5), 48 percent. Between 1950 and 1960 the greatest decrease in mortality is found in the ring for both males and females.

For white males 65 and over in the lowest socioeconomic class (SE 1) mortality actually increased between 1930 and 1960, by 23 percent. This is the only subcategory of the population which experienced an increase in mortality over the 30-year period and points to the need for more intensive epidemiological investigation— both biomedical and social. Mortality for white males 65 and over in each of the other socioeconomic groups declined, with the greatest decline evident in the second highest class (SE 4), 12 percent. White females over 65 registered a decrease in death rates in each of the socioeconomic groups, the highest decline occurring in the intermediate class (SE 3) and the lowest decrease in the lowest economic class (SE 1), 12 percent.

In contrast with the situation for whites, a definite pattern of changes in mortality over the 30-year period is evident for non-whites. For both nonwhite males and females under 65, and for nonwhite males over 65, the greatest decrease in mortality occurred in the highest socioeconomic class (SE 3); and the lowest decline in the lowest economic class (SE 1). Among nonwhite females 65 and over is found the only exception to this pattern; the greatest mortality decrease is found in the intermediate class (SE 2) and the smallest in the highest class (SE 3). The range of differences in changes in mortality by socioeconomic class, however, as among whites, is relatively narrow.

Finally, in respect to mortality changes over the 30-year period, white females have experienced greater decreases in mortality relative to white males than have nonwhite females relative to nonwhite males. But it is to be recalled that nonwhite mortality for both sexes has been and still is appreciably higher than white, although as will be shown below, the gap has narrowed.

A consistent pattern of change in infant mortality by socioeconomic status is evident between 1930 and 1960 for each color and sex subgrouping (Table 4.5). There was an inverse relationship between socioeconomic status and the percentage decrease in infant mortality over the 30-year period as a whole, more pronounced among whites than nonwhites. However, comparison of changes during the 1930-40 decade with changes during the 20-year period from 1940 to 1960 reveals quite different patterns by socioeconomic group (available data did not permit calculation of changes by socioeconomic level, 1940-50 and 1950-60). The inverse relationship between percentage decrease in infant mortality and socioeconomic level was very marked during the first decade, 1930-40; for example, the rate for white females in the lowest socioeconomic group declined by 59 percent as compared with a decline of only 12 percent for the highest socioeconomic group in the city. However, between 1940 and 1960 there was no consistent pattern by socioeconomic level in the changes in infant mortality, a not surprising finding given the fact that the overall decline in white infant mortality, for example, was quite small (11 percent for males and 19 percent for females) as compared with the sharp declines experienced during the preceding decade (51 percent for males and 49 percent for females).

Sex Differentials

For the country as a whole, among both whites and nonwhites for each age group, male mortality was considerably above female for every period considered (Table 4.7). Moreover, with not a single exception, the gap between male and female age-adjusted death rates increased over the 30-year period. The same pattern holds for the city of Chicago. In both the nation and the city the mortality gap

Table 4.7. Sex differentials in age-adjusted death rates, by color and socioeconomic group: Chicago Standard Metropolitan Statistical Area
(SMSA) and City of Chicago, 1930-1960

| Age and socioeconomic group[a] | Percent by which male rate exceeds female rate | | | | | | | |
| | White | | | | Nonwhite | | | |
	1960	1950	1940	1929-1931[b]	1960	1950	1940	1929-1931[b]
All ages								
United States............	64	48	32	21	36	25	17	9
Chicago SMSA............	62	49	---	---	37	34	---	---
City of Chicago......	64	52	34	24	38	36	34	23
SE 1 (low)........	78	60	36	30	45	35	40	22
SE 2..............	61	49	33	23	38	32	28	21
SE 3..............	63	39	26	20	21	34	34	23
SE 4..............	59	42	30	18	...	...	...	...
SE 5 (high).......	63	45	45	29	...	...	...	...
Ring (outside City)..	53	42	---	---	44	--*	---	---
Under 65 years								
United States............	88	68	43	25	36	24	15	6
Chicago SMSA............	79	71	---	---	33	25	---	---
City of Chicago......	87	72	45	30	32	27	26	18
SE 1 (low)........	83	76	46	33	35	28	35	17
SE 2..............	76	68	44	27	35	27	27	20
SE 3..............	79	55	37	27	19	17	18	14
SE 4..............	88	63	40	22	...	...	...	...
SE 5 (high).......	88	56	61	38	...	...	...	...
Ring (outside City)..	74	62	---	---	32	--*	---	---
65 years & over								
United States............	47	34	21	14	35	26	24	18
Chicago SMSA............	47	33	---	---	45	51	---	---
City of Chicago......	51	34	24	16	45	53	51	36
SE 1 (low)........	71	44	23	22	65	52	53	41
SE 2..............	51	33	20	16	43	40	34	23
SE 3..............	51	23	19	14	22	63	73	45
SE 4..............	43	28	23	13	...	...	...	...
SE 5 (high).......	48	36	29	19	...	...	...	...
Ring (outside City)..	39	29	---	---	67	--*	---	---

Source: Table 4.3   See Table 4.3 for notes a, b and --*.

between the sexes was greater for whites than for nonwhites. Finally,
not unexpectedly the sex mortality gap is greater among whites
under 65 than among whites 65 and over, but not too different
among the nonwhites in the two age groups.

For the two periods for which SMSA data are available, the sex
difference in mortality in the ring increased over time, and was
smaller than that for the nation or the city for whites, but not for
nonwhites. Among nonwhites under 65 in the ring the mortality gap
between males and females, although below that of the nation,

matched that of the city. Among nonwhites 65 and over, the sex mortality gap was considerably greater in the ring than for the nation and the city and, also, greater than that for any socioeconomic class within the city.

Among whites no regular pattern of sex differences in mortality by socioeconomic group is apparent. There is some tendency toward a U-shaped curve, with the sex gap in mortality greater in the lower and higher socioeconomic classes, but the pattern is not marked and the irregularities hold for both age groups. Among nonwhites more of a pattern is discernible. The smallest difference in male and female mortality is found in the highest socioeconomic group for each period for nonwhites under 65, and the greatest difference in the lowest class for three of the four time periods. Among nonwhites 65 and over, the greatest sex difference, in contrast, occurs in the highest socioeconomic class for three of the four periods, but for the fourth, 1960, the sex gap in mortality is smallest in the highest class.

Expectation of Life

Expectation of life at birth has consistently increased in the city of Chicago and in the ring of the SMSA over the time periods shown in Table 4.8.[5] This holds true for each color and sex group. In the city, the increase in longevity between 1930 and 1960 was much greater for nonwhites than for whites. Nonwhite female longevity increased by 19.4 years, nonwhite male by 18.2 years; white female by 10.2 years, and white male by 7.5 years. In 1960, however, white longevity was still well above nonwhite. White male expectation of life at birth in 1960, at 65.2 years was 4.3 years above that for nonwhite males; and white female average longevity at 72.0 years was 5.5 years above that of nonwhite females. Longevity in the metropolitan ring was above that in the city, both in 1950 and in 1960, for each color and sex group. The differences were larger for nonwhites than for whites in 1960, the only year for which nonwhite life tables could be calculated for the ring.

There was a well-defined positive relationship between expectation of life at birth and socioeconomic class, which, with few inversions, holds for each sex and color group. Among white males the difference in expectation of life at birth between the lowest and highest socioeconomic group diminished from 11.8 years in 1930 to 9.0 years in 1960 (taking the ring as the highest group in 1960). Among white females the class difference in longevity decreased

Table 4.8. Expectation of life at birth, by color, sex and socioeconomic group: Chicago Standard Metropolitan Statistical Area (SMSA) and City of Chicago, 1930-1960

Color, sex and socioeconomic group [a]	Expectation of life at birth $(\overset{o}{e}_0)$				Socioeconomic differences in $(\overset{o}{e}_0)$ [c]				Change in $(\overset{o}{e}_0)$ [d]			
	1960	1950	1940	1929-1931 [b]	1960	1950	1940	1929-1931	1930 to 1960	1950 to 1960	1940 to 1950	1930 to 1940
White males												
Chicago SMSA........	66.7	65.5	---	---	...	...	...	...	---	1.2	---	---
City of Chicago..	65.2	64.7	62.6	57.7	...	...	...	...	7.5	0.5	2.1	4.9
SE 1 (low)....	60.0	60.8	57.8	51.2	0	0	0	0	8.8	-0.8	3.0	6.6
SE 2.........	64.6	64.4	61.5	56.2	4.6	3.6	3.7	5.0	8.4	0.2	2.9	5.3
SE 3.........	66.5	67.0	64.2	59.2	6.5	6.2	6.4	8.0	7.3	-0.5	2.8	5.0
SE 4.........	67.9	67.4	65.3	61.2	7.9	6.6	7.5	10.0	6.7	0.5	2.1	4.1
SE 5 (high)...	67.4	68.8	65.3	63.0	7.4	8.0	7.5	11.8	4.4	-1.4	3.5	2.3
Ring of SMSA.....	69.0	67.7	---	---	9.0	6.9	---	---	---	1.3	---	---
White females												
Chicago SMSA........	73.1	71.3	---	---	...	...	...	...	---	1.8	---	---
City of Chicago..	72.0	70.7	67.1	61.8	...	...	...	...	10.2	1.3	3.6	5.3
SE 1 (low)....	67.7	67.8	62.7	56.4	0	0	0	0	11.3	-0.1	5.1	6.3
SE 2.........	71.2	70.3	66.0	60.2	3.5	2.5	3.3	3.8	11.0	0.9	4.3	5.8
SE 3.........	72.8	71.6	67.6	62.5	5.1	3.8	4.9	6.1	10.3	1.2	4.0	5.1
SE 4.........	73.8	72.1	69.2	64.4	6.1	4.3	6.5	8.0	9.4	1.7	2.9	4.8
SE 5 (high)...	73.6	73.4	70.2	67.2	5.9	5.6	7.5	10.8	6.4	0.2	3.2	3.0
Ring of SMSA.....	74.6	72.7	---	---	6.9	4.9	---	---	---	1.9	---	---
Nonwhite males												
Chicago SMSA........	61.3	58.5	---	---	...	...	...	...	---	2.8	---	---
City of Chicago..:	60.9	58.0	51.0	42.7	...	...	...	...	18.2	2.9	7.0	8.3
SE 1 (low)....	56.7	55.4	47.4	38.9	0	0	0	0	17.8	1.3	8.0	8.5
SE 2.........	59.9	58.8	51.2	40.7	3.2	3.4	3.8	1.8	19.2	1.1	7.6	10.5
SE 3 (high)...	65.1	62.1	53.6	47.6	8.4	6.7	6.2	8.7	17.5	3.0	8.5	6.0
Ring of SMSA.....	66.1	--*	---	---	9.4	--*	---	---	---	--*	---	---
Nonwhite females												
Chicago SMSA........	66.9	64.0	---	---	...	...	...	...	---	2.9	---	---
City of Chicago..	66.5	63.7	56.7	47.1	...	...	...	...	19.4	2.8	7.0	9.6
SE 1 (low)....	62.5	61.0	53.2	42.9	0	0	0	0	19.6	1.5	7.8	10.3
SE 2.........	65.1	64.4	56.8	45.4	2.6	3.4	3.6	2.5	19.7	0.7	7.6	11.4
SE 3 (high)...	68.1	67.4	59.1	51.7	5.6	6.4	5.9	8.8	16.4	0.7	8.3	7.4
Ring of SMSA.....	72.3	--*	---	---	9.8	--*	---	---	---	--*	---	---

Source: See text for sources of data and methods used to compute life tables. See Table 4.3 for notes a, b and --*.

[c] Computed by subtracting $\overset{o}{e}_0$ for SE group 1 from $\overset{o}{e}_0$ for each of the other groups.

[d] Computed by subtracting $\overset{o}{e}_0$ for beginning of period from $\overset{o}{e}_0$ for end of period.

from 10.8 years to 6.9 years. Among nonwhites there was no comparable decrease in class differences in longevity during the 30-year period.

Analysis of the changes in expectation of life at birth for the decades shown indicates, consistent with earlier observations, that the greatest gains in longevity were achieved in the earlier decades. In Chicago, as for the nation as a whole, mortality seemed to remain on a plateau during the fifties, and in some subcategories longevity actually decreased during the decade (white males in SE 1, SE 3, and SE 5; and white females in SE 1).

Actual differences in expectation of life by sex are shown for each color and socioeconomic group in Table 4.9. Among each color and socioeconomic class in the city, except for nonwhites in the highest socioeconomic group, the sex difference in longevity increased over

Table 4.9. Sex differentials in expectation of life at birth, by color and socioeconomic group: Chicago Standard Metropolitan Statistical Area (SMSA) and City of Chicago, 1930-1960

Color and socioeconomic group[a]	Sex differentials in $\overset{o}{e}_{o}$ (female minus male)			
	1960	1950	1940	1929-1931[b]
White, Chicago SMSA...........	6.4	5.8	---	---
City of Chicago............	6.8	6.0	4.5	4.1
SE 1 (low)..............	7.7	7.0	4.9	5.2
SE 2....................	6.6	5.9	4.5	4.0
SE 3....................	6.3	4.6	3.4	3.3
SE 4...................	5.9	4.7	3.9	3.2
SE 5 (high).............	6.2	4.6	4.9	4.2
Ring (outside City)........	5.6	5.0	---	---
Nonwhite, Chicago SMSA........	5.6	5.5	---	---
City of Chicago............	5.6	5.7	5.7	4.4
SE 1 (low)..............	5.8	5.6	5.8	4.0
SE 2....................	5.2	5.6	5.6	4.7
SE 3 (high).............	3.0	5.3	5.5	4.1
Ring (outside City)........	6.2	--*	---	---

Source: Table 4.8. See Table 4.3 for notes a, b and --*.

time. Among whites for each period there was a tendency for the sex difference to decrease as socioeconomic status increased, except for an upturn in the highest class. Among nonwhites a slight decline in the sex difference in longevity as socioeconomic status increased was evident from 1940 to 1960. In 1960, the sex difference among whites in the ring was below that for the city as a whole and for the highest socioeconomic class within the city. In contrast, the sex difference among nonwhites in the ring was above that for nonwhites in the city and in all socioeconomic groups.

5 / SOCIOECONOMIC DIFFERENTIALS BY CAUSE OF DEATH

In the preceding chapters differentials in mortality by various indexes of socioeconomic class have been presented for all causes of death combined. In this chapter analysis is made of socioeconomic differences in mortality by cause of death. Consideration of the cause of death helps to explain the differences previously noted and more explicitly directs attention to the way in which social and economic factors influence mortality through intervening variables— various disease entities resulting in death.

There is a voluminous literature on mortality from specific causes of death. No attempt is made here to review these materials, nor are the findings of the studies reviewed here analyzed from the perspective of the epidemiological literature on each cause of death. Such a review and analysis may be found in the monographs on particular causes of death that were undertaken as part of the APHA series of monographs on vital and health statistics. Two studies provided the basic data for this chapter, the 1960 Matched Records Study, discussed in Chapters 2 and 3 and Appendix A; and the 1950 Chicago Study based on areal indexes, discussed in Chapter 4. Each study provides an overview of socioeconomic differentials for selected general causes of death covering the entire range of causes on a comparable basis.

Education Differentials, United States, 1960[1]

Several considerations led to the selection of education as the most satisfactory of the several indexes of socioeconomic status available in the 1960 Matched Records Study. First, it is preferable to income for the reason elaborated in Chapter 2—the reverse causal path to which income is subject especially for men. Second, it is preferable to occupation because it applies with equal validity to retired men and working men, and to all women. Finally, it is not subject to variation over time in the lifespan of an individual as are both income and occupation.

The present distribution of all 1960 deaths in the United States by 23 selected causes of death is reported in Table 5.1; the corresponding numbers for each cause are given in Appendix Table A.14. The 23 categories include 19 unduplicated cause-of-death groups (Causes

Table 5.1. Percent distribution of white decedents 25 years and over by cause of death, by sex and age: United States, 1960

Cause of death (ISC codes)	White males			White females		
	25 & over	25-64 years	65 & over	25 & over	25-64 years	65 & over
ALL CAUSES..	100.0	100.0	100.0	100.0	100.0	100.0
1. Tuberculosis, all forms (001-019).............................	0.8	1.1	0.6	0.3	0.7	0.2
2. Malignant neoplasms, incl. lymph. & hematop. tissues (140-205)..	16.2	18.2	15.0	18.6	32.8	13.7
2a. of stomach (151)...	1.4	1.3	1.5	1.2	1.3	1.1
2b. of intestine & rectum (152-154).........................	2.3	2.2	2.4	3.2	4.3	2.9
2c. of lung, bronchus, & trachea (162,163)...................	3.6	5.3	2.7	0.8	1.6	0.5
2d. of breast (170)...	0.0	0.0	0.0	3.7	8.3	2.1
2e. of uterus, ovary, fallopian tube & broad ligament (171-175)	...	...	...	3.3	7.3	1.9
2f. of prostate (177).......................................	1.6	0.5	2.3	...	...	...
2g. Other malignant neoplasms................................	7.2	9.0	6.1	6.4	10.2	5.1
3. Diabetes mellitus (260)....................................	1.4	1.3	1.4	2.6	2.7	2.5
4. Major cardiovascular-renal diseases (330-334,400-468,592-594)..	60.4	50.7	66.0	61.9	38.8	69.9
4a. Vascular lesions affecting central nervous system (330-334)	10.2	5.1	13.2	14.9	8.0	17.2
4b. Rheumatic fever & chronic rheumatic heart disease (400-416)	1.0	1.9	0.5	1.4	3.7	0.7
4c. Arteriosclerotic & degenerative heart disease (420,422)....	39.8	37.1	41.3	33.2	19.4	38.0
4d. Hypertensive disease, with & without heart (440-447).......	3.5	2.3	4.2	5.9	3.6	6.7
4e. Other cardiovascular-renal diseases......................	5.9	4.3	6.9	6.5	4.1	7.3
5. Influenza & pneumonia, except pneumonia of newborn (480-493)...	3.3	2.4	3.8	3.3	2.3	3.6
6. Cirrhosis of liver (581)...................................	1.6	2.9	0.8	1.0	2.7	0.4
7. All accidents (800-962)....................................	4.8	8.8	2.4	3.2	4.8	2.6
7a. Motor-vehicle accidents (810-835).........................	2.0	4.1	0.7	1.0	2.7	0.4
7b. Accidents except motor vehicle (800-802,840-962)...........	2.8	4.7	1.7	2.2	2.1	2.3
8. Suicide (963,970-979)......................................	1.6	3.3	0.7	0.7	2.2	0.2
9. Other causes of death......................................	10.0	11.3	9.3	8.4	13.0	6.8

Source: Same source as columns (5) and (6), Table A.14.

1, 2a-2g, 3, 4a-4e, 5, 6, 7a-7b, 8), 3 major causes of death (Causes 2, 4, 7) and a residual (Cause 9).[2] Tabulations of deaths in the 1960 Matched Records Study were made for 41 causes of death, based on recommendations submitted by authors of eight of the monographs in the APHA series of monographs. The 23 causes for which data are reported in Tables 5.1 and 5.2, respectively, include those recommended causes which had sufficiently large numbers of deaths, and combinations of more detailed causes when numbers were small and the combined cause was thought to be meaningful. In addition, some recommended detailed causes with numbers too small for reliable estimates were not compiled at all.

For all white males 25 and over two general causes of death accounted for over three-fourths (76.6 percent) of all mortality in 1960 (see Table 5.1). Both of these were degenerative causes; one, major cardiovascular-renal diseases, comprised 60.4 percent of the deaths, and the other, malignant neoplasms including lymphatic and hematopoietic tissues, 16.2 percent. Accidents were the next most important cause of death for males, and this cause contributed only 4.8 percent of all mortality. The basket category "other causes of death" accounted for 10.0 percent of the mortality of males 25 and over, so that the combination of all the other cause categories shown accounted for less than 10 percent of adult male mortality.

For all white females 25 and over the same two degenerative causes of death accounted for over four-fifths of all mortality (80.5 percent) in 1960. Major cardiovascular-renal diseases accounted for 61.9 percent of adult female mortality and malignant neoplasms accounted for 18.6 percent. The next most important cause of death for white females was, as for males, "all accidents" and this cause contributed only 3.2 percent of all mortality. Since "other causes" constituted 9.4 percent of all adult female mortality, all the other categories of causes of death shown accounted for less than 7 percent of adult female deaths.

These major causes of death had differential impact by age for each sex. Among males 25 to 64, 50.7 percent of the deaths were attributable to major cardiovascular-renal diseases, whereas they accounted for 66.0 percent of all deaths of males 65 and over. In contrast, malignant neoplasms accounted for a larger proportion of the deaths of the younger males, 18.2 percent, than of the older males, 15.0 percent. Among females similar patterns obtained, with the major cardiovascular-renal diseases contributing more to the mortality of the older than the younger women, 69.9 as compared with 38.8 percent, and with the malignant neoplasms contributing more to the mortality of the younger than the older women, 32.8 as compared with 13.7 percent. But almost twice as many of the younger female deaths than the younger male deaths were attributable to malignancies, 32.8 percent as compared with 18.2 percent. Contrariwise, the cardiovascular-renal diseases accounted for a much greater proportion of the deaths to younger men than to younger women, 50.7 percent as compared with 38.8 percent. Interestingly enough, the contribution of each of these major causes was about the same among deaths to older men and older women. Cardiovascular-renal diseases accounted for 69.9 percent of all older female deaths and 66.0 percent of that of all older males. Malignancies contributed 13.7 percent of all older female mortality and 15.0 percent of that of older males. This discussion of the relative contribution of cardiovascular diseases and malignant neoplasms to male and female deaths in the younger and older ages should not be confused with measures of the incidence of death from these causes among the four sex-age groups. Male mortality from each cause exceeded female mortality at both age levels.

Education differentials in mortality rates for the 23 selected causes of death in the United States, May-August, 1960, are reported in Table 5.2 and portrayed graphically in Figure 5.1. These differentials

Table 5.2. Mortality ratios by years of school completed for selected causes of death, by sex and age, for the white population 25 years and over: United States, May-August, 1960

Cause of death (ISC codes) and years of school completed	White males			White females		
	25 & over	25-64 years	65 & over	25 & over	25-64 years	65 & over
ALL CAUSES...............................	1.00	1.00	1.00	1.00	1.00	1.00
Less than 8 years school................	1.02	1.14	1.01	1.16	1.31	1.10
Elementary, 8 years.....................	1.01	1.07	1.00	1.05	1.08	1.03
High school, 1-4 years..................	1.00	.97	.99	.90	.89	.94
College, 1 year or more.................	.89	.77	.98	.72	.80	.70
1. Tuberculosis, all forms (001-019)............	1.00#	1.00#	--[a]	--[a]	--[a]	--[a]
Less than 8 years school................	1.53#	1.84#	--[a]	--[a]	--[a]	--[a]
Elementary, 8 years.....................	1.17#	1.19#	--[a]	--[a]	--[a]	--[a]
High school, 1-4 years..................	.64#	.80#	--[a]	--[a]	--[a]	--[a]
College, 1 year or more.................	.39#	.21#	--[a]	--[a]	--[a]	--[a]
2. Malignant neoplasms, incl. lymph. & hematop. tissues (140-205)	1.00	1.00	1.00	1.00	1.00	1.00
Less than 8 years school................	1.04	1.09	.98	1.01	1.13	1.00
Elementary, 8 years.....................	1.04	1.12	.97	1.01	1.05	1.01
High school, 1-4 years..................	.95	.94	1.04	1.01	.94	1.04
College, 1 year or more.................	.92	.83	1.10	.93	.92	.89
2a. of stomach (151)......................	1.00	1.00	1.00	1.00	--[a]	--[a]
Less than 8 years school................	1.11	1.25	1.05	1.22	--[a]	--[a]
Elementary, 8 years.....................	1.05	1.07	1.04	1.03	--[a]	--[a]
High school, 1-4 years..................	1.00	.97	1.06	.94	--[a]	--[a]
College, 1 year or more.................	.55	.56	.56	.45	--[a]	--[a]
2b. of intestine & rectum (152-154).........	1.00	1.00	1.00#	1.00	1.00	1.00
Less than 8 years school................	1.06	1.19	1.00#	.98	1.23	.92
Elementary, 8 years.....................	1.03	.95	1.06#	1.10	1.11	1.11
High school, 1-4 years..................	.90	.91	.95#	1.02	.91	1.09
College, 1 year or more.................	.95	.98	.96#	.75	.74	.72
2c. of lung, bronchus & trachea (162,163)......	1.00	1.00	1.00	1.00	1.00#	--[a]
Less than 8 years school................	1.12	1.18	1.07	1.16	1.23#	--[a]
Elementary, 8 years.....................	1.01	1.14	.86	.94	.96#	--[a]
High school, 1-4 years..................	.99	.95	1.10	.92	.94#	--[a]
College, 1 year or more.................	.70	.61	.90	.97	.90#	--[a]
2d. of breast (170).......................	--[a]	--[a]	--[a]	1.00	1.00	1.00
Less than 8 years school................	--[a]	--[a]	--[a]	.83	.87	.85
Elementary, 8 years.....................	--[a]	--[a]	--[a]	1.01	.98	1.09
High school, 1-4 years..................	--[a]	--[a]	--[a]	1.05	1.03	1.01
College, 1 year or more.................	--[a]	--[a]	--[a]	1.18	1.11	1.28
2e. of uterus, ovary, fallopian tube & broad ligament (171-175)	...	...	...	1.00	1.00	1.00
Less than 8 years school................	...	...	...	1.16	1.42	.98
Elementary, 8 years.....................	...	...	...	.96	1.11	.81
High school, 1-4 years..................	...	...	...	.99	.88	1.25
College, 1 year or more.................	...	...	...	.77	.68	.98
2f. of prostate (177).......................	1.00	--[a]	1.00	...	...	...
Less than 8 years school................	.91	--[a]	.93	...	...	...
Elementary, 8 years.....................	.95	--[a]	.96	...	...	...
High school, 1-4 year..................	.86	--[a]	.78	...	...	...
College, 1 year or more.................	1.77	--[a]	1.87	...	...	...
2g. Other malignant neoplasms[b]............	1.00	1.00	1.00	1.00	1.00	1.00
Less than 8 years school................	.98	.99	.93	1.05	1.12	1.05
Elementary, 8 years.....................	1.06	1.14	.98	1.04	1.13	1.00
High school, 1-4 years..................	.98	.95	1.14	.93	.88	.97
College, 1 year or more.................	.98	.94	1.13	.98	1.00	.93
3. Diabetes mellitus (260).......................	1.00	1.00	--[a]	1.00	1.00#	1.00
Less than 8 years school................	1.06	1.03	--[a]	1.48	2.16#	1.29
Elementary, 8 years.....................	.90	.80	--[a]	.96	.96#	.93
High school, 1-4 years..................	1.09	1.24	--[a]	.77	.62#	.89
College, 1 year or more.................	.85	.71	--[a]	.42	.50#	.40
4. Major cardiovascular-renal diseases (330-334,400-468,592-594).	1.00	1.00	1.00	1.00	1.00	1.00
Less than 8 years school................	.99	1.06	1.00	1.18	1.38	1.12
Elementary, 8 years.....................	1.00	1.03	1.01	1.06	1.12	1.02
High school, 1-4 years..................	1.06	1.03	.99	.88	.86	.93
College, 1 year or more.................	.93	.80	.98	.63	.66	.65
4a. Vascular lesions affecting central nervous system (330-334)	1.00	1.00	1.00	1.00	1.00	1.00
Less than 8 years school................	1.07	1.17	1.06	1.14	1.44	1.09
Elementary, 8 years.....................	1.01	1.02	1.01	.99	.97	.99
High school, 1-4 years..................	.92	.90	.93	.95	.89	.98
College, 1 year or more.................	.86	.92	.83	.70	.71	.71

(continued)

Table 5.2. Mortality ratios by years of school completed for selected causes of death, by sex and age, for the white population 25 years and over: United States, May-August, 1960--(continued)

Cause of death (ISC codes) and years of school completed	White males			White females		
	25 & over	25-64 years	65 & over	25 & over	25-64 years	65 & over
4b. Rheumatic fever & chronic rheumatic heart disease (400-416)	1.00	1.00	--[a]	1.00	1.00	--[a]
Less than 8 years school	.91	.98	--[a]	.95	1.10	--[a]
Elementary, 8 years	1.08	1.12	--[a]	1.14	1.14	--[a]
High school, 1-4 years	1.07	1.04	--[a]	.96	.95	--[a]
College, 1 year or more	.90	.79	--[a]	.97	.87	--[a]
4c. Arteriosclerotic & degenerative heart disease (420,422)	1.00	1.00	1.00	1.00	1.00	1.00
Less than 8 years school	.95	1.01	.99	1.21	1.41	1.13
Elementary, 8 years	1.01	1.01	1.02	1.07	1.16	1.03
High school, 1-4 years	1.10	1.07	1.01	.86	.84	.92
College, 1 year or more	.93	.81	.98	.59	.59	.62
4d. Hypertensive disease, with & without heart (440-447)	1.00	1.00	1.00	1.00	1.00	1.00
Less than 8 years school	1.14	1.27	1.11	1.24	1.52	1.16
Elementary, 8 years	.91	1.05	.87	1.06	1.26	1.00
High school, 1-4 years	.89	.92	.88	.85	.75	.95
College, 1 year or more	.93	.71	1.09	.49	.59	.48
4e. Other cardiovascular-renal diseases	1.00	1.00	1.00	1.00	1.00	1.00
Less than 8 years school	.99	1.20	.96	1.14	1.27	1.09
Elementary, 8 years	1.00	1.06	.99	1.12	1.13	1.10
High school 1-4 years	1.02	.98	1.01	.82	.90	.82
College, 1 year or more	.99	.70	1.20	.75	.74	.79
5. Influenza & pneumonia, except pneumonia of newborn (480-493)	1.00	1.00#	1.00	1.00	--[a]	1.00#
Less than 8 years school	1.20	1.63#	1.12	1.14	--[a]	1.05#
Elementary, 8 years	.98	1.06#	.95	1.09	--[a]	1.05#
High school, 1-4 years	.81	.76#	.86	.89	--[a]	.99#
College, 1 year or more	.75	.63#	.84	.68	--[a]	.66#
6. Cirrhosis of liver (581)	1.00	1.00	--[a]	1.00	1.00	--[a]
Less than 8 years school	1.00	.96	--[a]	.88	1.03	--[a]
Elementary, 8 years	.99	1.08	--[a]	1.20	.93	--[a]
High school 1-4 years	.98	1.01	--[a]	.99	1.06	--[a]
College, 1 year or more	1.06	.94	--[a]	.90	.89	--[a]
7. All accidents (800-962)	1.00	1.00	1.00	1.00	1.00	1.00
Less than 8 years school	1.13	1.45	1.02	1.19	1.19	1.03
Elementary, 8 years	1.06	1.16	1.03	1.26	1.19	1.17
High school, 1-4 years	1.01	.92	1.14	.83	.90	.89
College, 1 year or more	.66	.64	.55	.77	.96	.59
7a. Motor-vehicle accidents (810-835)	1.00	1.00	--[a]	1.00	1.00	--[a]
Less than 8 years school	1.21	1.29	--[a]	1.02	1.04	--[a]
Elementary, 8 years	1.10	1.18	--[a]	1.18	1.26	--[a]
High school, 1-4 years	.98	.96	--[a]	.92	.89	--[a]
College, 1 year or more	.68	.70	--[a]	1.01	1.09	--[a]
7b. Accidents except motor vehicle (800-802,840-962)	1.00	1.00	1.00	1.00	--[c]	--[a]
Less than 8 years school	1.11	1.55	.99	1.30	--[c]	--[a]
Elementary, 8 years	1.06	1.15	1.07	1.27	--[c]	--[a]
High school, 1-4 years	1.03	.89	1.15	.77	--[c]	--[a]
College, 1 year or more	.63	.59	.53	.58	--[c]	--[a]
8. Suicide (963,970-979)	1.00	1.00	--[a]	--[a]	--[a]	--[a]
Less than 8 years school	1.29	1.25	--[a]	--[a]	--[a]	--[a]
Elementary, 8 years	1.21	1.28	--[a]	--[a]	--[a]	--[a]
High school, 1-4 years	.84	.89	--[a]	--[a]	--[a]	--[a]
College, 1 year or more	.69	.72	--[a]	--[a]	--[a]	--[a]
9. Other causes of death[d]	1.00	1.00	1.00	1.00	1.00	1.00
Less than 8 years school	1.18	1.44	1.05	1.17	1.38	1.08
Elementary, 8 years	1.01	1.08	.96	1.04	1.02	1.05
High school, 1-4 years	.85	.85	.89	.87	.87	.87
College, 1 year or more	.85	.72	1.09	.91	.93	.89

Source: Population Research Center, University of Chicago, 1960 Matched Records Study (see Appendix A).

Does not meet the reliability requirement that the Special Sample Survey of May-August deaths (which provided data for estimating characteristics of decedents not matched with census records) have at least five unmatched decedents reported in this sex-age-education subgroup of the population.

[a] Education differentials not computed because less than 150 matched Stage II deaths from this cause.

[b] For males, cause 2g includes cause 2d as well as cancer sites not listed in this table.

[c] Education differentials not computed because of excessively high inflation factor for unmatched NCHS Survey deaths.

[d] For females, cause 9 includes causes 1 and 8, in addition to causes not listed in this table.

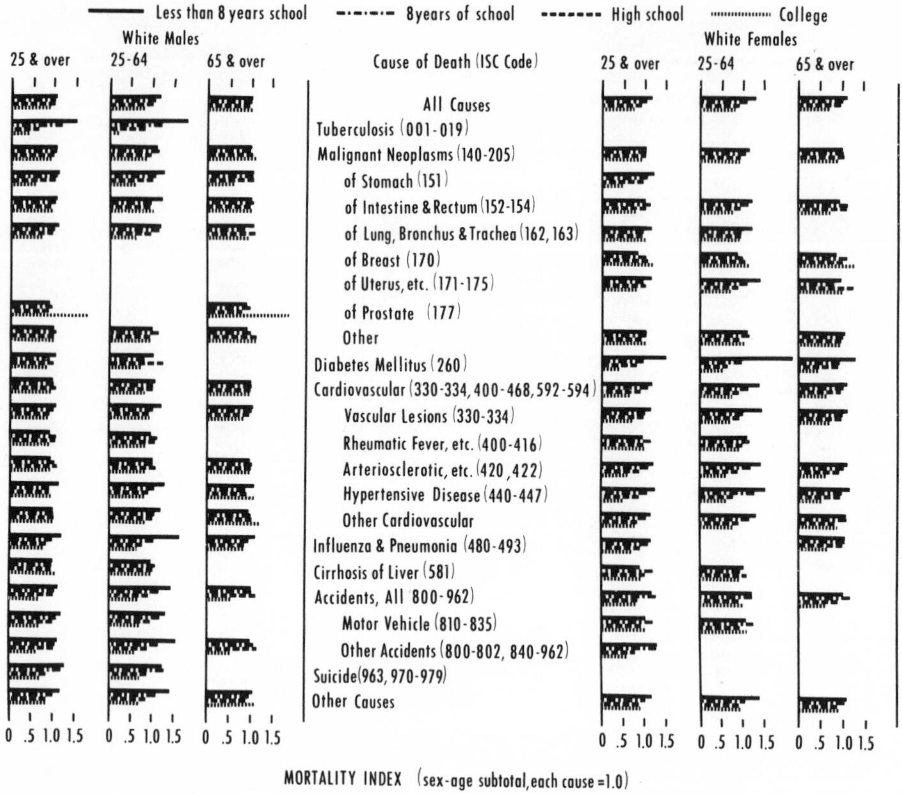

Figure 5.1. Mortality differentials by years of school completed, for selected causes of death by sex and age: United States white population, May-August 1960.

are summarized under four broad cause-of-death groupings in the sections that follow.

Major Cardiovascular-renal Diseases

The category "major cardiovascular-renal diseases," combining the five subcategories of causes of death shown, was inversely related to educational status for both white males and white females 25 to 64 years of age, although the relationship was stronger for females. White females 25 to 64 with the lowest education, less than elementary school, had a mortality index from this cause 2.1 times that of women with the highest education, one or more years of college. White males 25 to 64 with the lowest education had an index from this cause 1.3 times that of the highest educated males.

For the general category "major cardiovascular-renal diseases" the inverse pattern with education persisted for older females, those 65 and over, although it was obscured for older males by reason of varying patterns of specific forms of these diseases, as is indicated below. For the least educated older women the mortality index from this cause was 1.7 times that for the best educated older women.

Within the category "major cardiovascular-renal diseases" the most important specific cause of death of those shown, both for males and females, was "arteriosclerotic and degenerative heart disease." This cause of death accounted for 39.8 percent of all adult male deaths and 33.2 percent of the deaths of all adult females. For the younger persons 25 to 64, this cause of death was responsible for 37.1 percent of male, and 19.4 percent of female mortality. For the older persons, those 65 and over, this cause of death accounted for 41.3 percent of male mortality and 38.0 percent of female.

This most important of all the "specific" causes of mortality shown, for both males and females 25 to 64 years, was very definitely inversely related to education for females, and, with irregularity, also showed this relationship for males. For the least educated females mortality from this cause was 2.4 times that of the best educated females. For the lesser educated males mortality from this cause was 1.2 to 1.3 times that of the best educated. For the older males, those 65 and over, the inverse pattern tended to disappear, whereas for the older women the inverse pattern persisted. The death rate from arteriosclerotic and degenerative heart disease for the least educated older women was 1.8 times that of the best educated.

Next in importance to arteriosclerotic and degenerative heart disease in this general category of cause of death was "vascular lesions affecting the central nervous system." This cause accounted for 10.2 percent of all adult male deaths in 1960 and 14.9 percent of all deaths of adult females. Moreover, this cause of death contributed 13.2 percent of all mortality of the older men, those 65 and over, and 17.2 percent of deaths of the older women. It accounted, also, for 5.1 percent of all deaths of men 25 to 64, and 8.0 percent of the deaths of women of this age.

Vascular lesions affecting the central nervous system showed (with only one minor inconsistency for younger males) inverse patterns with education both for the younger and older males and females. Among both the younger and older males the least educated had mortality 1.3 times that of the best educated. Among the younger females the ratio of mortality of the least to the best educated was 2.0; and among the older women the ratio was 1.6.

Hypertensive disease accounted for 3.5 percent of all adult male and 5.9 percent of all adult female mortality. For older persons, those 65 and over, this cause of death contributed 4.2 percent of all deaths for males and 6.7 percent for females. For the younger persons, 25 to 64 years, this cause accounted for 2.3 percent of male and 3.6 percent of female deaths. Hypertensive disease was consistently inversely correlated with education for males 25 to 64 and for females both 25 to 64 and 65 and over. For the older males a U-shaped relationship obtained. Among the younger males mortality of the least educated was 1.8 times that of the best educated. Among the younger women the least educated had a mortality index 2.6 times that of the best educated. Among the older women mortality of the least educated was 2.4 times that of the best educated. Among the older males mortality indexes for the two intermediate education groups were about 20 percent below the indexes for the least educated and the best educated.

Rheumatic fever and chronic rheumatic heart disease accounted for only 1.0 percent of all adult male and 1.4 percent of all adult female mortality. But this cause contributed 3.7 percent of the deaths of younger women and 1.9 percent of those of younger men. It accounted for only 0.5 percent of the deaths of older men and 0.7 percent of those of older women.

This cause of death tended to be inversely related to education, with one inconsistency, both among men and among women 25 to 64. The numbers were small, however, and for persons 65 and over they were too small to report indexes. In the younger age group, the mortality of males with an elementary school education was 1.4 times that of the best educated group, but among those with the least education, less than elementary school, it was only 1.2 times that of the best educated. Females 25 to 64 showed a very similar pattern.

Finally, the category "other cardiovascular-renal diseases" also made a significant contribution to deaths for both sexes. In 1960, these residual cardiovascular causes accounted for 5.9 percent of all adult male and 6.5 percent of all adult female deaths. They were more important causes of death among the older than the younger members of each sex, accounting for 6.9 percent and 7.3 percent of the deaths of older males and females, respectively; and 4.3 percent and 4.1 percent of the deaths of the younger males and females.

The other cardiovascular-renal diseases showed a consistent inverse relationship with education for the younger males and for females of both ages. Curiously enough, the pattern was consistently positive for the older males. For both the least educated younger males and females, mortality from this residual category of cardiovascular-renal disease was 1.7 times that of the best educated. For the older females the death rate of the lesser educated was 1.4 times that of the best educated. For the older males the mortality of the least educated was 19 percent below that of the best educated.

Malignant Neoplasms

This category of causes of death includes seven subgroupings for which data could be shown, two of which, malignancies of the breast and uterus, are not applicable to males and one of which, prostatic carcinoma, is not applicable to females. For the general category, for males 25 to 64, there was an inverse relationship and for males 65 and over a positive relationship with education. For the younger women the inverse relationship obtained. However, differentials among the older women were, for the most part, limited to women with some college education, who had lower mortality than less educated women. For the less educated younger men mortality from malignant neoplasms was over 30 percent higher than that of the best educated. For the least educated younger women the death rate from this cause was 23 percent higher than that of the best educated. For the less educated older women mortality from malignancies was 12 to 16 percent above that of the best educated. In contrast with these inverse patterns, the mortality of the less educated older men was 11 percent below that of the best educated. The more specific causes of death help to explain the patterns of association of malignancies as a cause of death with education.

Males. Of the specific forms of malignant neoplasms shown those of the lung, bronchus, and trachea were the largest cause of death for males, accounting for 3.6 percent of all adult male deaths, 5.3 percent of males 25 to 64, and 2.7 percent of males 65 and over. This cause of death was inversely related with education for the younger males but showed no consistent pattern for the older. Among the least educated younger men mortality from cancer of the lung, bronchus, or trachea was almost twice (1.9 times) that of the best educated. Among the older men, unless sample variance is responsible, the irregular pattern suggests that factors other than education must account for the considerable variation shown.

Next in importance as a cancerous cause of death for males were malignancies of the intestine and rectum. This cause of death accounted for 2.3 percent of all adult male deaths, 2.2 percent of the deaths of younger males and 2.4 percent of those of older males. For the younger men, mortality from this cause of death among the least educated was 22 percent higher than among the best educated, although it should be noted that the mortality of males with intermediate education was below that of males with some college. For older males the data were unstable but there was an indication of a slight inverse relationship between this cause of death and education.

Cancer of the stomach accounted for 1.4 percent of all adult male deaths, 1.3 percent of those of the younger and 1.5 percent of those of the older males. For this cause of death the inverse pattern with education was quite pronounced. The mortality of the least educated younger males was more than twice that of the best educated, and the mortality of the less educated older males was almost twice that of the best educated.

In contrast with the inverse relationship with education shown for the other cancer sites, cancer of the prostate tended to show a positive relationship with education. The numbers were too small to show separately for males 25 to 64, but the pattern was evident for all adult males and for males 65 and over. For each of the less educated categories of males mortality from this cause of death was only about half that of the best educated males. This is a finding that definitely requires further investigation. One possible explanation may be that since the best educated males tend better to survive other causes of death they succumb to prostatic carcinoma as a degenerative cause of death which might kill off all males if they lived long enough. This hypothesis is suggested by the relatively high incidence of prostatic malignancy reported for older males in autopsies of death from other causes.

Among men the residual category "other malignant neoplasms" accounted for more cancer deaths than any of the specific sites reported. Of total adult male deaths 7.2 percent in 1960 were the result of this cause. For the younger men, those 25 to 64, 9.0 percent of all deaths were the result of this residual category and for the older men, those 65 and over, this cause of death accounted for 6.1 percent of all deaths.

Since the specific forms of malignant neoplasms show both an inverse and a positive relationship with education it should not be too surprising that this residual category of malignancies shows no consistent pattern. For the younger males an inverted U-pattern is suggested, with the highest death rate occurring among males who completed elementary school. It may be noted, however, that the two less educated groups of younger men had higher death rates than the two better educated. Among the older males there appeared to be a definite positive relationship with education, with the least educated men having a death rate 18 percent below the best educated. The two higher educated groups of older males definitely had higher death rates than the two lower educated.

Females. Of the specific forms of malignant neoplasms shown applicable to females, cancer of the breast and of the uterus, ovary, fallopian tube, and broad ligament were the major causes of death. Mammary carcinoma accounted for 3.7 percent of all adult female mortality and cancer of the uterus, etc., for 3.3 percent. Among the younger women cancer of the breast accounted for 8.3 percent of all deaths and cancer of the uterus, etc., for 7.3 percent. Among the older women cancer of the breast contributed 2.1 percent and cancer of the uterus, etc., 1.9 percent of all mortality.

The relationships between education and these major malignancy causes of female mortality are quite different. Whereas cancer of the uterus and related organs as a cause of death showed a definite and consistent inverse relationship with education for women 25 to 64, cancer of the breast showed a definite and consistent positive relationship for these younger women. Among the younger women the mortality of the least educated from malignant neoplasms of the uterus and related organs was 2.1 times that of the best educated women. In contrast, the death rate of the least educated younger women from mammary carcinoma was 22 percent below that of the best educated. The difference in these patterns of association with education appears to have a ready explanation. Obstetricians and gynecologists consulted have uniformly indicated that the positive relationship between mortality from cancer of the breast and education is undoubtedly attributable to the lesser childbearing and breast feeding of women of high socioeconomic status.

Among the older women, those 65 and over, the positive association between education and death from breast cancer persisted, although the pattern was irregular. The death rate of the least educated older women from this cause was one-third lower than that of the best educated. The inverse relationship between deaths from cancer of the uterus and related organs disappeared among the older women.

Cancer of the intestine and rectum was almost as important among women as cancer of the breast or cancer of the uterus and related organs. This cause accounted for 3.2 percent of the deaths of all adult females, 4.3 percent of the younger females and 2.9 percent of the older. Among the younger women this cause of death was inversely related with education, the mortality of the least educated being 65 percent higher than that of the best educated. Among the older women the relationship of this cause of death with education was that of an inverted U, with the highest mortality among the two intermediate education groups. All three of the less educated categories of older women, however, had considerably higher death rates from cancer of the intestine and rectum than did the best educated women.

Of the other specific forms of malignant neoplasms, those of the stomach accounted for only 1.2 percent of adult female deaths and those of the lung and related organs only 0.8 percent. Although small numbers make the data unstable it is clear that for cancer of the stomach there was an inverse relationship with education; for cancer of the lung an inverse pattern was also suggested.

Finally, for females as well as for males the residual category of "other malignant neoplasms" accounted for a relatively large proportion of deaths, 6.4 percent of those of all adult females, 10.2 percent of those of the younger females, and 5.1 percent of those of the older. As among the males this basket category of deaths from malignancies tended to lose its inverse relationship with education for women 25 to 64, although the two categories of lesser education show higher mortality than the two categories of higher education. Among the older women, in contrast with the positive association with education for older men, other malignant neoplasms showed an inverse relationship with education. The least educated older women had a death rate from these causes 12 percent above that of the best educated.

Accidents

Of the remaining causes of death, that is, causes other than malignant neoplasms and major cardiovascular-renal diseases, accidents, as has been noted, produced the most mortality for both men and women. For both sexes the death rate from "all accidents" was inversely related with education for persons 25 to 64 years of age, although the differentials are much greater for men than for women. For males this age the mortality from this cause of the least educated was more than twice (2.3 times) that of the best educated; and for females mortality of the least educated was 23 percent above that of the best educated. For older persons, those 65 and over, the inverse pattern tended to become irregular, although mortality of the three lesser educated groups of both males and females was much higher than that for the best educated groups.

Accidents, except motor vehicle, accounted for 2.8 percent of all adult male deaths and for 2.2 percent of the female. Such accidents accounted for more of the deaths of younger than of older men, 4.7 percent as compared with 1.7 percent. Among women this cause of death apparently was contrariwise, more important among the older than the younger, 2.3 as compared with 2.1 percent. Among all adult men and women accidents except motor vehicle were inversely related with education. The least educated younger men had a death rate from this cause over 2 1/2 times that of the best educated. The least educated women (all women 25 and over) had a death rate over twice that of the best educated women. There were too few cases to permit tabulation of this cause of death for the adult women subclassified by age. For the older men the pattern was irregular, but the three lesser educated groups all had mortality indexes roughly twice as high as the college educated.

Motor vehicle accidents accounted for 2.0 percent of all male and 1.0 percent of all female adult deaths. A larger proportion of the deaths for younger persons than for older persons of each sex were attributable to this cause. Among males, the proportions of deaths from this cause for the younger and older, respectively, were 4.1 and 0.7 percent; among females the corresponding percentages were 2.7 and 0.4 percent. The number of deaths to older men and women from motor vehicle accidents was too small to permit computation of education differentials. Among all adult males and those 25 to 64 there was a consistent inverse relationship with education, with the mortality of the least educated from this cause in each instance being about 1.8 times that of the best educated. Among the adult females the relationship between this cause of death and education was irregular.

Other Causes of Death

As has been indicated all other causes of death than those discussed above—cardiovascular-renal diseases, malignant neoplasms, and accidents—accounted for a relatively small proportion of deaths in 1960 for both men and women. Of the remaining causes the residual category "other causes of death" made the greatest contribution to both male and female mortality, accounting for 10.0 percent of all male and 9.4 percent of all female deaths. It should be observed that even for this residual category, however, there was a strong inverse relationship with education for the younger men and women. Among men 25 to 64 who died from this set of causes the least educated had a mortality index twice that of the best educated; among the women the death rate of the least educated was 48 percent above that of the best educated. For the older men a U-shaped pattern characterized this set of causes of death and education, with the best educated having the highest mortality. For the older women the two less educated groups had significantly higher mortality from these causes than did the two better educated.

Although the five other specific causes of death for which data are presented accounted for only a small proportion of the total deaths in 1960, 8.7 percent of the male and 7.6 percent of the female, some of these causes have the largest education differentials found in the study.

Of these five causes of death influenza and pneumonia were the most important for each sex. This cause accounted for 3.3 percent of all adult male and, also, of all adult female mortality and for each sex was a more important cause of death for the older than for the younger adults—for males 3.8 as compared with 2.4 percent, and for females 3.6 as compared with 2.3 percent. Both for all adult men and women there was a consistent inverse relationship between this cause of death and education. Among the adult men, mortality of the least educated was 1.6 times that of the best educated; and among comparable women 1.7 times. The differentials were much more pronounced among the younger men than the older men, with the mortality of the least educated being 2.6 times that of the best educated. The small numbers of deaths for the age subclassifications should be taken into account, however; and for women the numbers were too small to report results for the younger group.

Two of the remaining causes produced enough deaths to permit separate statistics by sex, namely, diabetes mellitus and cirrhosis of the liver. The former accounted for 1.4 percent of all male and 2.6 percent of all female deaths, the latter for 1.6 percent of male and 1.0 percent of female deaths. Diabetes mellitus showed no regular pattern of association with education for adult males but showed a consistent and high inverse pattern with education for adult females. Among adult females the least educated had a death rate from this cause 3.5 times that of the best educated. Cirrhosis of the liver showed no consistent pattern with education for either sex.

Finally, for the remaining two causes, tuberculosis and suicide, data can be presented, because of small numbers, only for males. Tuberculosis accounted for only 0.8 percent of adult male deaths in 1960, 1.1 percent of the younger deaths and 0.6 percent of the older. Suicide accounted for 1.6 percent of all adult male deaths, 3.3 percent of the younger and 0.7 percent of the older.

Both tuberculosis and suicide were highly associated with education as causes of death. The least educated adult males (25 and over) had a mortality index from tuberculosis almost four times (3.9) that of the best educated, and the differentials were even greater among the younger men. Similarly, mortality from suicide of the least educated adult men was almost twice that of the best educated. Both causes suffer from small numbers of deaths, and the results though clearly significant are subject to relatively high sampling variance.

Sex Differentials by Cause of Death

Differences in mortality between the sexes varied greatly by cause of death and by level of educational attainment (see Table 5.3). For all causes combined, the mortality of all adult males was 60 percent higher than that of all adult females, and the differential was much greater at the younger ages, 98 percent, than at the older ages, 43 percent. Among the younger age group, 25 to 64 years, there was relatively little variation in the sex differential, but for the older population male mortality was over twice as high as female mortality among the college educated, as compared with 1.3 to 1.5 times as high among the three less educated groups.

The pattern of sex differentials varied greatly by cause of death for the five causes reported on here.[3] Below age 65, male mortality from malignant neoplasms was only 8 percent higher than that of females, with little variation by education level. Above age 65, the differential was much greater, with male mortality exceeding female mortality by 64 percent in general, and by more than 100 percent in the best educated group.

Mortality from arteriosclerotic and degenerative heart disease showed excessively high male mortality at the younger ages—the

Table 5.3. Sex differentials in the mortality of the white population 25 years of age and over, for selected causes of death, by years of school completed and age: United States, May-August, 1960

Cause of death (ISC codes) and age	Total	Less than 8 years school	8 years school	High school 1-4 years	College 1 year or more
ALL CAUSES OF DEATH, TOTAL 25 AND OVER.....................	1.60	1.42	1.54	1.78	1.96
25-64 years...	1.98	1.74	1.95	2.15	1.89
65 & over...	1.43	1.32	1.38	1.49	2.03
2. Malignant neoplasms, incl. lymph. & hematop. tissues (140-205)...	1.36	1.39	1.39	1.28	1.35
25-64 years...	1.08	1.04	1.14	1.08	.98
65 & over...	1.64	1.61	1.58	1.65	2.02
4. Major cardiovascular-renal diseases (330-334,400-468,592-594)....	1.59	1.33	1.51	1.91	2.34
25-64 years...	2.58	1.98	2.36	3.08	3.16
65 & over...	1.34	1.21	1.32	1.43	2.02
4a. Vascular lesions affecting central nervous system (330-334)..	1.16	1.09	1.18	1.13	1.43
25-64 years...	1.33	1.09	1.41	1.35	1.72
65 & over...	1.12	1.09	1.15	1.06	1.32
4c. Arteriosclerotic & degenerative heart disease (420,422)......	1.93	1.53	1.82	2.49	3.08
25-64 years...	3.62	2.59	3.15	4.63	4.97
65 & over...	1.53	1.34	1.53	1.68	2.41
4d. Hypertensive disease, with & without heart (440-447).........	.91	.84	.79	.95	1.74
25-64 years...	1.24	1.04	1.03	1.52	1.49
65 & over...	.85	.81	.73	.79	1.91

Source: Population Research Center, University of Chicago, 1960 Matched Records Study. Sex differentials defined as ratio of mortality index for males to mortality index for females; causes selected have at least 350 matched Stage II decedents and 10 unmatched NCHS Survey decedents of each sex. (See Appendix A for definition of mortality index.)

mortality index for males 25 to 64 was over 3.5 times that for females of the same age—and this differential was much larger (5.0) in the best educated than in the least educated group (2.6). At the older ages, male mortality was 1.5 times that of females, with a much larger differential (2.4) for the best educated.

Hypertensive disease is the only cause reported here for which males had lower mortality than females, and this was true only for older males with less than a college education. Among the college educated, male mortality from this cause was 1.5 times as high as female mortality in the younger ages, and almost twice as high in the older ages.

Patterns of Mortality by Cause

For 15 of the 18 causes of death reported for males, and 14 of the 17 reported for females, there was an inverse relationship with education. Among men the inverse relationship for 4 of the 15 causes did not hold for all adult men, but only for younger men. Among the women this was true of 1 of the 14 causes of death inversely associated with education.

Especially significant is the fact that the inverse pattern obtained for 8 causes of death that accounted for 83 percent of all the deaths of adult males and females. These causes, with the percentages of all deaths resulting therefrom in 1960, are shown below:

Cause of Death	Males	Females
Arteriosclerotic & degenerative heart disease	39.8	33.2
Vascular lesions affecting central nervous system	10.2	14.9
"Other malignant neoplasms"	7.2	6.4
"Other cardiovascular diseases"	5.9	6.5
Hypertensive disease	3.5	5.9
Influenza and pneumonia	3.3	3.3
Malignant neoplasms of the lung, etc.	3.6	–
Malignant neoplasms of the uterus, etc.	–	3.3
"Other causes" (cause 9 in Table 5.2)	10.0	9.4
SUM	83.5	82.9

For two of the eight causes listed above for men—vascular lesions and influenza and pneumonia—the inverse pattern held for both younger (25-64) and older (65 and over) men; for the other causes the inverse relationship was limited to the younger males and did not hold for the older. For females all except one of the causes listed—malignant neoplasms of the uterus—showed an inverse relationship with education at the older as well as at the younger ages. In fact, the differences between the male and female patterns for the arteriosclerotic and "other cardiovascular" causes were responsible, to a great extent, for the larger education differentials among females than males for all causes of death combined. These two causes alone accounted for 46 and 40 percent, respectively, of the adult male and female deaths, and for each cause the difference between the pattern of education differentials for men and women was striking.

Also a significant finding was the positive relationship between education and cause of death for prostatic carcinoma for males and mammary carcinoma for females. As has been indicated above, there seems to be a ready explanation for the latter but a more obscure one for the former which merits research attention.

Socioeconomic Differentials, Chicago, 1950

Cause-of-death data were also available for the white population by socioeconomic status in Chicago in 1950, based on the areal indexes of class described in Chapter 4. In Table 5.4 these findings are compared with the education differentials for the United States in

1960 presented above. For deaths from all causes combined there was a high inverse relationship by socioeconomic status, as has already been observed (in Chapter 4) for each sex and both age groups in the city of Chicago in 1950. The same pattern was evident for the nation in 1960 except for males 65 and over, as noted in Chapter 2.

A similar inverse pattern held, in the main, for white persons 25 to 64 of each sex, as shown both in the city and in the nation for the following causes of death: tuberculosis; malignant neoplasms; diabetes mellitus; major cardiovascular-renal diseases; vascular lesions affecting the central nervous system; hypertensive disease, with and without heart disease; influenza and pneumonia, except pneumonia of newborn; and all accidents. The inverse relationship between socioeconomic status and mortality also held in both the city and the nation for females 25 to 64 who died from arteriosclerotic and degenerative heart disease. Among persons 25 to 64 years of age this inverse pattern did not hold only for males who died of arteriosclerotic and degenerative heart disease. In the city, the death rate for this cause in the lowest socioeconomic class was well above that of the other four classes, which did not show much variation; in the nation, men with the highest education had the lowest incidence of mortality from this cause, but the lower education groups did not show a gradient pattern.

As was to be expected, persons 65 and over of each sex experienced less variation in mortality by cause of death than their younger counterparts and also exhibited greater irregularity in pattern. Some persons in this group, however, did show an inverse gradient between class and mortality for some causes, especially the older females who died from major cardiovascular-renal diseases, especially hypertensive disease.

For each cause, except vascular lesions affecting the central nervous system, the variation in mortality by socioeconomic status was greater in the city than in the nation. But the fact that the city was divided into five socioeconomic groups whereas the nation was divided into only four was undoubtedly a factor in this pattern. The greatest relative differentials in mortality by socioeconomic status occurred in deaths from tuberculosis. In the city the death rate from tuberculosis was for males 25 to 64 almost three times as high in the lowest economic class as its average for the city (index 2.84); and in the nation almost twice as high (index 1.84). The two causes of death with the next greatest socioeconomic class differences for the

Table 5.4. Comparison of socioeconomic differentials in mortality in Chicago, 1950, with education differentials in mortality in the United States, May-August, 1960, for the white population 25 years and over, by sex and age, for selected causes of death

Cause of death (ISC codes), sex and age	Chicago--1950 mortality by socioeconomic group[a]					U.S.--1960 mortality by years of school completed[b]				Number of deaths	
	I (low)	II	III	IV	V (high)	Less than 8 years	8 years	High school 1-4 years	College 1 year or more	Chicago 1950	1960 U.S. matched Stage II (unweighted)
ALL CAUSES											
White males 25 & over.....	1.36	1.07	.89	.86	.79	1.03	1.01	1.00	.89	18,099	27,869
25-64 years.............	1.51	1.09	.87	.82	.70	1.15	1.06	.97	.77	9,333	18,194
65 & over...............	1.23	1.04	.92	.90	.89	1.01	1.00	.98	1.00	8,766	9,675
White females 25 & over...	1.25	1.09	.97	.91	.82	1.16	1.05	.90	.73	13,247	17,810
25-64 years.............	1.44	1.13	.93	.84	.73	1.30	1.08	.89	.81	5,292	10,089
65 & over...............	1.13	1.05	1.00	.95	.88	1.09	1.03	.94	.70	7,955	7,721
1. Tuberculosis, all forms (001-019)											
White males 25 & over.....	2.66	1.06	.53	.43	.39	1.53#	1.17#	.64#	.39#	623	231
25-64 years.............	2.84	1.04	.52	.45	.29	1.84#	1.19#	.80#	.21#	491	172
2. Malignant neoplasms, incl. lymph. & hematop. tissues (140-205)											
White males 25 & over.....	1.15	1.14	.94	.90	.82	1.04	1.04	.95	.92	3,104	5,080
25-64 years.............	1.27	1.19	.91	.84	.75	1.09	1.12	.94	.83	1,590	3,377
65 & over...............	1.04	1.09	.97	.98	.89	.98	.97	1.04	1.10	1,514	1,703
White females 25 & over...	1.07	.97	1.02	.95	.98	1.01	1.01	1.01	.93	2,600	4,664
25-64 years.............	1.15	1.02	.99	.91	.97	1.13	1.05	.94	.92	1,499	3,377
65 & over...............	.98	.92	1.05	1.01	1.00	1.00	1.01	1.04	.89	1,101	1,287
3. Diabetes mellitus (260)											
White females 25 & over...	1.33	1.08	1.02	.80	.78	1.48	.96	.77	.42	428	492
4. Major cardiovascular-renal diseases (330-334,400-468,592-594)											
White males 25 & over.....	1.30	1.04	.90	.90	.85	.99	1.00	1.06	.93	10,941	15,976
25-64 years.............	1.37	1.06	.89	.89	.79	1.06	1.03	1.03	.80	5,150	9,732
65 & over...............	1.25	1.02	.91	.90	.91	1.00	1.01	.99	.98	5,791	6,244
White females 25 & over...	1.24	1.11	.97	.92	.80	1.18	1.06	.88	.63	8,353	9,248
25-64 years.............	1.53	1.16	.91	.86	.62	1.38	1.12	.86	.66	2,535	4,055
65 & over...............	1.12	-1.08	.99	.94	.88	1.12	1.02	.93	.65	5,818	5,193
4a. Vascular lesions affecting central nervous system (330-334)											
White males 25 & over.....	1.09	1.04	.95	.96	.99	1.07	1.01	.92	.86	1,302	2,172
25-64 years.............	1.00	1.21	.98	.89	.87	1.17	1.02	.90	.92	508	1,016
65 & over...............	1.14	.93	.92	1.00	1.08	1.06	1.01	.93	.83	794	1,156
White females 25 & over...	.97	1.09	1.03	.95	.91	1.14	.99	.95	.70	1,454	2,004
25-64 years.............	1.07	1.21	1.04	.90	.70	1.44	.97	.89	.71	433	825
65 & over...............	.93	1.04	1.02	.98	1.00	1.09	.99	.98	.71	1,021	1,179
4c. Arteriosclerotic & degenerative heart disease (420,422)[c]											
White males 25 & over.....	1.19	1.01	.91	.95	1.00	.95	1.01	1.10	.93	5,040	11,176
25-64 years.............	1.20	.97	.93	.97	.98	1.01	1.01	1.07	.81	2,547	7,129
65 & over...............	1.18	1.05	.88	.93	1.02	.99	1.02	1.01	.98	2,493	4,047
White females 25 & over...	1.22	1.09	.96	.89	.89	1.21	1.07	.86	.59	2,954	5,041
25-64 years.............	1.50	1.22	.94	.78	.63	1.41	1.16	.84	.59	799	2,119
65 & over...............	1.12	1.05	.97	.93	.98	1.13	1.03	.92	.62	2,155	2,922
4d. Hypertensive disease, with & without heart (440-447)											
White males 25 & over.....	1.16	1.16	.96	.84	.80	1.14	.91	.89	.93	1,045	817
25-64 years.............	1.21	1.24	.90	.89	.71	1.27	1.05	.92	.71	433	422
65 & over...............	1.13	1.11	1.00	.80	.88	1.11	.87	.88	1.09	612	395
White females 25 & over...	1.30	1.11	.96	.96	.70	1.24	1.06	.85	.49	1,208	912
25-64 years.............	1.68	1.16	.82	.96	.57	1.52	1.26	.75	.59	404	370
65 & over...............	1.11	1.09	1.03	.96	.76	1.16	1.00	.95	.48	804	542
5. Influenza & pneumonia, except pneumonia of new born (480-493)											
White males 25 & over.....	1.99	1.21	.76	.57	.30	1.20	.98	.81	.75	382	450
7. All accidents (800-962)											
White males 25 & over.....	1.80	1.14	.81	.67	.48	1.13	1.06	1.01	.66	685	1,744
25-64 years.............	1.89	1.15	.80	.66	.44	1.45	1.16	.92	.64	481	1,497

Source: Population Research Center, University of Chicago, 1960 Matched Record Study for U.S. (see Appendix A) and 1950 analysis based on census tract data of socioeconomic status (see Chapter 4). Comparison limited to causes of death for which both Chicago and U.S. data were tabulated and for which there were at least 150 U.S. deaths matched with 1960 Stage II Census records and 350 Chicago deaths.

\# Does not meet reliability requirement specified in Table 5.2.

[a] Ratios of actual to expected deaths in which expected deaths were computed by applying age-specific death rates for all white males (or females) in Chicago in 1950 to the age composition of the 1950 population in each socioeconomic group. Therefore, the ratio for the white population of each sex-age group was 1.00.

[b] Education differentials are "relatives" in which the mortality index for each education subgroup is expressed as a ratio to the index for the sex-color-age group to which it belongs; therefore, the "relative" for the white population of each sex-age group is 1.00. See Appendix A for definition of the mortality index used.

[c] Chicago 1950 data refer to arteriosclerotic heart disease only (ISC Code 420) but this cause was 95.3 percent of the total for Codes 420 and 422 in the U.S. in 1960.

city were influenza and pneumonia (index of 1.99 for males 25 and over) and all accidents (index of 1.89 for males 25-64). The two causes of death in the nation with the next greatest socioeconomic differences in mortality were hypertensive disease for females 25-64 (index 1.52) and vascular lesions affecting the central nervous system, for females 25 to 64 (index 1.44).

Although the indexes of socioeconomic status are quite different, it is clear cut that large differentials are to be found in mortality by cause of death in Chicago as in the nation and that, by and large, the patterns of differences are similar.

6 / DIFFERENTIAL MORTALITY BY RACE, NATIVITY, COUNTRY OF ORIGIN, MARITAL STATUS, AND PARITY

This chapter summarizes mortality differentials by a number of "social" characteristics which, though related to socioeconomic status, are not generally considered a component of socioeconomic status as such. Death statistics by race, country of birth, and marital status are readily available because these items are reported on the legal death records. However, death rates calculated by relating deaths (tabulated by characteristics as reported on death certificates) to a base population (tabulated by characteristics as reported on census records) have been viewed with suspicion because of potential errors resulting from discrepancies in the reporting of these items on death certificates and census schedules.

The analyses of mortality by race, country of origin, and marital status in this chapter utilize the tabulations of deaths compiled by the National Center for Health Statistics for the three-year period 1959-61, supplemented by cross classifications (compiled from the 1960 Matched Records Study) which compare responses to these questions on 1960 death certificates and 1960 census schedules. The latter permits correction of the death rates for discrepancies in reporting on the two records and, incidentally, also provides some indication of the extent of error involved in using uncorrected rates.

The mortality ratios for ever-married women by parity (number of children ever borne) were derived from the 1960 Matched Records Study, as explained in Appendix A.

Nonwhite-White Differentials

Three sets of death rates by color, sex, and age were calculated for the United States, 1959-61, and the results are summarized in Table 6.1. Rate no. 1, the uncorrected rate reported in the first and fourth columns of the table, was calculated from uncorrected deaths for 1959-61 and population statistics for 1960, as compiled from the death certificates and 1960 census records by the National Center for Health Statistics and the Bureau of the Census, respectively. Rate no. 2 differs from rate no. 1 in that corrected deaths (classified by estimated census age) provided the numerators of the rates. The

Table 6.1. Nonwhite-white differentials in age-specific death rates, by sex: United States, 1959-61

Sex and age	White			Nonwhite			Percent by which nonwhite rate exceeds white rate		
	Uncorrected death rate per 100,000 pop.	Percent difference from #1 if:		Uncorrected death rate per 100,000 pop.	Percent difference from #1 if:		Uncorrected rate	Corrected for age reporting	Corrected for undercount
		Deaths corrected for age reporting	Pop. corrected for net undercount		Deaths corrected for age reporting	Pop. corrected for net undercount			
	#1	#2	#3	#1	#2	#3	#1	#2	#3
Males, all ages[a]	10.982	0.0 [b]	-2.8	11.503	0.3 [b]	-10.9	5	5 [b]	-4
Under five years	6.269	...	-2.0	12.366	...	-7.7	97	...	86
5-9 years	.537	-2.6	-2.4	.723	-1.5	-5.5	35	36	30
10-14 years	.516	-0.4	-2.5	.788	7.1	-5.3	53	64	48
15-19 years	1.252	-3.6	-3.8	1.658	-2.1	-12.5	32	35	21
20-24 years	1.669	6.7	-4.3	2.749	5.8	-17.5	65	63	42
25-29 years	1.521	4.4	-4.2	3.430	10.8	-19.7	126	139	89
30-34 years	1.732	2.7	-3.1	4.286	2.6	-18.0	147	147	109
35-39 years	2.534	7.5	-2.5	5.992	9.8	-14.5	136	141	107
40-44 years	4.170	5.8	-1.9	8.765	1.4	-12.8	110	101	87
45-49 years	7.093	1.9	-1.6	12.415	-5.5	-11.5	75	62	57
50-54 years	11.833	0.4	-3.6	19.162	-7.7	-17.8	62	49	38
55-59 years	17.846	0.7	-0.4	25.005	-9.5	-5.9	40	26	32
60-64 years	27.514	1.4	-3.0	40.538	-15.2	-9.7	47	23	37
65-69 years	40.507	0.1	-3.8	51.037	-8.1	-1.8	26	16	29
70-74 years	59.092	-2.2	-3.8	64.932	8.7	-1.8	10	22	12
75-79 years	86.987	0.5	-3.8	76.280	15.7	-1.8	-12	1	-10
80-84 years	135.443	-2.2	-3.8	110.174	21.7	-1.8	-19	1	-17
85 years & over	217.500	-2.8	-3.8	152.387	19.4	-1.8	-30	-14	-28
Females, all ages[a]	8.007	-0.1 [b]	-1.6	8.715	0.8 [b]	-8.1	9	10 [b]	2
Under 5 years	4.725	... [b]	-1.2	9.831	... [b]	-6.4	108	... [b]	97
5-9 years	.383	2.9	-1.6	.610	2.5	-4.9	59	59	54
10-14 years	.308	5.8	-1.3	.442	6.8	-4.1	44	45	39
15-19 years	.503	2.0	-2.6	.804	9.3	-10.1	60	71	48
20-24 years	.604	7.8	-2.3	1.358	16.6	-9.6	125	143	108
25-29 years	.716	20.8	-1.4	2.102	0.0	-8.7	194	143	172
30-34 years	.971	15.4	-0.6	3.078	13.4	-5.9	217	211	200
35-39 years	1.475	5.0	0.1	4.481	-3.5	-6.2	204	179	184
40-44 years	2.379	9.3	0.2	6.608	-1.4	-6.4	178	151	160
45-49 years	3.685	0.9	-0.7	9.194	-4.8	-8.4	149	125	130
50-54 years	5.603	0.9	-4.2	14.195	-21.0	-18.2	153	98	116
55-59 years	8.297	1.3	-1.6	19.518	-16.0	-10.0	135	95	115
60-64 years	13.622	2.6	-4.2	30.195	-22.1	-14.1	122	68	99
65-69 years	21.549	-1.7	-2.1	34.744	-1.2	-12.2	61	62	44
70-74 years	35.832	4.6	-2.1	47.425	19.0	-12.2	32	51	19
75-79 years	60.842	0.3	-2.1	58.792	16.1	-12.2	-3	12	-13
80-84 years	106.543	-8.0	-2.1	84.775	18.9	-12.2	-20	3	-29
85 years & over	194.777	-2.1	-2.1	128.712	39.4	-12.2	-34	-6	-41

Source: Rate #1 based on tabulations of 1959-61 deaths by characteristics reported on death certificates. Rate #2 based on deaths corrected for discrepancies in reporting of age on death certificates and census records for all matched Stage II deaths in the 1960 Matched Records Study (see text for details of correction procedure). Rate #3 based on uncorrected deaths and estimates of 1960 population corrected for net census undercounts by age, sex and color (Siegel, 1968). Population base for rates 1 and 2 was taken from 100-percent enumeration, 1960 Census of Population.

[a] Refers to general death rate (not standardized for age).

[b] Correction not available for this age group because tabulation comparing age responses on death certificates and census records excluded all persons under 1 year of age.

estimates of corrected deaths were prepared by the National Center for Health Statistics using cross classifications of census age by death certificate age for matched Stage II deaths in the 1960 Matched Records Study.[1] The net corrections made in rate no. 2 are shown for each five-year age interval in the second and fifth columns of Table 6.1. Rate no. 3 was calculated from uncorrected deaths and population statistics corrected for net census undercounts of the 1960 population by age, sex, and color as estimated by Siegel

(1968). The net corrections for net census undercount (including age misstatement and census underenumeration) in each five-year age interval are shown in the third and sixth columns of Table 6.1.

It should be noted at the outset that neither correction provides an estimate of true rates. However, together they provide useful information on the quality of data used to calculate death rates, as well as some indication of the likely range of error in the rates. The correction for age discrepancies (no. 2) ignores known errors resulting from census underenumeration, and the corrections for net census undercount (no. 3) are known to be deficient at the older ages and, in some ages, they also appear to be inconsistent with the documented age discrepancies. Rate no. 2 probably has reasonable corrections for discrepancies in age reporting on the two records. It is designed to measure the incidence of mortality by age as age is reported in the census record. In this rate both deaths and population are classified by census age, thus removing one source of error from uncorrected death rates, namely, differences in the reporting of age on the two records.[2] No correction is made for sex and color, which were reported virtually identically on both records. Rate no. 2 would be accurate if it could be assumed that census age was correctly reported, that there was no underenumeration in the census and no underregistration of deaths, and that the adjustments made to convert death certificate age to census age were correct.

Rate no. 3, on the other hand, relates deaths tabulated by death certificate age to population counts corrected for estimated net census undercounts by age, sex, and color. Siegel's estimates of net census undercounts are considered reasonably reliable at the younger ages but increasingly subject to error as age increases. Moreover, because the undercounts include both underenumeration and age misstatement—and the two cannot be separated with the methods used by Siegel—the corrections applied to deaths in rate no. 2 cannot be used in conjunction with the correction applied to the population base in rate no. 3. Rate no. 3 would be accurate if it could be assumed that: (1) the estimated census undercounts were accurate and the corrected population derived from them was accurately classified by age, sex, and color; and (2) death registration was complete and responses on the death certificates represented correct age, sex, and color of decedents.

The percentage differences between each set of corrected rates and the uncorrected death rates suggest that with few exceptions—notably females 25-34 years of age—age-specific death rates for white males and females are reasonably accurate. However, death rates for nonwhites are clearly subject to substantial error. The estimated net census undercounts for nonwhites results in *decreases* of 10 to 20 percent in corrected death rates (no. 3) for a substantial number of age groups, and discrepancies in the reporting of age on death and census records result in *increases* of 16 to 40 percent in corrected death rates (no. 2) above age 75. The poor quality of the nonwhite data, in combination with the smaller though not always negligible errors in white data, made it very difficult to measure accurately nonwhite-white differentials in death rates, as is evident in the percentage differences reported in the last three columns of Table 6.1. In evaluating these proportionate differences between nonwhite and white rates it should be remembered that the very large relative differentials at the younger ages—especially for males 20-44—are based on very small absolute differences in age-specific death rates; that is, the number of deaths involved in the large percentage differences between nonwhite and white rates at the younger ages is very small indeed, compared to the numbers involved in the much smaller proportionate differences at the older ages, when death rates are high and absolute differences between nonwhite and white rates much larger (and, incidentally, both positive and negative because the mortality curves for whites and nonwhites apparently "cross" at some point above age 70).

The evidence on the "crossing" of the white and nonwhite mortality is especially difficult to evaluate. In the uncorrected rates both the male and the female curves cross at age 75; that is, nonwhite death rates are higher than white death rates below age 75 but lower than white rates after age 75. When corrected for age reporting, the nonwhite and white curves do not cross until the last open-ended age interval, 85 and over, and this might be due to older age of whites than nonwhites, on the average, in this age interval. When corrected for net census undercounts, however, the male curves for nonwhites and whites cross at age 75 in a similar fashion to the uncorrected rate, and the female curves cross at age 75 even more noticeably than in the uncorrected rate. However, the weakness of the census undercounts at the older ages has already been noted, and it is possible that the age patterns above age 65 are more adequately reflected by rate no. 2 than by rate no. 3. In this connection it should be noted that estimates of net census undercount were not available by age above age 65 (they were assumed to be constant above age 65 in corrected rate no. 3), and also that the comparisons of age response on death certificates and matched census records showed a very high overreporting of age for nonwhites on the census records (if it is assumed that the death certificate age is more accurate than the census age).

Nonwhite-white differentials in age-adjusted death rates are summarized in Table 6.2, in terms of the percentage by which the rate for nonwhites exceeds the rate for whites.

Table 6.2. Nonwhite-white differentials in age-adjusted death rates, by sex and age: United States, 1959-61

Sex and rate	All ages	Under 35	35-64 years	65 & over
Males				
Rate #1 (uncorrected).....................	25	89	59	-4
Rate #2 (corrected for age reporting).....	27	92	45	6
Rate #3 (corrected for undercount)........	20	73	45	-2
Females				
Rate #1 (uncorrected).....................	48	112	141	3
Rate #2 (corrected for age reporting).....	50	111	99	21
Rate #3 (corrected for undercount)........	34	100	119	-8

Source: Same as Table 6.1. Death rates standardized by the direct method, using 10-year age intervals and the 1960 total United States population as standard.

The correction for discrepancies in age reporting (rate no. 2) has relatively little effect on the nonwhite-white differential for all ages combined, but correction for net census undercounts reduces the differential substantially. For example, the uncorrected rate for nonwhite males, all ages, was 25 percent higher than the same rate for white males, as compared with a difference of 20 percent when the index was corrected for net census undercounts. Among females, the color differential was reduced from an uncorrected rate that was 48 percent higher for nonwhites than for whites, to a 34 percent difference after correction for net census undercounts. The greater mortality of nonwhites was much higher at the younger ages than at the older ages, and the crossing of the age-specific mortality curves at age 75 in rate no. 3 resulted in lower nonwhite than white mortality in the age-adjusted indexes for males and females 65 and over when corrected for net census undercounts. When corrected for age discrepancies only (no. 2), the color differential was the reverse, the rate for nonwhite males 65 and over being 6 percent higher than the rate for white males, and the rate for nonwhite females 65 and over 21 percent higher than the comparable rate for white females.

Although it seems clear that the nonwhite-white differentials in mortality covering all ages are more accurately measured by rate no. 3 than by rate no. 2 or 1—simply because corrections for net census undercounts are much greater for nonwhites than for whites—the choice between the two corrections is not so clear for the three broad age groups. Age misclassification can play an important role in this choice, and little is known about "true age" despite the considerable amount of evidence available on discrepancies in the reporting of age on different records for the same person. More specifically, it is difficult to judge the relative accuracy of age-adjusted rates no. 2 and no. 3 for ages 65 and over, and to determine if and when the age-specific mortality curves for nonwhites and whites "cross."

This leads to the conclusion that the nonwhite-white differential based on rate no. 3, all ages, gives the "better" estimate of average greater mortality among nonwhite males and females, without much assurance that the same rate also provides better estimates of age-specific differences between nonwhite and white mortality. Comparison of the corrections made in age-specific death rates no. 2 and no. 3 reveals inconsistencies[3] that are difficult to reconcile but which do suggest that for some ages rate no. 2 (corrected for age reporting) may be "better" than rate no. 3.

It is to be emphasized, however, that with the best correction possible, the age-adjusted death rate (over all ages combined) of nonwhite males was 20 percent greater than white, and that of nonwhite females 34 percent greater than white.

Differentials by Race

Nonwhites in the United States, although predominantly Negro, include a number of other racial groups that are identified in official tabulations of vital statistics and census enumerations. Because of the small numbers of deaths each year among the so-called minor nonwhite races and the questionable accuracy and comparability of age and race reporting on death certificates and census records, deaths for the three-year period 1959-61 were used to calculate age-adjusted mortality indexes by race, with corrections for discrepancies in the reporting of race on death certificates and census

Table 6.3. Mortality indexes by race and sex: United States, 1959-61

Sex and race	Uncorrected mortality indexes[a]				Corrected mortality index (indirect method)[b] 5 years & over	Uncorrected death rate children under 5	Infant mortality rate (1960)[c]
	Direct standardization			Indirect stand., 5 years & over			
	35-64 years	65 years & over	5 years & over				
Males.......	1.3170	1.1917	1.2368	1.2416	1.2416	.007064	.029332
White...........	1.2480	1.1964	1.2126	1.2149	1.2157	.006216	.026005
Nonwhite........	1.9688	1.1299	1.4452	1.5244	1.5155	.012130	.047880
Negro..........	2.0663	1.1442	1.4869	1.5704	1.5554	.012376	.049123
Other..........	1.1003	.9605	1.0456	1.0526	1.1059	.009303	.034383
Indian[d]......	1.5941	.9302	1.2704	1.3949	1.5097	.013834	.051750
Japanese.....	.6452e	.8558e	.7859	.7871	.8066	.004427e	.017195e
Chinese......	--e	--e	1.2673	1.2820	1.3424	--e	--e
Females.....	.7009	.8433	.7913	.7957	.7957	.005464	.022586
White...........	.6193	.8415	.7600	.7683	.7681	.004713	.019638
Nonwhite........	1.4650	.8483	1.0666	1.1075	1.1098	.009795	.038456
Negro..........	1.5202	.8575	1.0916	1.1314	1.1324	.009986	.039434
Other..........	.7117	.6747	.7015	.7056	.7304	.007530	.027592
Indian[d]......	1.0449	.7762	.9148	.9721	1.0498	.011530	.041407
Japanese.....	.4341e	.5837e	.5305	.5067	.5192	.003339e	.013325e
Chinese......	--e	--e	.6167	.5914	.6968	--e	--
Both sexes..	1.0000	1.0000	1.0000	1.0000	1.0000	.006278	.026040
White...........	.9246	1.0005	.9717	.9722	.9725	.005480	.022906
Nonwhite........	1.7084	.9809	1.2471	1.3052	1.3022	.010965	.043211
Negro..........	1.7795	.9899	1.2770	1.3358	1.3294	.011183	.044318
Other..........	.9423	.8465	.9032	.9095	.9511	.008431	.031053
Indian[d]......	1.3140	.8551	1.0920	1.1847	1.2810	.012689	.046557
Japanese.....	.5376e	.7402e	.6701	.6633	.6797	.003904e	.015317e
Chinese......	--e	--e	1.1003	1.0764	1.1502	--e	--e

[a] Each directly standardized index is equal to the ratio of the uncorrected age-adjusted death rate (standardized by the direct method, 1960 total U.S. as standard) for the sex-race subgroup to the same rate for the total U.S. population, 1959-61. The indirectly standardized index is the ratio of actual deaths (reported deaths, 1959-61) to expected deaths for the sex-race subgroup, in which expected deaths were computed by applying uncorrected age-specific death rates for the total U.S., 1959-61, to the 1960 age composition of the sex-race subgroup; it is equivalent to the ratio of the uncorrected age-adjusted death rate (computed by the indirect method, with 1959-61 total U.S. as standard) for the sex-race subgroup, 1959-61, to the same rate for the total U.S. population, 1959-61. Population base for rates taken from tabulations based on 25-percent sample, 1960 Census. All indexes standardized using 8 age groups over age 5: 5-14, 15-24, 25-34, ..., 75 & over.

[b] Actual deaths for numerators of this indirectly standardized index are deaths classified by "estimated census race"; these estimates were derived by correcting race of decedents reported on death certificates for discrepancies between the reporting of race on death certificates and census records (see text for details of estimation procedure). Expected deaths for denominators are same as for uncorrected index, indirect method.

[c] Infant deaths (under 1 year), divided by live births. Based on vital statistics data for one year only, 1960.

[d] Indexes for Indians adjusted for an estimated excess count of 14,000 Indians 55 to 59 years old in the 25 percent sample statistics in the 1960 Census (see Donald S. Akers and Elizabeth A. Larmon, "Indians and Smudges on the Census Schedule," unpublished). This excess was assumed to be equally distributed between males and females.

[e] Index or rate not calculated because numbers judged too small for reasonable estimates.

records.[4] No corrections have been made for net census undercounts because estimates of undercounts were available only for whites and nonwhites, as mentioned earlier. For the United States as a whole, the nonwhite undercounts could be applied to Negroes. This adjustment has not been made by race for two reasons: (1) the net effect of the correction would be the same for Negroes as for nonwhites, and can be inferred from Tables 6.1 and 6.2 and the previous analysis for nonwhites; and (2) the correction could not be made for the other racial groups.

Mortality indexes for racial groups are presented in Table 6.3. The corrected indexes were standardized by the indirect method because data were not available to make corrections for race reporting separately for each age group. The indirectly standardized indexes are limited to persons 5 and over because the race comparison of response tabulation used to correct the indexes (see note 4)

Table 6.4. Race differentials in mortality, by sex: United States, 1959-61

Sex and race	Uncorrected mortality indexes[a]				Corrected mortality index (indirect method)[b] 5 years & over	Uncorrected death rate children under 5	Infant mortality rate (1960)[c]
	Direct standardization			Indirect stand., 5 years & over			
	35-64 years	65 years & over	5 years & over				
Males							
White...........	0	0	0	0	0	0	0
Nonwhite........	58	-6	19	25	25	95	84
Negro..........	66	-4	23	29	28	99	89
Other..........	-12	-20	-14	-13	-9	50	32
Indian[d]......	28	-22	5	15	24	123	99
Japanese.....	-48[e]	-28[e]	-35	-35	-34	-29[e]	-34[e]
Chinese......	--	--	5	6	10	--	--
Females							
White...........	0	0	0	0	0	0	0
Nonwhite........	137	1	40	44	44	108	96
Negro..........	145	2	44	47	47	112	101
Other..........	15	-20	-8	-8	-5	60	41
Indian[d]......	69	-8	20	27	37	145	111
Japanese.....	-30[e]	-31[e]	-30	-34	-32	-29[e]	-32[e]
Chinese......	--	--	-19	-23	-9	--	--
Both sexes							
White...........	0	0	0	0	0	0	0
Nonwhite........	85	-2	28	34	34	100	89
Negro..........	92	-1	31	37	37	104	93
Other..........	2	-15	-7	-6	-2	54	36
Indian[d]......	42	-15	12	22	32	132	103
Japanese.....	-42[e]	-26[e]	-31	-32	-30	-29[e]	-33[e]
Chinese......	--	--	13	11	18	--	--

Source: Table 6.3. Race differentials indicate the percent by which the mortality index or rate for each race exceeds (or, if negative, is less than) the same index or rate for whites.

Notes a to e: Same as Table 6.3.

excluded infants under 1. For this reason, death rates for children under 5 and infant mortality rates are reported separately in the last two columns of Table 6.3. The size and pattern of the race differentials are summarized in Table 6.4, in terms of the percent difference between the mortality index for each race and the index for whites.

Perhaps the most striking finding is the very low mortality of the Japanese, which has also been documented in other studies (Gordon, 1957 and 1967; Hechter and Borhani, 1965). The corrected indexes for Japanese males and females 5 and over were about one-third lower than the corresponding indexes for white males and females, respectively, and only one-half as large as the corrected indexes for Negro males and females. The Japanese also had infant and child mortality rates one-third below the white rates, and two-thirds below the Negro.

Negroes had the highest mortality of any of the racial groups, with corrected indexes 28 and 47 percent above the white indexes for males and females, respectively. The Negro-white differentials are very similar to the "uncorrected" nonwhite-white differentials in Table 6.2, which is to be expected, since they comprised 92 percent of the nonwhites in 1960. Indians had the next highest mortality, with corrected indexes 24 and 37 percent higher than the white indexes for males and females 5 and over, respectively. Chinese males had a corrected mortality index about 10 percent higher than the same index for white males, but the index for Chinese females was 9 percent below that for white females.

The correction for discrepancies in the reporting of race on death certificates and census records has very little effect on the mortality indexes for whites, all nonwhites, Negroes, and Japanese (see Table 6.3). The comparison of race responses for matched decedents showed very few discrepancies for these race categories. The corrections did significantly change the indexes for Indians and Chinese, however.

Sex differentials in mortality for the several racial groups are presented in Table 6.5. The Chinese have exceptionally high differences between male and female mortality, but this may be due, in part at least, to the high sex ratio among the Chinese, indicating a large group of nonfamily males who may be subject to higher mortality than the male family members, by reason either of lower socioeconomic status or of some other factor, perhaps nonfamily status itself, which would be consistent with the findings on marital

Table 6.5. Sex differentials in mortality, by race: United States, 1959-61

Race	Uncorrected mortality indexes[a]				Corrected mortality index (indirect method)[b] 5 years & over	Uncorrected death rate children under 5	Infant mortality rate (1960)[c]
	Direct standardization		Indirect stand., 5 years & over				
	35-64 years	65 years & over	5 years & over				
All races......	88	41	56	56	56	29	30
White...........	102	42	60	58	58	32	32
Nonwhite........	34	33	35	38	37	24	25
Negro..........	36	33	36	39	37	24	25
Other..........	55	42	49	49	51	24	25
Indian[d]......	53	20	39	43	44	20	25
Japanese.....	49[e]	47[e]	48	55	55	33[e]	29[e]
Chinese......	--	--	105	117	93	--	--

Source: Table 6.3. Sex differential indicates the percent by which the mortality index or rate for males exceeds the same index or rate for females.

Notes a to e: Same as Table 6.3.

status differentials in mortality reported later in this chapter. In any case, the Chinese are the only racial group reported in Table 6.5 which has an abnormal sex ratio.

Data are not available to ascertain directly the extent to which racial differences in mortality may be due to social and economic differences. However, the following information on median family income indicates that socioeconomic status may account for some of the race differentials observed in mortality:

Race	Median Family Income, 1959
Indian	$2,728
Negro	3,047
White	5,893
Chinese	6,207
Japanese	6,842

Family income is clearly highest among the Japanese, and next highest among the Chinese. The corrected mortality indexes rank in inverse order to the median family income ranking of the racial groups, except for the Indians, whose exceptionally low income is no doubt related to the "reservation" residence of many Indians. In other words, the race differentials, in general, are consistent with the inverse relationship between mortality and socioeconomic status as measured by average family income (see Chapter 2).

The implications of race differentials in mortality have also been summarized in terms of life expectancies computed from the uncorrected age-specific death rates for whites, all nonwhites, Negroes, and Japanese, the racial groups which needed no correction for discrepancies in race reporting. Expectation of life at birth, at age 25 and at age 55 are shown for these groups in Table 6.6.[5]

The life expectancy at birth of Japanese females was over 80 years and that of Japanese males over 74 years, or about 6 years longer than the life expectancy of white males and females. Negroes had life expectancies at birth 6 and 7 years less than those for white males and females, although part of this was due to high census undercounts for Negroes. This pattern of differentials held for expectation of life at ages 25 and 55 as well. Life expectation at age 25 was 51.9 years for Japanese males compared with 45.7 years for whites and 41.3 years for Negroes. For females life expectation at age 25 was 57.2 years for Japanese, 51.9 years for whites and 46.3 years for Negroes. Hence at age 25 Japanese males enjoyed an expectation of life 10.6 years above that of Negroes and 6.2 years above whites. Similarly, at age 25 Japanese females could look forward to 10.9 more years of life than Negro females and 5.3 more years than white.

At age 55 differences among the three races in life expectation narrowed. Japanese males at age 55 had an expectation of life of 24.2 years compared with 19.5 years for whites and 18.4 years for

Table 6.6. Expectation of life at selected ages, by sex and race: United States, 1959-61

Sex and race	Expectation of life ($\overset{o}{e}_x$)			Difference from $\overset{o}{e}_x$ for whites		
	At birth	At age 25	At age 55	At birth	At age 25	At age 55
Males						
White.....	67.6	45.7	19.5	0	0	0
Nonwhite..	61.8	41.8	18.7	-5.8	-3.9	-0.8
Negro...	61.3	41.3	18.4	-6.3	-4.4	-1.1
Japanese	74.4	51.9	24.2	6.8	6.2	4.7
Females						
White.....	74.7	51.9	24.3	0	0	0
Nonwhite..	67.7	46.7	22.4	-7.0	-5.2	-1.9
Negro...	67.2	46.3	22.1	-7.5	-5.6	-2.2
Japanese	80.4	57.2	29.2	5.7	5.3	4.9

Source: Abridged life tables calculated from uncorrected age-specific death rates based on reported deaths as compiled by National Center for Health Statistics and on population statistics tabulated from the 25-percent sample, 1960 Census of Population. See text for explanation of procedure used to calculate life tables.

Negroes. Japanese females at age 55 had a life expectancy of 29.2 years compared with 24.3 years for whites and 22.1 years for Negroes. Thus, at age 55 Japanese males had an advantage of 5.8 years of life remaining over Negroes and 4.7 years over whites. Japanese females at age 55 had an advantage of 7.1 years of life remaining over Negro females and 4.9 years over whites. Regional variations in differential mortality by race are discussed in Chapter 7.

Nativity Differentials

Differences in mortality between the native white and foreign-born white population 35 years of age and over are shown for the nation in 1960 in Table 6.7. The figures reported indicate the percentage differences between age-adjusted death rates of foreign-born whites and native whites, both uncorrected (calculated from death and population statistics as compiled from death certificates and census

Table 6.7. Nativity differentials in mortality for the white population 35 years of age and over, by sex: United States, 1959-61

Sex and age	Nativity differentials in age-adjusted death rates standardized by:[a]			
	Direct method		Indirect method	
	Uncorrected	Corrected	Uncorrected	Corrected
White males 35 & over...	5	-4	7	-2
35-64 years........	-5	-13	-1	-10
65 & over..........	11	1	11	1
White females 35 & over.	19	5	25	11
35-64 years........	10	-2	13	3
65 & over..........	22	8	22	8

Source: Uncorrected differentials based on age-adjusted death rates calculated from deaths classified by nativity, color, sex and age as tabulated from death certificate characteristics by National Center for Health Statistics, and population tabulations from the 1960 Census of Population as compiled by the Bureau of the Census; deaths to persons for whom nativity was not reported on the death certificate were excluded from these calculations, a procedure which has the effect, in the ratios presented here, of assuming that they were distributed proportionately by nativity. Corrected differentials based on age-adjusted death rates calculated from deaths corrected for discrepancies in the reporting of nativity on death certificates and census records following procedures explained in the text.

[a] Nativity differentials indicate the percent by which the age-adjusted death rates for foreign-born whites exceeded (or, if negative, were less than) corresponding rates for native whites. The total 1960 U.S. population was used as the standard population for both the direct and indirect methods.

schedules) and corrected for discrepancies between the reporting of nativity on the two records.[6] In this case, comparisons based on uncorrected death rates are very misleading.

For example, correction of the age-adjusted rate for discrepancies in nativity reporting actually reversed the difference in mortality between native and foreign born white males. Whereas uncorrected rates standardized by the direct method indicate that mortality for foreign born was 5 percent higher than for native males 35 and over, corrected mortality for foreign born was 4 percent lower than for natives. Using the indirect method of standardization, mortality for foreign born males 35 and over was 7 percent higher than for natives; corrected it was 2 percent lower than for natives. (Results obtained by both direct and indirect standardization techniques are reported here because the former exercises more rigid control over age composition but the latter was the only method that could be used in the analysis of mortality differentials by country of birth among the foreign born [because adjustments for discrepant responses were not available by age], and it seemed advisable to have comparable measures for nativity and country of birth differentials.)

For females, correction of the age-adjusted death rate resulted in sharp decreases in the size of the nativity differential. Foreign-born females 35 and over experienced 19 percent higher mortality with the uncorrected data and 5 percent higher mortality when deaths were corrected for discrepant reporting of nativity. With indirect standardization, mortality of foreign born white females 35 and over was 25 percent greater than of white; corrected the differential dropped to 11 percent.

For males 35 to 64, with direct standardization, the foreign-born death rate, which was 5 percent below that for natives using uncorrected data, changed to 13 percent below the native rate when corrected. Using indirect standardization, the differential changed from one percent below to 10 percent below. Comparable changes for males 65 and over using the direct and indirect methods were from 11 percent higher mortality for foreign born to one percent higher.

For women 35 to 64 correction of the directly standardized death rates changed mortality for the foreign born from 10 percent higher than for natives to 2 percent lower, and correction of the indirectly standardized rates changed foreign-born mortality from 13 percent higher to 3 percent higher. For women 65 and over correction of both the directly and indirectly standardized rates changed the differential from 22 percent higher for the foreign born to 8 percent higher.

Three general conclusions are suggested by the nativity differentials in Table 6.7. First, death rates for native and foreign-born whites based on "uncorrected" deaths and population data as collected and published in the census and vital statistics reports are subject to considerable error. Second, in the age group 35-64 the mortality of foreign-born white males was significantly below that of native white males, whereas there was only a slight difference between the mortality of foreign-born and native white females. Above age 65, there was very little difference between native and foreign-born white males, but foreign-born white females experienced higher death rates than native white females.

Table 6.8. Mortality ratios for foreign-born population 35 years of age and over, by country of birth and sex: United States, 1959-61

Country of birth	Mortality ratios							
	Males				Females			
	35 & over (un-corrected ratios)	Corrected ratio			35 & over (un-corrected ratios)	Corrected ratio		
		35 & over	35-64 years	65 & over		35 & over	35-64 years	65 & over
Total foreign born...	1.00	1.00	1.00	1.00	1.00	1.00	1.00	1.00
United Kingdom.....	.91	1.01	1.11	.98	.84	.96	.92	.95
Ireland...........	1.41	1.15	1.23	1.13	1.42	1.23	1.25	1.21
Norway...........	.92	.91	.96	.89	.91	.91	.80	.90
Sweden...........	.97	.94	.99	.93	.96	.94	.82	.91
Germany..........	1.00	.99	.89	1.01	.98	1.01	.78	1.03
Austria..........	1.22	1.10	1.11	1.10	1.21	1.02	1.03	1.02
Poland...........	1.07	1.15	1.04	1.17	1.07	1.06	1.21	1.03
Czechoslovakia.....	.95	1.03	.94	1.04	1.00	1.06	1.00	1.06
Hungary..........	.97	.90	1.02	.88	.93	1.06	1.25	1.02
Yugoslavia........	1.01	1.08	1.00	1.09	.88	.94	.86	.97
Lithuania.........	1.22	1.18	.99	1.20	1.16	1.04	1.34	.99
Finland...........	1.17	1.19	1.09	1.19	1.08	1.08	1.12	1.05
USSR.............	1.07	1.05	1.12	1.03	1.12	1.15	1.12	1.17
Italy............	.90	.90	.88	.90	.95	.94	.91	.95
Canada...........	1.06	1.07	1.12	1.05	.97	.97	.99	.97
Mexico...........	.88	.88	.93	.87	.98	.96	1.29	.90
All other countries	.93	.94	.95	.95	.86	.87	.88	.88

Source: Mortality ratios were calculated from age-adjusted death rates standardized by the indirect method using the 1960 total U.S. population as standard, with rates for total foreign born set equal to 1.00. Uncorrected ratios based on tabulations of 1959-61 deaths and 1960 population as compiled by NCHS and Bureau of the Census from characteristics reported on each record. Corrected ratios based on estimates of deaths corrected for discrepancies in reporting of country of birth on death certificates and 1960 Census records (see text for details of correction procedure and limitations of data available for correction).

Differentials by Country of Birth of Foreign Born

Differentials in age-adjusted death rates, 1959-61, by country of birth of the foreign-born population are shown in Table 6.8, both uncorrected and corrected for discrepant reporting of country of birth on death certificates and census records. Unfortunately, however, the corrections made for discrepancies in reporting of country of birth are subject to an unknown bias because the cross classification (compiled by the National Center for Health Statistics) comparing country of birth on the two records included only those matched decedents in the 1960 Matched Records Study who were reported as foreign-born white in the 1960 census records. Consequently, corrections could not be made for discrepancies in both nativity and country of birth simultaneously, a potentially serious limitation because there was a sizeable relative underreporting of foreign born in the 1960 census, as indicated by the following figures: 12,255 of the matched decedents were reported as foreign white on both records, 1,282 as native white on their census record and foreign white on their death certificate, and only 212 reported as foreign white on their census record and native white on their death certificate. Therefore, the correction of 1959-61 deaths by country of birth as reported on the census records fails to deflate the reported numbers of deaths of foreign born for those decedents who were reported as foreign born on their death record but as native in the census, and this group may well be highly selective of particular countries. The direction of the bias, given the correction procedure used,[7] is toward rates that are too high in general for the foreign born and perhaps substantially overstated for particular countries.

In consequence it is felt that no detailed reliable conclusions can be drawn on differential mortality of the foreign born by country of birth. The data are presented primarily to compare uncorrected with "partially corrected" differentials, as a warning against accepting uncorrected differentials at face value. One might infer that the relatively low "corrected" mortality of the foreign born with origins in Norway and Sweden is probably accurately indicated, at least in direction, because of what is known from other sources. Similarly, one might infer that the relatively high mortality of the foreign born with origins in Eastern European countries is probably indicative of the true situation. On the other hand, the relatively high mortality of the foreign born originating in Canada and the relatively low mortality of the foreign born in Mexico, Italy, and Hungary may reflect problems of reporting more than differentials in death rates.

Marital Status Differentials

The official death statistics for the United States have consistently indicated that married persons have lower death rates than do those who have never married or whose marriages have been broken by divorce or death (e.g., see Bureau of Census, July 1945; NCHS, May 1956 and December 1970). Analysts have just as consistently pointed out the difficulties of separating the effect of marital status itself on mortality from the effect of selection by marriage (the more fit are more likely to marry) as well as from the influence of socioeconomic factors with marriage (e.g., see NCHS, July 1945, p. 44; Shurtleff, 1956, p. 654; Sheps, 1961, p. 547; Berkson, 1962). The same analysts have also listed discrepancies in the reporting of marital status on death certificates and census records as possibly responsible for part of the differences in mortality by marital status. The 1960 Matched Records Study provided an opportunity to evaluate the effect of the latter—discrepant reporting—on observed marital status differentials.

In this report, emphasis will be placed on a brief summary of the pattern of marital status differentials in mortality in the United States from 1940 to 1960 and, for 1960, an evaluation of the effect of discrepancies in the reporting of marital status on death certificates and census records. Table 6.9 reports uncorrected age-adjusted death rates by marital status for 1940, 1949-51, and 1959-61, based on tabulations of deaths and population as compiled by the NCHS and the Bureau of the Census; and in addition, corrected death rates for 1959-61 based on estimates of deaths corrected for discrepancies in the reporting of marital status on the death certificates and census records.[8] In the last four columns of the table, the age-adjusted rates are converted to percentage differences from corresponding rates for married persons.

Three general conclusions follow from these data. First, with minor exceptions—chiefly among persons 65 and over—there was no consistent increase or decrease in the size of "uncorrected" marital status differentials during the 20-year period. Second, the uncorrected rates in 1960 exaggerated the higher mortality of widowed and divorced persons by substantial amounts. Third, marital status differentials were much larger for men than women.

Among white males 15 and over, the 1960 uncorrected age-adjusted death rate for married persons was exceeded by 52 percent for single persons, by 75 percent for the widowed, and by 122 per-

Table 6.9. Age-adjusted death rates by marital status, color and sex: United States, 1940, 1949-51, 1959-61 (per 1,000 population)

Sex, color and age	Uncorrected age-adjusted death rate			Corrected age-adjusted death rate 1959-61	Percent difference from rate for married persons			
					Uncorrected rate			Corrected rate 1959-61
	1940	1949-51	1959-61		1940	1949-1951	1959-1961	
WHITE MALES								
15 & over......	15.279[a]	11.908	11.516	11.516				
Single......	18.501[a]	16.468	15.270	16.286	38	56	52	58
Married.....	13.436[a]	10.581	10.065	10.279	0	0	0	0
Widowed.....	22.556[a]	16.945	17.604	16.751	68	60	75	63
Divorced....	29.117[a]	21.772	22.297	18.055	117	106	122	76
35 & over......	23.090	20.582	19.983	19.983				
Single......	27.779	28.459	26.338	28.132	36	55	50	57
Married.....	20.476	18.342	17.549	17.960	0	0	0	0
Widowed.....	31.673	27.474	28.220	27.124	55	50	61	51
Divorced....	42.891	36.911	37.951	30.951	109	101	116	72
35-64 years...	11.875	10.589	9.747	9.747				
Single......	16.624	16.725	14.430	15.284	59	80	69	75
Married.....	10.437	9.311	8.546	8.739	0	0	0	0
Widowed.....	19.488	17.199	16.636	15.533	87	85	95	78
Divorced....	24.886	22.342	24.079	20.095	138	140	182	130
65 & over......	78.322	69.797	70.393	70.395				
Single......	82.717	86.249	84.975	91.403	18	37	37	44
Married.....	69.913	62.818	61.879	63.373	0	0	0	0
Widowed.....	91.680	78.074	85.277	84.206	31	24	38	33
Divorced....	31.564	108.659	106.259	84.410	45	73	72	33
WHITE FEMALES								
15 & over......	11.698[a]	7.807	6.818	6.817				
Single......	11.989[a]	8.309	7.361	7.556	13	17	23	20
Married.....	10.613[a]	7.097	5.968	6.279	0	0	0	0
Widowed.....	13.682[a]	9.728	8.366	7.970	29	37	40	27
Divorced....	18.748[a]	10.878	8.502	7.640	77	53	42	22
35 & over......	17.689	13.651	12.012	12.012				
Single......	18.093	14.316	12.690	13.030	13	16	21	18
Married.....	15.974	12.364	10.499	11.071	0	0	0	0
Widowed.....	19.554	15.395	13.633	13.212	22	25	30	19
Divorced....	28.179	18.571	14.368	12.971	76	50	37	17
35-64 years....	8.096	5.952	4.835	4.835				
Single......	8.487	6.619	5.828	6.038	12	19	32	34
Married.....	7.595	5.540	4.426	4.515	0	0	0	0
Widowed.....	9.815	7.663	6.231	5.866	29	38	41	30
Divorced....	11.306	7.939	6.842	6.198	49	43	55	37
65 & over......	64.935	51.563	47.363	47.358				
Single......	65.402	52.220	46.484	47.461	14	14	15	9
Married.....	57.242	45.971	40.407	43.358	0	0	0	0
Widowed.....	67.519	53.475	50.089	49.388	18	16	24	14
Divorced....	111.272	70.935	51.435	46.322	94	54	27	7
NONWHITE MALES								
15 & over......	22.253[a]	15.843	14.624	14.624				
Single......	28.685[a]	25.676	18.672	19.796	55	95	58	57
Married.....	18.559[a]	13.142	11.805	12.583	0	0	0	0
Widowed.....	39.299[a]	28.504	25.888	22.243	112	117	119	77
Divorced....	37.714[a]	26.078	23.730	19.123	103	98	101	52
35 & over......	31.291	26.055	24.485	24.487				
Single......	39.966	42.753	30.835	32.897	52	98	56	56
Married.....	26.350	21.609	19.739	21.112	0	0	0	0
Widowed.....	50.658	42.780	40.816	36.514	92	98	107	73
Divorced....	52.981	41.883	39.823	32.858	101	94	102	56

(continued)

Table 6.9. Age-adjusted death rates by marital status, color and sex: United States, 1940, 1949-51, 1959-61 (per 1,000 population)--(continued)

Sex, color and age	Uncorrected age-adjusted death rate			Corrected age-adjusted death rate	Percent difference from rate for married persons			
					Uncorrected rate			Corrected rate
	1940	1949-51	1959-61	1959-61	1940	1949-1951	1959-1961	1959-61
35-64 years....	22.651	18.299	15.693	15.696				
Single......	29.919	32.946	22.070	22.734	57	120	76	67
Married.....	19.073	14.988	12.569	13.633	0	0	0	0
Widowed.....	42.266	35.320	30.663	25.790	122	136	144	89
Divorced.....	38.969	29.531	29.175	25.437	104	97	132	87
65 & over....	73.840	64.249	67.788	67.782				
Single......	89.447	91.052	74.001	82.950	44	68	34	43
Married.....	62.191	54.220	55.046	57.942	0	0	0	0
Widowed.....	91.987	79.519	90.826	89.330	48	47	65	54
Divorced....	121.987	102.717	92.260	69.402	96	89	68	20
NONWHITE FEMALES								
15 & over......	19.373[a]	12.978	10.615	10.615				
Single......	23.555[a]	15.479	11.185	12.241	41	42	37	40
Married.....	16.684[a]	10.905	8.140	8.756	0	0	0	0
Widowed.....	24.407[a]	18.054	14.748	13.730	46	66	81	57
Divorced....	27.905[a]	15.162	10.980	9.940	67	39	35	14
35 & over......	27.144	21.508	18.113	18.113				
Single......	32.823	25.148	18.473	20.501	41	41	35	39
Married.....	23.268	17.874	13.712	14.789	0	0	0	0
Widowed.....	32.730	27.696	23.945	22.940	41	55	75	55
Divorced....	40.782	24.601	18.359	16.534	75	38	34	12
35-64 years....	20.469	15.590	11.656	11.656				
Single......	24.598	19.746	13.043	14.060	46	58	41	42
Married.....	16.840	12.465	9.255	9.928	0	0	0	0
Widowed.....	26.887	22.437	17.416	16.384	60	80	88	65
Divorced....	25.075	17.309	12.803	10.479	49	39	38	6
65 & over......	60.015	50.658	49.910	49.913				
Single......	73.330	51.753	45.211	52.220	34	16	27	35
Married.....	54.921	44.512	35.662	38.730	0	0	0	0
Widowed.....	61.505	53.592	56.104	55.227	12	20	57	43
Divorced....	118.133	60.512	45.716	46.351	115	36	28	20

Source: Uncorrected rates based on tabulations of deaths and population as compiled by NCHS and Bureau of the Census from characteristics reported on each record. Corrected rates based on estimates of deaths corrected for discrepancies in reporting of marital status on death certificates and census records (see text for details of correction procedure). Age-adjusted death rates calculated by direct method, using total 1940 U.S. population as standard. Rates for 1959-61 (corrected and uncorrected) standardized over 5-year age groups from ages 15-19 to 85 and over; rates for 1940 and 1949-51 standardized over 5-year age groups except for ages 25 to 64 years, within which 10-year age intervals were used.

[a] Refers to persons 20 and over rather than 15 and over.

cent for divorced persons. When corrected for discrepancies in the reporting of marital status, the rate for single persons was 58 percent higher than that for married persons; the rate for widowed, 63 percent higher; and the rate for divorced, 76 percent higher. Among white females 15 and over, the rates for single, widowed, and divorced women exceeded that for married women by 23, 40, and 42 percent, respectively, before correction; and by 20, 27, and 22 percent after correction.

Among nonwhite males 15 and over, the 1960 rates for single, widowed, and divorced men exceeded that for married men by 58, 119, and 101 percent, respectively, before correction, and by 57, 77,

Table 6.10. Percent difference between corrected and uncorrected mortality indexes by marital status, color, sex and age: United States, 1959-61

Color and age	Single		Married		Widowed		Divorced	
	Males	Females	Males	Females	Males	Females	Males	Females
White								
15 & over.......	7	3	2	5	-5	-5	-19	-10
35 & over.......	7	3	2	5	-4	-3	-18	-10
35-64 years..	6	4	2	2	-7	-6	-17	-9
65 & over....	8	2	2	7	-1	-1	-21	-10
Nonwhite								
15 & over.......	6	9	7	8	-14	-7	-19	-9
35 & over.......	7	11	7	8	-11	-4	-17	-10
35-64 years..	3	8	8	7	-16	-6	-13	-18
65 & over....	12	16	5	9	-2	-2	-25	1

Source: Table 6.9. Percent difference indicates the percent by which the corrected mortality index exceeds (or is less than, if negative) the uncorrected mortality index.

and 52 percent after correction. Among nonwhite females, the 1960 rates for single, widowed, and divorced women were 37, 81, and 35 percent higher than that for married women before correction, and 40, 57, and 14 percent higher after correction.

The reasons for the marked decreases in the mortality of the widowed and divorced as a result of correcting for discrepancies in the reporting of marital status are evident in Table 6.10, which shows the percentage difference between corrected and uncorrected rates for 1959-61. For example, among white males, the rate for married persons increased by 2 percent as a result of correction, and the rate for divorced persons decreased by 17 to 21 percent, depending on the age group. Among white females, correction for discrepant reporting increased the death rate for married persons by 2 to 7 percent and decreased the rate for widowed by 9 to 10 percent. Among nonwhite males and females there were similar changes as a result of correction.

In all the color-sex-age groups in Table 6.10, correction for discrepant reporting decreased the death rates for the widowed and divorced and increased the death rates for single and married persons. In some cases the increase was larger for single than for married persons, in which case the corrected differential is larger than the uncorrected differential (for example, white males 15 and over); in other cases the increase was larger for married than for single.

It is apparent from Tables 6.9 and 6.10 that discrepancies in the reporting of marital status on the death certificates and census records do introduce substantial errors in marital status differentials. For example, among white females 35 and over, the corrected 1960 death rate for divorced persons was only 17 percent higher than the corrected rate for married persons, as compared with a 37 percent difference between their uncorrected rates. Similarly the difference between corrected rates for widowed and married nonwhite males 15 and over was only 52 percent, as compared with 101 percent before correction. It is also true, however, that sizeable differences remain after corrections for discrepant reporting of marital status.

Parity Differentials

A number of researchers have indicated a particular interest in the effect of high fertility on the mortality of women. Because of the known negative associations between completed fertility (parity) and education, it seemed advisable to standardize for education as well as for age when computing mortality ratios for ever-married women of different parities. The results are reported in Table 6.11. "Ever-married" women include all women except those classified as "never-married" in the census.

Among ever-married women 45-64 years old, whose childbearing

Table 6.11. Mortality ratios for ever-married white women 45 years of age and over, by number of children ever borne: United States, May-August, 1960

Number of children ever borne (parity)	Standardized for age			Standardized for age and education		
	45 & over	45-64 years	65 & over	45 & over	45-64 years	65 & over
Ever-married white women.....	1.00	1.00	1.00	1.00	1.00	1.00
No children...............	1.01	1.04	1.00	1.03	1.07	1.02
1 child...................	.95	1.02	.94	.97	1.04	.95
2 children................	.98	.92	1.02	1.00	.94	1.03
3 children................	.95	.89	.97	.95	.89	.98
4 children................	1.01	.99	1.01	1.00	.96	1.01
5 or 6 children...........	1.00	1.11	.97	.98	1.05	.95
7 or more children........	1.12	1.24	1.09	1.08	1.14	1.06

Source: Population Research Center, University of Chicago, study based on matching death certificates with 1960 Census records (see Appendix A). The mortality ratios in this table measure the range of parity differentials in mortality within each broad age group of ever-married white women. They were derived from the two sets of mortality indexes--one standardized for age only, and the second standardized for both age and education level--described in Appendix A, section 3g, by setting the index for each age subgroup equal to 1.00.

has been virtually completed, the mortality ratios show a marked J-shaped pattern as the number of children ever borne increases. The age-standardized ratio decreases from 1.04 for women with no children to 0.89 for women with 3 children and then increases sharply to 1.24 for women with 7 or more children, a differential of 39 percent between the highest and lowest ratios. When standardized for age and education simultaneously, the J-pattern remains although not quite as pronounced, with the mortality ratio for women with 7 or more children being 28 percent higher than the ratio for women with 3 children.

Similarly, for women 65 and over there is a tendency for the J-shaped pattern to appear but there are fluctuations in the data reflecting, no doubt, problems of reporting and recall as well as the increasing one of other factors in mortality as time since childbearing increases. The impact of the data for women 65 and over affects, of course, the pattern for all women 45 and over which includes them.

These data suggest that very high fertility per se—independent of socioeconomic status—may shorten a woman's life. The lower mortality for women with 2 to 4 children than for women of lower parity is subject to more debate, but it may reflect the presence, in the low parities, of women who are subfecund or sterile, conditions which may be related to poor health and higher mortality. It may also reflect the higher mortality of women by reason of mammary carcinomas, which appear to be associated with no or low childbearing (see Chapter 5). These findings certainly point to the need for more intensive investigation of the effect of heavy childbearing on female mortality.

7 / GEOGRAPHIC DIFFERENTIALS AND SOCIOECONOMIC CORRELATES

Geographic variations in mortality in the United States have been described in numerous studies, but little headway has been made in the identification of factors responsible for the marked geographic differences in death rates that have been observed (Sauer, 1970; Sauer and Brand, 1971). In some of these studies, attention has been directed to the relationship between geographic variations in mortality and variations in socioeconomic indexes of the areas (for example, see Altenderfer, 1947; Wiehl, 1948; Hamilton, 1955).

The relationship between geographic variation in death rates and variation in average socioeconomic level of the geographic areas has been used in some studies to isolate geographic differentials *independent of* their differences in average socioeconomic level, and in other studies to document the existence of socioeconomic differentials in mortality by indirect inference. The former interest can be pursued by correlating death rates for geographic areas with one or more socioeconomic indexes for the areas (in which case the "unexplained variation" is independent of socioeconomic factors) *or* by calculating for the geographic areas death rates standardized by one or more socioeconomic factors. In the United States, for example, standardization of death rates by color (as well as age) would substantially reduce the variation in age-adjusted death rates among the states. The second interest—in socioeconomic differentials—can be pursued either by correlation of death rates and socioeconomic indexes (in which case the "explained variation" documents the existence of socioeconomic differentials) *or* by aggregating small geographic areas into a number of socioeconomic levels using a socioeconomic index as the basis for ranking and aggregating the areas. Studies of the latter type were the subject of Chapter 4. This chapter has two major objectives: (1) a description of geographic variations in mortality in the United States based on tabulations of 1959-61 deaths by geographic divisions, by states, and by 121 economic subregions into which the nation is divided; and (2) investigation of the extent to which geographic variations are associated with variations in average socioeconomic level of these geographic areas.

Differentials by Geographic Division—Metropolitan and Nonmetropolitan

Mortality differentials were calculated for whites and nonwhites by sex, by geographic division, and by metropolitan-nonmetropolitan residence using age-adjusted death rates. The pattern of differentials which emerged, in general, conforms with findings for earlier periods (e.g., Wiehl, 1948; Sauer, 1962 and 1970).

Division Differentials by Sex

Three of the nine geographic divisions had male mortality above the national level (the South Atlantic [SA], 5 percent, the Middle Atlantic [MA], 4 percent; and East South Central [ESC], 2 percent). Four divisions had below average male mortality (West North Central [WNC], 8 percent, Pacific [Pac], 5 percent, and the West South Central [WSC] and Mountain [Mo], each 3 percent). The remaining two divisions, New England (NE) and East North Central (ENC), had about the average level of male mortality (deviating from the average by not more than 1 percent). Three divisions had above average female mortality (MA, 8 percent; ESC, 4 percent; and SA, 3 percent); and four divisions were below the national level of female mortality (WNC, 11 percent; Pac, 9 percent; WSC and Mo, each 7 percent). As for males, the New England and East North Central divisions experienced about average mortality for females (Table 7.1).

For males the three divisions with above average mortality (MA, SA, and ESC) remained above average for each of the three categories of metropolitan status shown. Similarly, the four divisions with below average mortality (WNC, WSC, Mo, and Pac) remained below the national level for each category of area by metropolitan status. The remaining divisions with average mortality (NE and ENC) remained close to the average for each metropolitan residence category, varying by a maximum of 3 percent (3 percent above for nonmetropolitan counties in NE and 3 percent below for nonmetropolitan counties in ENC). Similarly, for females the four divisions with above national levels of mortality with only two exceptions (nonmetropolitan counties in ENC and metropolitan counties with no central city in SA, each 1 percent below) were above average in each of the metropolitan residence categories; and the four divisions with below average mortality remained below average for every category of metropolitan residence.

For males the highest positive deviation from national average mortality occurred in metropolitan counties with no central city in the East South Central division (13 percent above); and the highest negative deviation was in nonmetropolitan counties in the West North Central division and the metropolitan counties with no central cities in the Mountain division (9 percent below). For females the highest positive deviation from national mortality occurred in the metropolitan counties with no central city in the East South Central division (12 percent above); and the highest negative deviation in the metropolitan counties with no central city in the Mountain division (12 percent below).

Division Differentials for Whites

For white males, mortality was above national levels in two divisions (MA, 5 percent, and NE, 2 percent), and below the national level in five divisions (WNC, 7 percent; WSC, 4 percent; and ESC, Mo, and Pac, each 2 percent). In the remaining two divisions white male mortality was at about the national level (ENC and SA). In both divisions with above average male mortality (NE and MA) age-adjusted death rates remained above average or at about average (only 1 percent deviation) for each metropolitan status area. In only three of the five divisions with below average mortality, however, did the below average pattern hold for each category of metropolitan residence (WNC, WSC, and Pac); reversals in the pattern of below average mortality occurred in the other two divisions (ESC and Mo). In the East South Central division white male mortality rose to 11 percent above average in metropolitan counties with no central city; and in the Mountain division it rose to 2 percent above the average in nonmetropolitan counties. In the two divisions with average white male mortality (ENC and SA) the age-adjusted death rates remained at near average for each of the metropolitan residence categories, the highest deviation being 3 percent for nonmetropolitan counties in the South Atlantic division.

The highest relative mortality for white males by metropolitan residence occurred in the metropolitan counties with no central city in the East South Central states (11 percent above the national average), a division with below average male mortality; and the lowest relative mortality occurred in metropolitan counties with no central city in the Mountain division (9 percent below the national average).

For white females three divisions had mortality above the national level (MA, 9 percent; NE, 4 percent; and ENC, 3 percent); and the remaining six divisions had below average mortality (WSC, 11 percent; WNC, 8 percent; SA, Mo, and Pac, each 5 percent; and ESC, 3 percent). The three divisions with above average white female mortality (NE, MA, ENC) remained above the national level for each category of metropolitan residence except for metropolitan counties with no central city in New England and the East North Central division, where they were average or about average. In three of the six divisions with below average mortality (WNC, WSC, Pac) each of the metropolitan residence categories was also below average; and in the other three divisions (SA, ESC, and Mo), the greatest variation above average was 8 percent for metropolitan counties with no central city in the East South Central division. The other deviations from below average female mortality did not exceed 1 percent. The highest relative age-adjusted death rate for white females occurred in nonmetropolitan counties in the Middle Atlantic states (11 percent above the national level), and the lowest, in the metropolitan counties with no central city in the West South Central states (12 percent below the national level).

Division Differentials for Nonwhites

For nonwhite males four divisions experienced mortality above the national level (SA, 10 percent; MA, 5 percent; WNC, 4 percent; ESC, 3 percent); four divisions experienced below average nonwhite mortality (Pac, 24 percent; Mo, 9 percent; WSC, 6 percent; and NE, 2 percent); and the remaining division experienced about average mortality (ENC, 1 percent below). In only one of the four divisions with above average nonwhite male mortality (SA) did the age-adjusted death rate remain above average in each category of metropolitan residence. The greatest deviation below average, however, was only 4 percent, for metropolitan counties with no central city in the West North Central division. The other deviations below average did not exceed 2 percent. The highest relative nonwhite male mortality was in metropolitan counties without a central city in the East South Central division (16 percent above the average); the lowest was in the metropolitan counties with no central city in the Pacific states (26 percent below the average).

For nonwhite females mortality was above the national level in three divisions (SA, 7 percent; ESC, 6 percent; WNC, 5 percent); and below the national level in four divisions (Pac, 26 percent; Mo, 11 percent; WSC and NE, 5 percent). In the remaining two divisions, mortality was at about the national level (MA and ENC).

For nonwhite females the three divisions with above average mortality (WNC, SA, and ESC) experienced above average mortality for each of the metropolitan residence categories. Similarly, without exception, the four divisions with below average mortality (NE, WSC, Mo, and Pac) remained below average for each of the metropolitan categories. The two divisions with about average non-white female mortality (MA and ENC) fluctuated above and below average in different metropolitan categories, with the greatest nega-tive deviation being 7 percent below for nonmetropolitan counties in the East North Central division and the greatest positive deviation being 2 percent for metropolitan counties with a central city in the Middle Atlantic division. The highest relative nonwhite female mortality was in metropolitan counties with no central city in the East South Central states (24 percent above average); and the lowest was in metropolitan counties with a central city in the Pacific states (29 percent below average).

Division Patterns

It is apparent that there were considerable differences in age-adjusted mortality by geographic division that tend to hold for each of the three categories of metropolitan residence. It is apparent also that divisional differences obtained for both whites and nonwhites of each sex. In summary of the above analysis the following patterns emerged. In the New England and Middle Atlantic divisions mortality was above average for whites of each sex and was below average or average for nonwhites except for nonwhite males in the Middle Atlantic states. In the South Atlantic and East South Central divisions mortality was above the national level for nonwhites of each sex and below or at the national level for whites of each sex. In the West North Central, South Central, Mountain, and Pacific divisions, both white and nonwhite mortality for each sex was below average, except for nonwhite females in the West North Central division, where mortality was above average. In the East North Central division nonwhite mortality for each sex and white male mortality was about average but nonwhite female mortality was above that for the nation.

Table 7.1. Differentials in age-adjusted death rates by geographic division and metropolitan-nonmetropolitan residence, by color and sex: United States, 1959-61

Sex and geographic division	Total					White					Nonwhite				
	Total	Metropolitan counties			Non-metro-politan counties	Total	Metropolitan counties			Non-metro-politan counties	Total	Metropolitan counties			Non-metro-politan counties
		All	With central city	No central city			All	With central city	No central city			All	With central city	No central city	
GEOGRAPHIC DIFFERENTIALS[a]															
Males, United States	1.00	1.00	1.00	1.00	1.00	1.00	1.00	1.00	1.00	1.00	1.00	1.00	1.00	1.00[b]	1.00
New England	1.00	.98	.98	.99	1.03	1.02	1.00	.99	1.00	1.05	.98	.97	.98	--[b]	.95
Middle Atlantic	1.04	1.03	1.05	1.02	1.05	1.05	1.03	1.04	1.01	1.08	1.05	1.04	1.05	1.00	.98
East North Central	1.00	1.01	1.01	1.00	.97	1.00	1.02	1.01	1.00	.99	.99	.99	.98	1.02	.86
West North Central	.92	.97	.98	.94	.91	.93	.97	.98	.95	.92	1.04	1.03	1.04	.96	1.05
South Atlantic	1.05	1.02	1.04	1.01	1.08	1.00	.98	.98	.99	1.03	1.10	1.11	1.12	1.09	1.09
East South Central	1.02	1.05	1.03	1.13	1.03	.98	1.01	.98	1.11	1.00	1.03	1.07	1.05	1.16	.99
West South Central	.97	.98	.98	.98	.97	.96	.98	.97	.97	.97	.94	.99	.99	.96[b]	.91
Mountain	.97	.94	.94	.91	1.00	.98	.97	.96	.91	1.02	.91	.92	.92	--[b]	.91
Pacific	.95	.94	.94	.95	.97	.98	.97	.96	.96	.99	.76	.75	.75	.74	.78
Females, United States	1.00	1.00	1.00	1.00	1.00	1.00	1.00	1.00	1.00	1.00	1.00	1.00	1.00	1.00[b]	1.00
New England	.99	.99	.98	.97	1.00	1.04	1.03	1.01	.99	1.05	.95	.95	.95	--[b]	.81
Middle Atlantic	1.08	1.07	1.09	1.04	1.06	1.09	1.09	1.10	1.04	1.11	1.01	1.01	1.02	.97	.96
East North Central	1.00	1.02	1.02	1.01	.99	1.03	1.03	1.03	1.01	1.03	1.00	1.01	1.00	.98	.93
West North Central	.89	.93	.93	.95	.90	.92	.94	.94	.93	.93	1.05	1.03	1.03	1.04	1.06
South Atlantic	1.03	1.01	1.02	.99	1.08	.95	.94	.92	.96	1.00	1.07	1.10	1.10	1.08	1.04
East South Central	1.04	1.05	1.04	1.12	1.08	.97	.96	.94	1.08	1.01	1.06	1.10	1.09	1.24	1.03
West South Central	.93	.94	.94	.93	.95	.89	.91	.90	.88	.92	.95	.99	.98	1.00[b]	.92
Mountain	.93	.90	.90	.88	.96	.95	.94	.92	.91	1.00	.89	.88	.88	--[b]	.88
Pacific	.91	.90	.90	.92	.92	.95	.94	.94	.92	.96	.74	.72	.71	.79	.79
METROPOLITAN DIFFERENTIALS[c]															
Males, United States	...	1.05	1.07	.97	1.00	...	1.05	1.07	.99	1.00	...	1.01	1.01	.95[b]	1.00
New England	...	1.00	1.01	.93	1.00	...	1.00	1.01	.94	1.00	...	1.04	1.05	--[b]	1.00
Middle Atlantic	...	1.03	1.06	.94	1.00	...	1.01	1.03	.93	1.00	...	1.07	1.09	.97	1.00
East North Central	...	1.09	1.10	1.00	1.00	...	1.08	1.09	1.00	1.00	...	1.15	1.15	1.12	1.00
West North Central	...	1.12	1.15	1.01	1.00	...	1.10	1.13	1.02	1.00	...	.99	1.01	.86	1.00
South Atlantic	...	.99	1.02	.91	1.00	...	.99	1.01	.95	1.00	...	1.03	1.04	.94	1.00
East South Central	...	1.07	1.07	1.07	1.00	...	1.06	1.05	1.10	1.00	...	1.08	1.07	1.10	1.00
West South Central	...	1.06	1.07	.98	1.00	...	1.05	1.06	.99	1.00	...	1.10	1.10	1.01[b]	1.00
Mountain	...	.99	1.01	.88	1.00	...	1.00	1.01	.89	1.00	...	1.02	1.03	--[b]	1.00
Pacific	...	1.03	1.03	.96	1.00	...	1.03	1.03	.96	1.00	...	.97	.97	.90	1.00
Females, United States	...	1.05	1.06	.99	1.00	...	1.05	1.07	1.03	1.00	...	.99	1.00	.94[b]	1.00
New England	...	1.04	1.04	.96	1.00	...	1.03	1.03	.96	1.00	...	1.16	1.16	--[b]	1.00
Middle Atlantic	...	1.06	1.09	.96	1.00	...	1.04	1.06	.96	1.00	...	1.04	1.06	.94	1.00
East North Central	...	1.09	1.11	1.01	1.00	...	1.05	1.07	1.00	1.00	...	1.08	1.08	.99	1.00
West North Central	...	1.09	1.10	1.04	1.00	...	1.06	1.07	1.03	1.00	...	.96	.97	.92	1.00
South Atlantic	...	.99	1.01	.90	1.00	...	.99	.99	.99	1.00	...	1.04	1.05	.97	1.00
East South Central	...	1.02	1.02	1.02	1.00	...	1.00	.99	1.09	1.00	...	1.06	1.06	1.13	1.00
West South Central	...	1.04	1.05	.97	1.00	...	1.04	1.04	.99	1.00	...	1.07	1.07	1.02[b]	1.00
Mountain	...	.99	1.00	.91	1.00	...	.99	.99	.93	1.00	...	.99	1.00	--[b]	1.00
Pacific	...	1.03	1.04	.99	1.00	...	1.03	1.04	.99	1.00	...	.90	.90	.93	1.00

Source: Age-adjusted death rates calculated (by direct method, using total 1960 United States population as standard) from age-specific death rates for 1959-61 provided by National Center for Health Statistics.

[a] Geographic differentials calculated as ratios of age-adjusted death rate for each geographic division to corresponding death rate for United States.

[b] Not calculated because total nonwhite population was less than 10,000.

[c] Metropolitan differentials calculated as ratios of age-adjusted death rate for each category of metropolitan-nonmetropolitan classification to corresponding death rate for nonmetropolitan counties.

In general, these divisional patterns obtained for counties classified by type of metropolitan residence, although exceptions occurred. The above analysis obscures differentials in mortality by type of metropolitan residence, which are next examined.

Metropolitan-Nonmetropolitan Differentials

Mortality differentials by type of metropolitan residence were calculated for each geographic division, by sex and color, using the age-adjusted death rates of nonmetropolitan counties as the base (Table 7.1, lower panel). In the nation as a whole, the mortality of all males and all females in metropolitan areas was 5 percent above the level of mortality in nonmetropolitan counties. For both males and females, in all but two of the divisions (SA and Mo) metropolitan mortality was above the level of nonmetropolitan mortality, with the greatest difference found in the West North Central division (12 percent above the nonmetropolitan level for males and 9 percent for females); and also 9 percent above for females in the East North Central division. In three other divisions (ENC, ESC, and WSC) metropolitan mortality for males was more than 5 percent above nonmetropolitan mortality. For females, only the Middle Atlantic division, in addition to the two above, had a metropolitan-nonmetropolitan differential larger than that for the nation.

For each sex in all divisions, mortality in metropolitan counties with a central city was higher than in nonmetropolitan counties. For each sex mortality in metropolitan counties without a central city was equal to or above that in nonmetropolitan counties in only three divisions (ENC, WNC, and ESC).

For both males and females in 8 of the 9 divisions, metropolitan counties with a central city had higher mortality than metropolitan counties without a central city. The single exception was in the East South Central division, where for each sex, although mortality was higher in metropolitan than in nonmetropolitan counties, there was no difference in mortality between metropolitan counties with, and those without, a central city.

For the members of each sex the largest metropolitan-nonmetropolitan differences in mortality were in the Middle West (ENC and WNC). For men the two highest relative mortality levels were in the metropolitan counties with a central city in the West North Central division (15 percent higher) and in the East North Central division (10 percent higher). For women the two highest relative mortality levels were in the same divisions but in reverse order, 11 percent and 10 percent higher, respectively. The lowest relative mortality levels for each sex were in the Mountain and South Atlantic divisions. For men the lowest relative mortality was in the metropolitan counties without a central city in the Mountain division (12 percent below) and next lowest in the South Atlantic division (9 percent below). For women the lowest relative mortality was also in metropolitan counties without a central city in the same divisions but in reverse order, 10 percent below and 9 percent below, respectively.

Patterns of differentials in mortality by type of metropolitan residence differed appreciably for whites and nonwhites. For the nation as a whole the mortality level in metropolitan counties with a central city was 7 percent above that in nonmetropolitan counties for whites of each sex. In contrast, the mortality level for nonwhites in metropolitan counties with a central city was equal to or about the same (1 percent higher for male nonwhites) as that in nonmetropolitan areas. Among whites the mortality level in metropolitan counties without a central city was above that in nonmetropolitan counties for females (3 percent above) and about the same for males (1 percent below). Among nonwhites, in contrast, the mortality level in metropolitan counties without a central city was below that in nonmetropolitan counties for each sex (6 percent below for nonwhite women and 5 percent below for nonwhite men). That is, it appears that for nonwhites the suburban and exurban areas in general offer conditions conducive to relatively lower mortality than do either metropolitan counties with central cities or nonmetropolitan counties. This generalization, while descriptive of the situation for the nation as a whole, does not apply to the individual divisions, among which there is considerable variation.

For white males the general pattern of differentials described above for all males holds without an exception. For white females, however, there was some deviation from the pattern of differentials for all females. In three of the divisions (SA, ESC, and Mo) the mortality level in metropolitan counties with a central city was below that in nonmetropolitan counties. Otherwise, the pattern of differentials for white women matched that for all women.

The pattern of metropolitan-nonmetropolitan differentials in mortality for nonwhites differed from that for whites. For nonwhite males the mortality level in metropolitan counties with a central city was above that in nonmetropolitan counties in all divisions except the Pacific; and the mortality level in metropolitan counties without a central city was above that in nonmetropolitan counties in three of the seven divisions for which the nonwhite data were adequate (ENC, ESC, WSC). In the other four divisions (MA, WNC, SA, and Pac) the level of mortality in the metropolitan counties without a central city was below that in nonmetropolitan counties. The two highest levels of mortality relative to that in nonmetropolitan areas for nonwhite males were in the ENC division, in metropolitan counties with a central city (15 percent above) and in metropolitan counties without a central city (12 percent above). The lowest relative mortality for nonwhite men was in the metropolitan counties without a central city in the West North Central division (14 percent below) and in the Pacific division (10 percent below).

For nonwhite females the level of mortality in metropolitan counties with a central city was above that of nonmetropolitan areas in six of the nine divisions; in only two was this mortality level lower (WNC and Pac); and in one (Mo) it was equal. In five of the seven divisions for which the data were adequate, the mortality level of nonwhite women in metropolitan counties without a central city was below that in nonmetropolitan counties. The two divisions in which the mortality level was higher in metropolitan counties without a central city than in nonmetropolitan counties were both in the South (ESC and WSC).

For nonwhite females the highest mortality levels relative to that in nonmetropolitan counties were in metropolitan counties with a central city in New England (16 percent above) and in metropolitan counties without a central city in the East South Central division (13 percent above). The lowest relative nonwhite female mortality was in the metropolitan counties with a central city in the Pacific division (10 percent below) and in the metropolitan counties without a central city in the West North Central division (8 percent below).

In summary, it is evident that for the nation as a whole and in almost all divisions mortality was higher in metropolitan counties with a central city than in nonmetropolitan counties for each sex. This pattern held for white males in all divisions and in six of the nine divisions for white females. In six of the nine divisions mortality in metropolitan counties without a central city was below that in nonmetropolitan areas for each sex, a pattern which held without exception for whites of each sex. For whites the areas with highest relative mortality were in the metropolitan counties with central cities in the East North Central and West North Central divisions, and in the metropolitan counties without a central city in the East South Central division.

For nonwhites, whose mortality level was above that of whites, the areas of highest relative mortality were for males in the metropolitan counties with central cities in the East North Central, in the West South Central and in the Middle Atlantic divisions; and for females in the metropolitan counties with central cities in the New England, the East North Central and the West South Central divisions. Mortality levels were also relatively high for nonwhite women in the metropolitan counties with a central city in the Middle Atlantic and East South Central divisions.

For nonwhite men pockets of relatively high mortality were also found in the metropolitan counties without central cities in the East North Central and East South Central divisions; and for nonwhite women in the East South Central division.

In light of the higher mortality levels of nonwhites the finding that nonwhite mortality levels were relatively lower in metropolitan counties without central cities indicates that in suburbia and exurbia in metropolitan areas, with notable exceptions in most of the South, nonwhites were experiencing relatively salutary living conditions.

Region Differentials by Race

Mortality indexes were calculated by region for each of the racial groups for which uncorrected death rates were not subject to distortion as a result of discrepancies in the reporting of race on death certificates and census records. In Chapter 6 it was shown that corrections for discrepant reporting of race on the two records had virtually no effect on the mortality indexes for whites and nonwhites and, among nonwhites, for Negroes and Japanese. Similar corrections did significantly change the mortality indexes for Indians (American) and Chinese, however. Because available data did not permit separate corrections for each region, this analysis of geographic differences in mortality by race is limited to four subgroups: whites, nonwhites, Negroes, and Japanese. Small numbers limit the geographic analysis to the four major regions shown in Table 7.2.

The analysis of geographic differentials in mortality by color (white and nonwhite), as well as analyses of geographic variations in nonwhite-white differentials in mortality, is greatly affected by geographic variations in the racial composition of the nonwhite population, especially in the West (Table 7.3). Although Negroes

Table 7.2. Race differentials by regions and region differentials by race: United States, 1959-61

Region	Male				Female			
	White	Non-white	Negro	Japa-nese	White	Non-white	Negro	Japa-nese
Race differentials[a]								
United States..........	0	32	36	-32 [c]	0	52	55	-33 [c]
Northeast............	0	33	37	-- [c]	0	43	46	-- [c]
North Central........	0	34	35	-36 [c]	0	53	55	-58 [c]
South................	0	36	37	-- [c]	0	65	66	-- [c]
West.................	0	8	27	-29	0	26	42	-27
Region differentials[b]								
United States..........	3	26	10	-1 [c]	6	28	16	-4 [c]
Northeast............	7	32	15	-- [c]	14	29	17	-- [c]
North Central........	1	24	7	-10 [c]	6	29	16	-40 [c]
South................	2	29	10	-- [c]	0	31	17	-- [c]
West.................	0	0	0	0	0	0	0	0

[a] Percent difference between mortality ratio for each race and the mortality ratio for whites, same sex and region. Mortality ratios were calculated as ratios of actual to expected deaths in which expected deaths were obtained by multiplying 1960 age-specific death rates for the total United States by the 1960 age composition of each sex-race subgroup in each region.

[b] Percent difference between mortality ratio for each region and the mortality ratio for West, same sex and race.

[c] Not calculated because less than 10,000 population of given sex and race.

constituted 92.1 percent of nonwhites in the nation, they made up only 36.2 percent of nonwhites in the Mountain division and only 51.1 percent in the Pacific division. In the former, 55.2 percent of nonwhites were Indians and in the latter 20.4 percent were Japanese. Since Indian mortality was relatively high (but below Negro) and Japanese mortality was relatively low (lower than white) the "non-

Table 7.3. Percent distribution of nonwhite population by race: United States, 1960

Geographic division	Negro	Indian	Japanese	Chinese	Other
United States......	92.1	2.6	2.3	1.2	1.8
New England............	91.2	2.3	1.3	3.2	2.0
Middle Atlantic.........	96.4	0.7	0.5	1.6	0.8
East North Central......	97.1	1.1	0.8	0.5	0.5
West North Central......	87.0	10.4	1.0	0.6	1.0
South Atlantic..........	98.7	0.8	0.1	0.1	0.3
East South Central......	99.5	0.2	0.1	0.1	0.1
West South Central......	96.8	2.6	0.2	0.2	0.2
Mountain...............	36.2	55.2	5.1	1.8	1.7
Pacific.................	51.1	4.4	20.4	7.6	16.5

Source: Bureau of the Census, 1960 Census of Population, Vol. I, Pt. 1, Table 56 (from 100% enumeration).

white" category can be very misleading in analyses by geographic area.

In the lower panel of Table 7.2 regional differentials in mortality are shown, with the mortality index for each sex and race in the West (the region of lowest mortality) as a standard.

For white males in the country as a whole, the mortality level was 3 percent higher than in the West. Similarly, nonwhite male mortality was 26 percent higher, Negro 10 percent higher, and Japanese 1 percent lower. For white females in the nation the mortality level was 6 percent higher than that in the West, and, for other females, 28 percent higher for nonwhites, 16 percent higher for Negroes, and 4 percent lower for Japanese. The relatively lower regional differentials for Negroes than for nonwhites should not obscure the fact that Negro mortality in the nation as a whole was higher than that for nonwhites (see top panel in Table 7.2 discussed below).

For males the highest level of mortality relative to that in the West was found for each race in the Northeast. For white males mortality in the Northeast was 7 percent above the level in the West, for nonwhites 32 percent above, and for Negroes 15 percent above. Too few Japanese were in the Northeast to permit analysis. The lowest relative mortality for males was in the North Central region, where for whites the level was only 1 percent above that in the West, for nonwhites 24 percent above, for Negroes 7 percent above, and for Japanese 10 percent below. It is noteworthy that the South had a lower level of Negro male mortality than the Northeast, although it was above that in the North Central region.

The pattern of regional mortality differential for females differed from that for males. Although the highest level of mortality for white women was in the Northeast (14 percent above) as for white men, there was relatively little variation in mortality level by region for nonwhite and for Negro women. Only a 2 percentage-point variation occurred for nonwhite women and a 1 percentage-point variation for Negro women. It is striking, however, that the mortality level of Japanese women in the North Central region was 40 percent below that in the West.

Race Differentials by Region

Using the mortality index of whites as a standard for each region, mortality differentials were obtained for each race. These differentials are presented in the upper panel of Table 7.2. Immediately apparent is the fact (obscured in the lower panel of the table) that Negro mortality levels were higher than nonwhite. For the nation, Negro male mortality was 36 percent above white, whereas nonwhite mortality was 32 percent above. In contrast Japanese male mortality was 32 percent below white. Among females, Negro female mortality for the nation was 55 percent above white, nonwhite 52 percent above, and Japanese 33 percent below.

Although the gap between Negro and white mortality was smallest in the West (27 percent above for males and 42 percent above for females), it is evident that there was relatively little variation among the regions in Negro-white differentials. Except in the West, Negro male mortality was more than one-third, and Negro female mortality was from about one-half to two-thirds above the white level. Even in the West Negro female mortality was over two-fifths above the white level. The varying racial composition of nonwhites is apparent in the very small difference between white and nonwhite mortality in the West, especially for males.

In contrast, Japanese mortality for each sex was well below the white level in each of the regions for which sufficient numbers of Japanese made calculations possible. It is evident that the advantage of the Japanese over whites was greater for each sex in the North Central region (36 percent below for males and 58 percent below for females). In the West, where Japanese were most numerous, the gap between Japanese and white mortality was the smallest, but nevertheless great (29 percent below for males and 27 percent below for females).

As indicated for the nation in Chapter 6, mortality levels by race were inversely associated with median family income level in each region (Table 7.4). Without exception Japanese family income in each region, as in the nation as a whole, exceeded white family income, which, in turn, was higher than Negro family income.

Mortality Differentials by States and Economic Subregions

Age-adjusted death rates were calculated for 1960 (1959-61) by states and by economic subregions. Frequency distributions of the rates are presented in Table 7.5. The detailed data for the economic subregions are given in Appendix Table B.1 and for the states in Tables B.2 to B.4. Figure B.1 in Appendix B is an outline map showing the boundaries of the 119 economic subregions into which

Table 7.4. Median family income by race and region:
United States, 1960

Region	Median family income, 1959		
	White	Negro	Japanese
United States.........	$5,893	$3,047	$6,842
Northeast...........	6,318	4,366	7,189
North Central......	5,994	4,267	7,381
South..............	5,009	2,380	4,745
West...............	6,444	4,484	6,839

Source: 1960 Census of Population, Vol. I,
Pt. 1, Tables 95 and 103; Subject Report PC(2)-1C,
Tables 14 and 16.

the United States (excluding Alaska and Hawaii) was subdivided for the 1960 census. These subregions do not necessarily conform to state boundaries, as can be seen in Figure B.1, Appendix B, which also shows state boundaries in those cases where subregion boundaries cut across state lines.[1]

Table 7.5. Distribution of age-adjusted death rates by states and economic subregions: United States, 1959-61

Age-adjusted death rate[a] (per 1,000 population)	Economic subregions				States					
	Total white	Total nonwhite	White		Total white	Total nonwhite	White		Nonwhite	
			Male	Female			Male	Female	Male	Female
4.5- 4.9.............	-	-	-	27	-	-	-	8	-	-
5.0- 5.4.............	-	-	-	48	-	-	-	20	-	-
5.5- 5.9.............	-	-	-	35	-	-	-	16	-	-
6.0- 6.4.............	12	-	-	8	2	-	-	4	-	1
6.5- 6.9.............	41	-	-	1	15	-	-	-	-	3
7.0- 7.4.............	39	-	-	-	22	-	-	-	-	1
7.5- 7.9.............	23	2	4	-	8	1	-	-	-	4
8.0- 8.4.............	3	4	26	-	-	2	8	-	-	8
8.5- 8.9.............	1	7	30	-	1	-	13	-	-	8
9.0- 9.4.............	-	12	35	-	-	8	17	-	1	6
9.5- 9.9.............	-	20	15	-	-	5	8	-	1	7
10.0-10.4.............	-	12	6	-	-	9	1	-	5	2
10.5-10.9.............	-	11	2	-	-	7	1	-	4	1
11.0-11.4.............	-	19	1	-	-	5	-	-	4	1
11.5-11.9.............	-	11	-	-	-	2	-	-	7	-
12.0-12.4.............	-	-	-	-	-	3	-	-	7	1
12.5-12.9.............	-	1	-	-	-	-	-	-	4	-
13.0-13.4.............	-	-	-	-	-	-	-	-	4	-
13.5-13.9.............	-	1	-	-	-	1	-	-	4	-
14.0-15.4.............	-	-	-	-	-	-	-	-	2	-
Q_1 = 1st quartile.......	6.68	9.45	8.45	4.99	6.85	9.45	8.65	5.08	10.90	8.05
Q_2 = median.............	7.07	10.14	8.95	5.26	7.15	10.30	9.05	5.33	11.83	8.80
Q_3 = 3rd quartile.......	7.40	11.09	9.38	5.64	7.39	11.00	9.40	5.65	12.75	9.55
Number of areas[b]........	119	100[b]	119	119	48	43[b]	48	48	43[b]	43[b]

[a] Calculated by direct method, using total 1940 population of United States as standard.

[b] The United States is divided into 119 economic subregions excluding Alaska and Hawaii; Appendix Table B.1 reports the death rates for each subregion and Figure B.1 is an outline map of the subregions. Subregions or states having less than 10,000 white or nonwhite population (males plus females) are excluded from the distributions.

States

Considering mortality by states, first, it may be noted (Table 7.5 and Appendix Tables B.2 to B.4) that age-adjusted death rates for all whites ranged from 6.4 deaths per 1,000 persons to 8.6. Only one state (Nevada) had a white death rate above 7.8. In contrast, nonwhite age-adjusted death rates by state ranged from 7.8 to 13.7 (for the 43 states with large enough nonwhite populations to calculate rates). In only three states did nonwhite mortality at the lower range overlap with white mortality at the upper range.

White male age-adjusted death rates ranged from 8.5 to 10.8. In contrast nonwhite male mortality ranged from 9.0 to 15.4. The median white male death rate was 9.05 compared with 11.83 for nonwhite males. White female age-adjusted death rates ranged from 4.7 to 6.1 as compared with the range of from 6.4 to 12.0 for nonwhite females. The median death rate for white women was 5.33 compared with 8.80 for nonwhite women. Thus, nonwhite mortality not only was well above the levels of white for each sex but also was spread over a much wider range.

Economic Subregions

The age-adjusted death rates for the 119 economic subregions show in greater area detail, of course, the actual geographic variations in white and nonwhite mortality for ecological and epidemiological purposes (see Figures 7.1 to 7.6). Considering first the frequency distribution of age-adjusted death rates by economic subregions it is evident that, as for states, death rates were much lower for whites than for nonwhites and their range was much smaller. White death rates by economic subregions ranged from 6.1 to 8.9, whereas those for nonwhites ranged from 7.5 to 13.8. The median death rate for whites was 7.07 as compared with 10.14 for nonwhites.

White population, total. Because of small numbers and also because the data for nonwhites are confounded by the heterogeneous racial composition of the nonwhite population the distribution of age-adjusted death rates by economic subregion is analyzed by sex only for whites (Table 7.5). White male death rates ranged from 7.5 to 11.2. In contrast, white female death rates ranged from 4.5 to 6.9. It is evident that there was no overlap in the distribution of white male and female death rates by economic subregion. The median death rate of males was 8.95 compared with 5.26 for females.

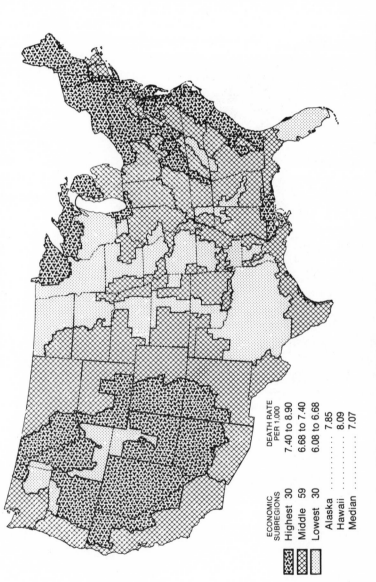

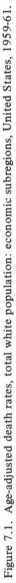

ECONOMIC
SUBREGIONS

DEATH RATE
PER 1,000

Highest 30 .... 7.40 to 8.90

Middle 59 .... 6.68 to 7.40

Lowest 30 .... 6.08 to 6.68

Alaska 7.85

Hawaii 8.09

Median 7.07

Figure 7.1. Age-adjusted death rates, total white population: economic subregions, United States, 1959-61.

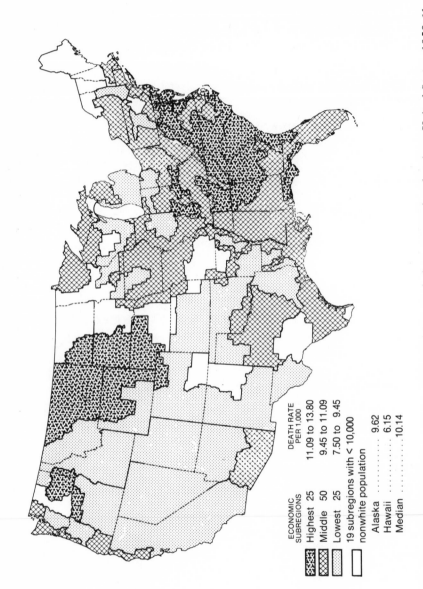

Figure 7.2. Age-adjusted death rates, total nonwhite population: economic subregions, United States, 1959-61.

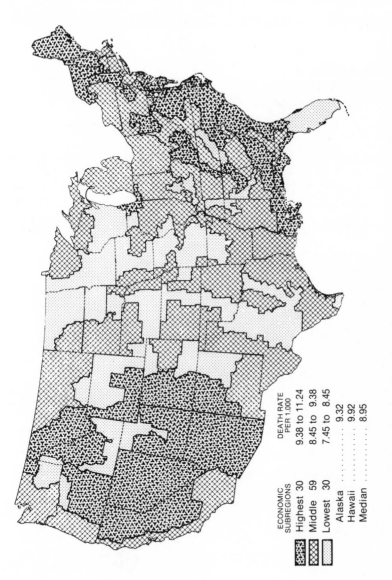

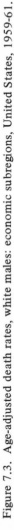

ECONOMIC SUBREGIONS	DEATH RATE PER 1,000
Highest 30	9.38 to 11.24
Middle 59	8.45 to 9.38
Lowest 30	7.45 to 8.45
Alaska	.... 9.32
Hawaii	.... 9.92
Median	.... 8.95

Figure 7.3. Age-adjusted death rates, white males: economic subregions, United States, 1959-61.

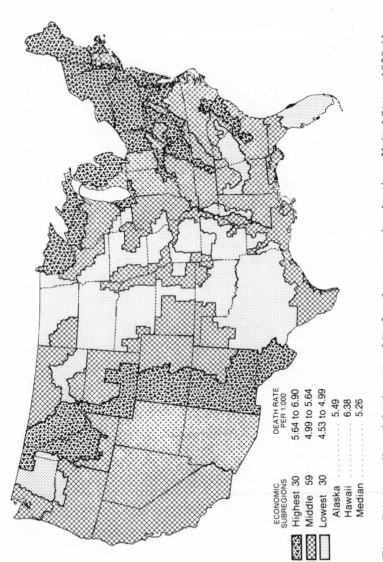
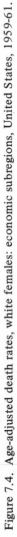

Figure 7.4. Age-adjusted death rates, white females: economic subregions, United States, 1959-61.

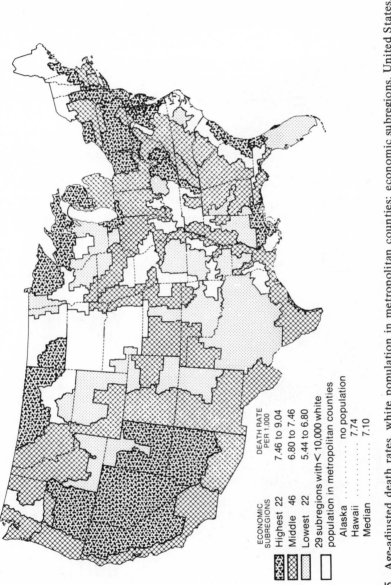
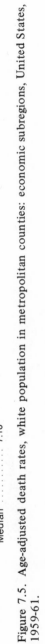

Figure 7.5. Age-adjusted death rates, white population in metropolitan counties: economic subregions, United States, 1959-61.

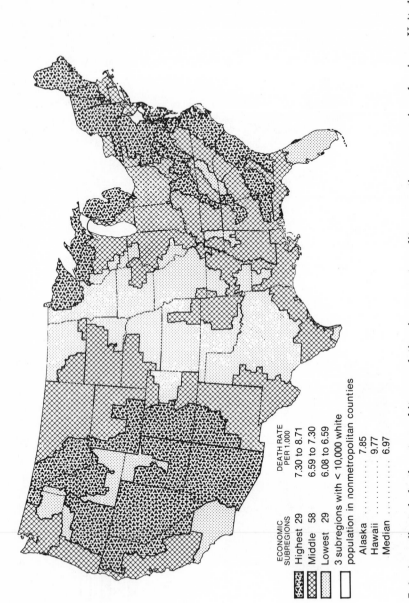

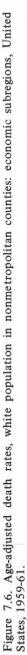

ECONOMIC
SUBREGIONS

Highest 29

Middle 58

Lowest 29

DEATH RATE
PER 1,000

7.30 to 8.71

6.59 to 7.30

6.08 to 6.59

3 subregions with < 10,000 white
population in nonmetropolitan counties

Alaska 7.85
Hawaii 9.77
Median 6.97

Figure 7.6. Age-adjusted death rates, white population in nonmetropolitan counties: economic subregions, United States, 1959-61.

In Figure 7.1 age-adjusted death rates for the total white population are mapped by economic subregion.[2] It is apparent that the highest mortality was clustered in well-definable areas. The 30 economic subregions with the highest death rates (7.40 to 8.90) were concentrated in a contiguous area in Northeastern United States (except for parts of Massachusetts, Connecticut, and Rhode Island and parts of Southeastern Pennsylvania and Northern Maryland) through the Central Appalachian Ridge and Valley (subregion 26), the Southern Appalachian Coal Mining (31) and the Southern Blue Ridge Mountains (33) economic subregions. A second cluster of high mortality was found in the Virginia-North Carolina Coastal Plain (21), the North Carolina Tidewater (22), and the South Carolina-Georgia Upper Coastal Plain (36) and South Carolina-Georgia Atlantic Flatwoods (37) subregions. A third high mortality area was in the Central Gulf Coast (58) subregion. A fourth high mortality area was in the Northern Woods (66) subregion cutting across Northern Michigan, Wisconsin, and Minnesota. A fifth area of high mortality was concentrated in the Southern Lake Michigan Industrial Conurbation (64) in Illinois and Indiana. Finally, a sixth area of high mortality, the largest in area but not in population, was in the Rocky Mountain (109) and the Western Desert, Semi-Desert, and Mountain (113) subregions encircling but not including the Snake River Valley, Wasatch Front and Utah Valley (112) subregion and excluding, also, the Palouse-Columbia River Basin (110). The high mortality in parts of the Southwest was of course attributable, in part, to the in-migration of persons in bad health seeking more favorable climate.

The thirty economic subregions with lowest age-adjusted death rates (6.08 to 6.68) were also well clustered. They included a broad band in central United States running north to south from the Red River Valley (89) and the North Dakota Central Plateau (90) down to Texas, including at the southern end the following economic subregions: Edwards Plateau (100); Grand Prairie and West Cross Timbers (96); Texas Blackland (97); Texas-Louisiana Timbered (79); and the Arkansas-Louisiana-Texas Coastal Plain (80). This concentration of low mortality areas was broken by a contiguous area with intermediate mortality levels which they surrounded, ranging from north to south from the Central Missouri River Valley (85) in Minnesota to the Ouachita Mountains (81) in Oklahoma. Also in the subregions with lowest white mortality were the following: the Florida Peninsula (39); the Southern Blue Ridge Mountains (33); the Alabama Upper Coastal Plain (56); the Tennessee-Mississippi Fall

Line Slopes and Pine Hills (60); Palouse-Columbia River Basin (110); and Snake River Valley, Wasatch Front, and Utah Valley (112).

The white population in the remainder of the nation experienced mortality of intermediate level (6.68 to 7.40).

Nonwhite population, total. The geographic pattern of nonwhite mortality differs significantly from that of the white (Figure 7.2). The 25 economic subregions with the highest nonwhite age-adjusted death rates (11.09 to 13.80) were concentrated in the main in two large clusters with some lesser high mortality pockets.

The major concentration of highest nonwhite mortality was in a contiguous area embracing most or large parts of the following states: New Jersey, Maryland, Virginia, West Virginia, Kentucky, Tennessee, North Carolina, South Carolina, Georgia, Alabama, and Mississippi. Within this broad area comprising most of the old South and the border states, only the Central Virginia Piedmont (20), the Virginia-North Carolina Coastal Plain (21), and the North Carolina Upper Coastal Plain (24) subregions did not fall into the areas of highest mortality, each of these economic subregions having had intermediate death rates (9.45 to 11.09).

The other major concentration of high nonwhite mortality rates was located in the Western South Dakota, Northwest Nebraska, and Southeast Montana subregion (104); the Southwest North Dakota and Northern Montana Plains (105); and the Upper Platte River, Yellowstone Valley, and Big Horn Basin (106). Whereas the non-whites in the South were predominantly Negro the nonwhites in this concentration were mainly Indians or members of other races.

Other areas with high nonwhite mortality were in the Florida Flatwoods (40), the Lower Wabash and Ohio Valley (51), the Ohio-Indiana Flatlands (46), the Palouse-Columbia River Basin (110), and the Northern Pacific Coast and Northern Puget Sound (118) subregions.

The relatively large land area in the West with lowest nonwhite mortality (age-adjusted death rates from 7.50 to 9.45) contains relatively few Negroes and heterogeneous other races, making any analysis with available data potentially misleading in view of the marked differences in mortality by race. But all of the areas of lowest nonwhite mortality merit more intensive ecological and socioeconomic, epidemiological investigation for possible clues which might be useful in the reduction of high nonwhite death rates.

Finally, it may be noted that nonwhite mortality in the north, although much higher than white, in general fell into the intermediate levels of nonwhite age-adjusted death rates (9.45 to 11.09) and were below the nonwhite mortality levels in the South Atlantic and East South Central states.

White population, by sex. Male and female age-adjusted death rates for whites show considerable variation in geographic pattern by economic subregions. In general, the subregions of highest white female mortality covered a smaller land area than did subregions of highest white male mortality; and the subregions of lowest female mortality were more concentrated than those for males.

Whereas the economic subregions of highest white female mortality in the northeastern section of the nation very closely resembled the subregions of highest total white mortality, those for males were much more restricted and excluded most of New York state and Pennsylvania. On the other hand, the subregions of highest white male mortality covered a much larger proportion of the south Atlantic seaboard and Gulf Coast than did the subregions of highest female mortality.

Furthermore, whereas the highest white female mortality followed the pattern of highest total white mortality in the Northern Woods, this subregion was not an area of highest mortality for males. Contrariwise, whereas highest white male mortality closely resembled the pattern for highest total white mortality in the West, those for females included less than half of the western high mortality subregions. The overlap in female and male highest mortality subregions included the Rocky Mountain (109) subregion and then extended into the Trans Pecos and Southern New Mexico (100) subregion, where males had intermediate mortality. Both sexes had high mortality in the Southern Lake Michigan Industrial Conurbation (64).

The subregions of lowest white female mortality were more concentrated than those of white males in the central areas of the nation. They also included the Southern Piedmont (42) subregion, which had an area of intermediate mortality for men.

White population, metropolitan and nonmetropolitan. With few exceptions, the economic subregions of highest and lowest mortality for whites in nonmetropolitan counties matched the map for total white mortality. The differences were too minute to detail here, although they merit ecological and epidemiological attention.

The areas of highest mortality for whites in metropolitan counties (age-adjusted death rates from 7.46 to 9.04) covered a smaller land area and departed significantly from the geographic pattern of total and nonmetropolitan mortality. The areas of highest metropolitan mortality included a much smaller part of the Northeast than either highest total white or white nonmetropolitan mortality. For one thing, most of Maine, New Hampshire, Vermont, and upstate New York did not contain metropolitan counties. The areas of high metropolitan mortality in the Northeast were confined from north to south to the following subregions: New England Secondary Industrial (2); Hudson Valley (6); New York City and Environs (5); Lehigh Valley (12); Philadelphia (13 and 14); and the South Jersey Coast, Delmarva Peninsula, and Virginia Peninsula (15). From east to west the highest metropolitan mortality in the Northeast included the following subregions: Northern Allegheny Mountains (17); Central Appalachian Ridge and Valley (26); Pittsburgh Steel and Bituminous Fuel (27); and Northeastern Ohio-Northwestern Pennsylvania (28). In addition, almost contiguous to the north, the Western Lake Plains-Ontario Shore (9) was also a high metropolitan mortality subregion and, to the south, the Southern Appalachian Coal Mining (31) subregion.

In the South the subregions with highest white metropolitan mortality were the South Carolina-Georgia Atlantic Flatwoods (37) and the Central Gulf Coast (58) subregions. Adjacent to Lake Michigan, subregions of highest metropolitan mortality were the Southern Lake Michigan Industrial Conurbation (64) and the Northern Woods (66). Toward the west there were two areas of highest metropolitan mortality. One was the Southwest North Dakota and Northern Montana Plains (105). The other was a much larger land area including the following economic subregions: Western Desert, Semi-Desert and Mountain (113); and the California Central Valley (116).

The subregions with the lowest white metropolitan mortality were smaller and not as concentrated as the subregions with lowest white nonmetropolitan mortality. The largest contiguous area in the central-south part of the country included the following economic subregions: Ozark Plateau (73); Middle Arkansas Valley and Ozark Slopes (74); Arkansas-Louisiana-Texas Coastal Plain (80); Wichita Prairies (94); Central Oklahoma (95); Grand Prairie and West Cross Timbers (96); Texas Blackland (97); Edwards Plateau (100); Texas-Oklahoma Rolling Plains (101); Southern High Plains (102); and

Southeast Colorado and Northeast New Mexico (107). To the east of this concentration of lowest white metropolitan mortality were almost contiguous, the Alabama Upper Coastal Plain (56) and the Mississippi-Alabama Piney Woods and Southern Brown Loan (59) subregions. To the east and south the Florida Peninsula (39) was also a subregion of lowest metropolitan mortality.

Other concentrations of lowest white nonmetropolitan mortality were to the west of Lake Michigan in the following subregions: Eastern Wisconsin (65); Upper Mississippi River Hill Lands (68); Corn Belt-Dairy Transition (69); and Red River Valley (89). Other economic subregions with lowest white metropolitan mortality were: Upper Platte River, Yellowstone Valley and Big Horn Basin (106); Snake River Valley, Wasatch Front, and Utah Valley (112); and to the far east the Kentucky Bluegrass (45), and North Carolina Upper Coastal Plain (24) subregions.

Correlates of Geographic Differentials

In the course of three separate studies of mortality undertaken at the Population Research Center, University of Chicago, correlations between death rates for geographic areas and socioeconomic indexes for the same areas were analyzed in order to evaluate the extent to which the geographic variations in death rates could be accounted for by differences in average socioeconomic level or other characteristics of the areas. Because they were undertaken in three different studies, with varying degrees of financial support and different objectives, the variables for each analysis were selected independently and the detail of the multiple variable analysis carried out varied considerably, as is evident in the findings summarized below.

States and Economic Subregions

Variations in age-adjusted death rates, 1959-61, among the 48 states and the 119 subregions—excluding Alaska and Hawaii—are summarized in the frequency distributions shown in Table 7.5. For the white population the range of variation was rather small. For example, the interquartile range (Q_1 to Q_3) of the white death rates was only 0.72 in the distribution by economic subregions, indicating that one-half of the subregions had age-adjusted death rates between 6.68 and 7.40. Among the nonwhites, however, the range of

Table 7.6. Simple correlation coefficients between age-adjusted death rates and selected characteristics, for 48 states and 119 economic subregions: United States, 1959-61

Dependent variable, color and sex	Independent variables									
	X_1	X_2	X_3	X_4	X_5	X_6	X_7	X_8	X_9	X_{10}
	Median years school	Median income or earnings, males	Median family income	Percent metropolitan or in central cities	Percent nonwhite	Percent Negro	Percent Japanese (of nonwhite)	Pop. per square mile	Percent employed in manufacturing	M.D.'s per 100,000 pop.
ECONOMIC SUBREGIONS										
All males, all ages......X_A	-.35	-.17	...	.17	.73	...	...	...	.26	...
White.................X_A	.04	.03	...	.25	...	...	...	...	.35	...
Nonwhite..............X_A	-.30	-.30	...	.06	...	...	...	...	-.01	...
All females, all ages....X_A	-.46	-.20	...	.16	.73	...	...	...	.34	...
White.................X_A	-.14	.31	...	.28	...	...	...	...	.55	...
Nonwhite..............X_A	-.31	-.32	...	-.11	...	...	...	...	-.13	...
STATES										
All males, all ages......X_A	-.38	...	-.13	.06	.64	.63	...	.13	.28	-.08
White.................X_A	.06	.23	.30	.12	...	...	...	...	...	...
Nonwhite..............X_A	-.36	-.44	-.40	-.32	...	...	-.32	...	...	...
All males, 25-64 years...X_C	-.48	...	-.31	.05	...	.75	...	.02	.15	-.20
White.................X_C	.03	.05	.11	.15	...	...	...	...	...	...
Nonwhite..............X_C	-.53	-.47	-.49	-.34	...	...	...	...	...	...
All males, 65 & over.....X_B	.01	...	.45	.19	...	.03	...	.52	.64	.43
White.................X_B	.05	.43	.52	.15	...	...	...	...	...	...
Nonwhite..............X_B	.22	.12	.16	.22	...	...	...	...	...	...
All females, all ages....X_A	-.52	...	-.14	.06	.70	.71	...	.31	.45	-.00
White.................X_A	-.20	...	.54	.17	...	...	...	...	...	...
Nonwhite..............X_A	-.45	...	-.41	-.36	...	...	-.53	...	...	...
All females, 25-64 years.X_C	-.52	...	-.28	.06	...	.83	...	.13	.26	-.14
White.................X_C	.02	...	.66	.32	...	...	...	...	...	...
Nonwhite..............X_C	-.59	...	-.49	-.34	...	...	...	...	...	...
All females, 65 & over...X_B	-.20	...	.31	.11	...	.11	...	.62	.72	.40
White.................X_B	-.30	...	.44	.06	...	...	...	...	...	...
Nonwhite..............X_B	.08	...	.03	-.02	...	...	...	...	...	...
Infant mortality rate....X_D	-.52	...	-.61	-.16	...	.75	...	-.26	-.26	-.52
White.................X_D	-.02	...	-.27	.11	...	...	...	...	...	...
Nonwhite..............X_D	-.49	...	-.59	-.51	...	...	-.13	...	...	...

Source: For states, all variables are reported in Appendix Tables B.2 to B.4. For economic subregions, the dependent variables are reported in Table B.1; the independent variables were obtained from special tables prepared by the Bureau of the Census for Donald J. Bogue who made them available to us.

... Data not available, not calculated or not applicable.

LIST OF VARIABLES

X_A, X_B, X_C Age-adjusted death rates, 1959-61, calculated by direct method, 1940 total U.S. population as standard.

X_D Infant mortality rate (deaths per 1,000 live births), U.S., 1960.

X_1 Median years of school completed (by sex and color). For economic subregions this median was standardized for age.

X_2 For economic subregions: median earnings of all employed males in 1959 (not available by color). For states: median personal income, in 1959, of males with personal income (by color).

X_3 Median family income in 1959 (by color for states, not available at all for subregions).

X_4 For economic subregions: percent of population in metropolitan counties (by color). For states: percent of population in central cities of urbanized areas (by color).

X_5 Percent nonwhite, of total population.

X_6 Percent Negro, of total population (not available for subregions).

X_7 Percent Japanese, of nonwhite population (not available for subregions).

X_8 Population per square mile of land area (total only).

X_9 Percent employed in manufacturing industries, of all employees (total only).

X_{10} Number of active non-Federal physicians per 100,000 civilian population (not available for subregions).

variation in death rates was much greater, the interquartile range being 1.64 (from 9.45 to 11.09).

The extent to which these geographic differences in mortality can be accounted for by variations in selected socioeconomic characteristics of the states and economic subregions is examined in Table 7.6, in terms of simple correlation coefficients. These correlations are "ecological correlations," in that they measure the association between variations in average death rates and in average levels of income, education, etc., of large areas (states and economic subregions) with heterogeneous populations. They are not measures of the relationship between mortality and income, or between mortality and education among individuals, and they are not intended as approximations to such relationships. Rather, the ecological correlations are used to measure the extent to which geographic variations in mortality can be accounted for by variations in average levels of other variables in the states and subregions.

First, it may be noted that the correlations between mortality and the socioeconomic indexes for persons 25-64 years old are in many cases strikingly different from those for persons 65 and over. This is not surprising in view of the marked differences in patterns of differential mortality for these two age groups, which has already been noted in Chapters 1 to 5. In fact, the correlation between death rates for persons 25-64 and persons 65 and over is quite low, as is evident in the following intercorrelations (r) between selected pairs of dependent variables for the 48 states.

r between death rate for ages 25-64 and for ages 65 and over

all males	0.32
all females	0.33

r between death rate for all ages and for ages 25-64

all males	0.94
all females	0.92

r between death rate for all ages and for ages 65 and over

all males	0.59
all females	0.65

r between death rates for males and females

25-64 years	0.95
65 and over	0.87

r between infant mortality and death rate for all ages

all males	0.61
all females	0.56

r between death rates for whites and nonwhites, all ages

all males	0.17
all females	0.04

Among the 48 states, the correlation between the age-adjusted death rate for ages 25-64 and the rate for ages 65 and over was only 0.32 and 0.33 for males and females, respectively, indicating that only 10 percent (0.32 and 0.33 squared) of the geographic variations in death rates for persons 25-64 years of age was associated with variations in death rates for persons 65 and over. Correlations between white and nonwhite rates for the states were even lower. For males only 3 percent of the geographic variation in white death rates was associated with variations in nonwhite death rates (r = 0.17) and for females less than 1 percent (r = 0.04).[3] On the other hand, death rates for ages 25-64 correlated quite highly with those for all ages (0.94 for males and 0.92 for females), as did death rates for males and females of the same age (0.95 for males and females 25-64, and 0.87 for males and females 65 and over). Infant mortality rates correlated only moderately with the age-adjusted death rate for all ages (0.61 for males and 0.56 for females).

The proportion of the population that was nonwhite (or Negro) accounted for more of the geographic variations in mortality among states and subregions than did any of the other socioeconomic variables for which data are reported in Table 7.6. For example, among states the proportion of the population that was Negro accounted for 56 to 69 percent of the variation in death rates of all persons 25-64 (r = 0.75 for males, 0.83 for females), and 40 to 50 percent of the variations in death rates for all ages combined (r = 0.63 for males, 0.71 for females), but it had almost no effect on variations in death rates for persons 65 and over. This was to be expected, of course, because, as was shown in Chapter 6, the death rates for whites and nonwhites cross at the older ages; that is, nonwhite ratios become lower than white rates at some point above age 70.

The correlations of median education level (X_1) and median family income (X_3) with age-adjusted death rates for the 48 states were quite varied, and in some cases were of opposite direction to the relationships between mortality and education or between mortality and income which were found to exist among individuals (see Chapter 2). For all males and females 25-64, median years of school completed was negatively related to the death rate (r from −0.48 to −0.52), but for ages 65 and over the correlations tended to disappear. For nonwhite males and females 25-64, similar negative relationships were observed (r = −0.53 to −0.59); again for ages 65 and over the correlation with education level became negligible. Among whites, however, the simple correlations between education and mortality were very low and inconsistent in direction.

Median family income showed somewhat weaker negative correlations with death rates of states than did median education level. Moreover, when the proportion Negro (X_6) was held constant the correlation was positive ($r_{A3.6}$ = 0.37 for males all ages and 0.47 for females all ages), indicating that with percent Negro controlled, the death rates of states tended to increase with increasing average income levels of states. These positive partial correlations for the total population are consistent with the positive simple correlations between mortality and income levels of states for the white population in both age groups in Table 7.6. Except for ages 65 and over, the correlation between mortality and income was negative and moderately high among nonwhites (r from −0.40 to −0.49).

Variations in percent Negro and median family income together account for 47 to 62 percent of the variation in death rates among the states ($R_{A.36}$ = 0.69 for all males and 0.78 for all females, all ages).

For persons 65 and over, variations in death rates by states were positively related to median family income (r_{B3} = 0.45 for all males, 0.31 for all females), positively related to density of population (r_{B8} = 0.52 for males, 0.62 for females), to percent of workers employed in manufacturing (r_{B9} = 0.64 for males, 0.72 for females), and to the per capita number of physicians ($r_{B(10)}$ = 0.43 for males, 0.40 for females). All of this suggests that death rates of older persons, especially, are high in densely populated industrial cities, which also have higher than average income.

Census Tracts (Chicago, 1950)

Age-adjusted death rates for census tracts in the city of Chicago in 1950 have been correlated with several socioeconomic indexes for the tracts.[4] The three indexes used as independent variables were: (1) median family income of all families in the tract, (2) percentage of the dwelling units in the tract that were in substandard condition, and (3) percentage of the census tract's population that was Negro. The age-adjusted death rates were standardized by the direct method, using the 1950 total population of Chicago as standard. In 1950, the city of Chicago was divided into 935 census tracts. After excluding tracts with small or "atypical" populations, which might distort the observed correlations, three samples of census tracts were selected for this analysis.[5] The random sample of 115 tracts for the entire city was selected to represent correlations between age-adjusted death rates of the total population of each tract and the three socioeconomic indexes for the tract. The sample of 84 tracts having 90 percent or more white population was selected to approximate correlations between white death rates and socioeconomic indexes. Finally, the 55 tracts having 90 percent or more Negro population included all the tracts in this category which were not excluded from the analyses for reasons cited in note 5; correlations based on these tracts are intended to approximate correlations between Negro death rates and socioeconomic indexes. The smaller numbers of tracts in the correlation analyses for males and females resulted from the exclusion of additional tracts because the number of male (or female) deaths fell below the required minimum (see note 5).

The correlations in Table 7.7 reveal a strong inverse relationship between total death rates and median family income for census tracts ($r = -0.64$), a strong positive association between total death rates and the proportion of dwelling units in substandard condition ($r = 0.72$), and a positive association between total death rates and the percent of the population that is Negro ($r = 0.54$).

The negative association between mortality and median family income was stronger among total Negroes ($r = -0.68$) than among total whites ($r = -0.46$); only slightly stronger among Negro males (-0.64) than among white males (-0.56), but substantially stronger among Negro females (-0.57) than among white females (-0.21). The positive associations between death rates and the proportion of substandard dwelling units in census tracts were a little larger, but the pattern was similar, with a stronger positive correlation among Negroes than among whites, especially for females.

The partial correlation coefficients in the first column of Table 7.7 indicate the extent to which the relationship between mortality and the three socioeconomic indexes were independent of each other in Chicago in 1950. The proportion of substandard dwelling units had the strongest *independent* relationship to mortality; its correlation with mortality being 0.61 with percent Negro held constant and 0.48 with both income and percent Negro held constant. The correlation between median family income and mortality decreased from -0.64 to -0.46 when percent Negro was held constant and was further reduced, to −0.16, when percent substandard dwelling units was also held constant. The correlation between the death rate and percent Negro was reduced from 0.54 to 0.18 when *both* income and substandard dwelling units were held constant.

These relationships are in marked contrast to those found in Table 7.6. Geographic variations in death rates for states and economic subregions—much larger areas with much more heterogeneous populations than census tracts—were most closely associated with variations in the proportion of the population that was nonwhite or Negro. Correlations between median family income and death rates were much smaller for states and economic subregions, and for whites the association was positive rather than negative.[6] With census tracts as units and Chicago as the universe, the negative association between income and mortality held for whites as well as for nonwhites. This, of course, was not unexpected, given the marked inverse relationship between mortality level and socioeconomic status among whites in the Chicago socioeconomic data analyzed in Chapter 4, which were derived by combining census tracts into socioeconomic groups on the basis of median family income for the tracts.

The multiple correlations in Table 7.7 show that about 56 percent (the square of R 1.234) of the variation in death rates among census tracts in Chicago was accounted for by the three independent variables combined; about 55 percent by median family income and the proportion of substandard dwelling units combined; about 41 percent by median family income alone, and 52 percent by percent substandard units alone. Among white males and among nonwhite males and females, more or less comparable proportions of the variation in death rates could be accounted for by income and substandard dwelling units. Among white females, however, the correlations were considerably weaker. For example, only 12 percent of the variation in white female death rates was accounted for by variations in median family income and percent substandard dwelling units combined.

Standard Metropolitan Statistical Areas (SMSA's)

In the 1960 census, 212 metropolitan agglomerations were identified as Standard Metropolitan Statistical Areas (SMSA's). Population data for these areas were published in the 1960 census reports, and the tabulations of 1959-61 deaths prepared by the National Center

Table 7.7. Simple, partial, and multiple correlations among age-adjusted death
rates, median family income, and proportion of dwelling units in substandard condition, based on census tracts: City of Chicago, 1950

Correlation coefficient	Sample of tracts for entire city (N=115)	Sample of tracts with 90 percent or more white population			Tracts with 90 percent or more Negro population		
		Total (N=84)	Male (N=69)	Female (N=69)	Total (N=55)	Male (N=44)	Female (N=44)
Simple correlation							
r_{12}··········	-.64	-.46	-.56	-.21	-.68	-.64	-.57
r_{13}··········	.72	.52	.63	.34	.69	.61	.62
r_{23}··········	-.72	-.55	-.55	-.55	-.88	-.85	-.85
r_{14}··········	.54	...	...	...	...	...	...
Partial correlation							
$r_{12.3}$········	-.25	-.24	-.33	-.04	-.20	-.29	-.10
$r_{13.2}$········	.49	.36	.46	.27	.27	.15	.31
$r_{12.4}$········	-.46	...	...	...	...	...	...
$r_{13.4}$········	.61	...	...	...	...	...	...
$r_{14.2}$········	.24	...	...	...	...	...	...
$r_{14.3}$········	.26	...	...	...	...	...	...
$r_{12.34}$········	-.16	...	...	...	...	...	...
$r_{13.24}$········	.48	...	...	...	...	...	...
$r_{14.23}$········	.18	...	...	...	...	...	...
Multiple correlation							
$R_{1.23}$········	.74	.56	.68	.34	.71	.65	.63
$R_{1.234}$········	.75	...	...	...	...	...	...

Source: Population Research Center, University of Chicago (see Chapter 4
for sources of basic data). Procedures followed in selecting the samples of
tracts are explained in the text of Chapter 7.

LIST OF VARIABLES

Dependent variable: X_1 = age-standardized death rate, total population
Independent variables: X_2 = median family income, all families
X_3 = percent of dwelling units in substandard condition
X_4 = percent of total population that was Negro
Number of tracts: N = number of census tracts in sample

for Health Statistics included deaths and age-adjusted death rates for
201 metropolitan areas. The 201 areas were identical to the census
SMSA's except for the New England states, where SMSA's were
defined on the basis of townships instead of counties. For the death
statistics, the New England SMSA's were redefined on the basis of
counties, and the total number was reduced from 212 to 201.

Relationships between variations in age-adjusted death rates among
the SMSA's and 23 independent variables were analyzed in a series of
multiple regression analyses. Some of the results are presented in
Table 7.8. The regressions reported in this table were selected to
include: (1) those which accounted for the most variation in death

rates among SMSA's; (2) the simplest regression in which only income, education, and size of area were the basic independent variables (with the addition of percent Negro in the total population); (3) the additional effects of more control variables (percent of population in central city, density, percent in manufacturing industries), an air pollution index, and two housing indexes (substandard condition of housing units and crowding). Definitions of the variables included in Table 7.8 follow:

X_1 Log of population of SMSA, 1960

X_2 Percent of population living in central city (cities) of SMSA, 1960 (separately for total, white, nonwhite)

X_3 Density of central city of SMSA, 1960 (population per square mile)

X_4 Percent of employed persons working in manufacturing industries, 1960

X_5 Percent of occupied housing units in substandard condition, 1960 (separately for total, white, nonwhite)

X_6 Percent of housing units with 1.01 or more persons per room, 1960 (separately for total, white, nonwhite)

X_7 Median family income (separately for all families, white families, nonwhite familes)

X_8 Median years of school completed (separately for total, white, and nonwhite persons 25 and over)

X_9 Percent of population 25 and over who completed 1 year or more of college (separately for total, white, nonwhite)

X_{10} Geometric means of micrograms of suspended particulate matter per cubic meter of air, 1960

X_{11} Number of days with maximum temperature of 90°F or more, 1960

X_{12} Percent Negro, of total population, 1960

The simple correlation coefficients for all males and females show a positive association between their death rates in SMSA's and the proportion of the SMSA population that was Negro (0.55 for males, 0.56 for females), a slightly weaker negative association between death rates and education level (−0.33 and −0.36 for males, −0.48 and −0.49 for females, depending on the measure of education used), and a relatively low correlation (0.28 for males, 0.32 for females) between death rates and the percent of housing units in substandard condition. Correlations for the other variables are too low to be substantively important. The multiple regressions show very similar results. In the case of the three variables mentioned above, their independent effects—as measured by the Beta coefficients in Table 7.8—are very little different from their gross correlations. It may also be noted that the low negative correlation between median family income and mortality (-0.21 for males, -0.20 for females) reverses itself into a very low positive independent effect in the multiple regression coefficients. The highest multiple correlation coefficient (R) for males was 0.76, in regression no. 5, indicating that about 58 percent (R^2) of the variation in male death rates among the SMSA's was accounted for by the combination of independent variables in this regression. The highest multiple R for all females was 0.85, indicating that about 72 percent of the variation in female death rates was accounted for by these variables (also regression no. 5).

About 53 percent of the variation in white female death rates was accounted for by the independent variables in regression no. 5 ($R = 0.73$), but the proportion for white males was much less, only 18 percent ($R = 0.43$). The most important independent variable in this regression was education level as measured by percent of persons who completed 1 year or more of college, which had a Beta coefficient of -0.54 for both males and females. The simple correlation coefficients showed moderate positive gross associations between death rates for white females and the density and industrial variables ($r = 0.46$ and 0.49).

The patterns of relationship were different for nonwhites. Two of the socioeconomic indexes, family income and education level, were negatively associated with variations in death rates among the SMSA's, and the housing indexes were positively associated. The simple correlation coefficients for males were -0.40 (income and mortality), -0.44 (median education and mortality), and 0.36 (substandard housing and mortality). For females, the correlations were -0.30 (with income), -0.43 (with median education) and $+0.36$ (with substandard housing). In all, about 42 percent of the variation among SMSA's in death rates of nonwhite males and females was accounted for by the independent variables in regression no. 4, which produced the largest multiple R.

The lack of substantively important correlations between the air pollution indexes (X_{10} and another index not reported here) does not necessarily imply that these variables may not be related to variations in the level of mortality. However, with the very limited

Table 7.8. Simple correlation coefficients and multiple regression and correlation coefficients based on regressions of age-adjusted death rates on selected characteristics, for 201 Standard Metropolitan Statistical Areas (SMSA's): United States, 1959-61

Color, sex and regression	X_1 Total population, SMSA (logarithm)	X_2 % of population in central city [a]	X_3 Population per sq. mile, central city	X_4 % employed in manufacturing industries	X_5 % of occup. units in substandard condition [a]	X_6 % of units with 1.01 or more persons per room [a]	X_7 Median family income 1959 [a]	X_8 Median years school completed [a]	X_9 % of pop. 25 & over with 1 or more years college [a]	X_{10} Density of particulate matter	X_{11} No. of days with temperature over 90°F	X_{12} % Negro, of total pop.	Multiple R
All males													
Simple correlation, r	.160	-.116	.187	.052	.277	.087	-.209	-.361	-.331	.030	.035	.546	...
β coefficients, Reg. #1	.137	..	..	..	..	..	.049	..	-.340	..	..	.550	.652
Reg. #2	.113	..	..	..	..	..	.130	-.345	..	..	..	.529	.636
Reg. #3	-.019	-.199	.104	.041	.169	..	..	..	..	.167	.012	.610	.727
Reg. #4	-.013	-.179	.032	-.124	..	..	.025	-.319	..	.163	-.043	.592	.757
Reg. #5	.027	-.174	.026	-.148	..	-.045	-.037	..	-.322	.184	.012	.626	.763
All females													
Simple correlation, r	.216	-.172	.315	.256	.321	.097	-.196	-.492	-.483	.072	-.074	.561	...
β coefficients, Reg. #1	.176	..	..	..	..	..	.109	..	-.513	..	..	.582	.768
Reg. #2	.139	..	..	..	..	..	.239	-.531	..	..	..	.551	.744
Reg. #3	-.069	-.061	.243	.139	.227	..	..	..	..	.149	-.157	.657	.795
Reg. #4	-.076	-.040	.152	-.066	..	..	.050[b]	-.396	..	.142	-.219	.651	.833
Reg. #5	.023	-.053	.157	-.079	..	.112	--[b]	..	-.402	.153	-.209	.654	.850
White males													
Simple correlation, r	.197	-.152	.229	.144	-.028	-.136	.053	-.207	-.301	.035	-.059	...	...
β coefficients, Reg. #1	.182	..	..	..	..	..	.075	..	-.338	..	..	...	.376
Reg. #2	.173	..	..	..	..	..	.090	-.264	..	..	..	...	.306
Reg. #3	-.060	-.168	.159	.040	-.040	..	..	..	..	.069	.172	...	.255
Reg. #4	-.010	-.143	.103	-.108	..	..[b]	.077	-.286	..	.035	.150	...	.326
Reg. #5	.028	-.124	.071	-.288	..	--[b]	.183	..	-.541	.021	.191	...	.432
White females													
Simple correlation, r	.312	-.323	.460	.486	.108	-.131	.098	-.477	-.545	.176	-.316	...	...
β coefficients, Reg. #1	.268	..	..	..	..	..	.172	..	-.621	..	..	...	.663
Reg. #2	.223	..	..	..	..	..	.282	-.627	..	..	..	...	.629
Reg. #3	-.028	-.100	.265	.121	.054	..	..	..	..	.169	-.241	...	.596
Reg. #4	.023	-.065	.164	-.126	..	..	.090	-.459	..	.136	-.298	...	.683
Reg. #5	.063	-.088	.191	-.186	..	.217	.142	..	-.542	.102	-.323	...	.726
Nonwhite males													
Simple correlation, r	-.095	-.265	-.015	-.115	.364	.220	-.402	-.440	-.225	-.012	.026	...	...
β coefficients, Reg. #1	.170	..	..	..	..	..	-.458	..	-.158	..	..	...	.451
Reg. #2	.199	..	..	..	..	..	-.229	-.362	..	..	..	...	.482
Reg. #3	.075	.045	.153	.005	.741	..	..	..	..	-.033	-.219	...	.581
Reg. #4	.014	-.009	.068	-.119	..	..	-.411	-.531	..	.211	-.482	...	.665
Reg. #5	-.039	.058	.312	.124	..	.190	-.772	..	-.053	.093	-.234	...	.628
Nonwhite females													
Simple correlation, r	-.154	-.246	-.083	-.024	.355	.318	-.296	-.433	-.308	.062	.105	...	...
β coefficients, Reg. #1	.023	..	..	..	..	..	-.254	..	-.259	..	..	...	.389
Reg. #2	.061	..	..	..	..	..	.065	-.512	..	..	..	...	.440
Reg. #3	-.075	-.039	.086	.064	.534	..	..	..	..	.138	-.014	...	.532
Reg. #4	-.054	.066	.013	-.099	..	..	-.096	-.744	..	.341	-.268	...	.645
Reg. #5	-.165	-.013	.192	.126	..	.299	-.416	..	-.049	.190	-.084	...	.547

Source: Age-adjusted death rates from tabulations of 1959-61 deaths compiled by the National Center for Health Statistics. Independent variables from published reports 1960 Census of Population except X_{10} from U.S. Public Health Service, Division of Air Pollution, Air Pollution Measurements of the National Sampling Network, Analyses of Suspended Particulates, 1957-1961 (Washington: Government Printing Office, 1962), Table 2.3; and X_{11} from U.S. Weather Bureau, Climatological Data--National Summary, Annual 1960, pp. 22-31. Regressions #1 and #2 based on 201 SMSA's for total population and white population, and on 100 SMSA's for nonwhite population. Regressions 3, 4 and 5 based on 119 areas for total population and white population (because variables X_{10} and X_{11} were available only for these areas), and on 82 areas for the nonwhite population. The nonwhite regressions excluded SMSA's with less than 5,000 nonwhite males or females, or with less than 90 percent of its nonwhite males or females classified as Negro.

.. Variable not included in regression.

[a] Variable computed separately for total population, white population, and nonwhite population for use in total, white and nonwhite regressions, respectively.

[b] This variable inadvertently omitted when regression was run on computer.

pollution statistics available on a comparable basis for SMSA's in 1960, and with confounding factors such as the mobility of the population from one area to another and varying lengths of exposure at the levels indicated in the 1960 measures that were available for the SMSA's, the results obtained in this gross approach to the effect of pollution on mortality were not unexpected.

8 / SUMMARY AND IMPLICATIONS

The failure of the United States further to reduce death rates since the early 1950's, especially in the light of the lower mortality achieved by less affluent nations, constitutes a serious challenge and raises embarrassing questions about the quality of life, including the delivery of medical services, in the nation. Moreover, the large differentials in age-adjusted death rates by various indexes of socio-economic status cast serious doubt on the professed equality of opportunity that presumably has characterized this nation from its inception; for differences in mortality may be taken as a significant indication of differences among the socioeconomic levels of the population in life styles and in the potential to cope with the forces that affect life itself—the ability to survive.

Over the years mortality has declined by reason of a number of factors, including increased productivity, higher standards of living, decreased internecine warfare, environmental sanitation, personal hygiene, public health measures, and modern medicine climaxed by the advent of the pesticides and chemotherapy. Programs aimed at the reduction of death rates have been primarily based on biomedical epidemiology and biomedical ameliorative programs. This analysis of socioeconomic differentials in mortality may be viewed as document-ation of the need for increasing attention to socioeconomic epi-demiology. The evidence indicates that further reductions in death rates in the United States may be achieved more readily through programs designed to improve the socioeconomic conditions of the disadvantaged elements of the population than through further advances in biomedical knowledge. It has become increasingly mani-fest that the biomedical knowledge already available is not effec-tively within the grasp of the lower socioeconomic components of the population of the nation. Medical services based on extant biomedical knowledge are not being adequately delivered to the disadvantaged in the United States.[1] But this is but one of the many factors in the deleterious life styles of the lower socioeconomic classes that augment the forces leading to their higher mortality. Other factors, as has been indicated above, some of which affect the availability of medical services, include such items as education, income, occupation, residential location, and all the elements making up the total life style associated with these indexes of the status and role of the person in society.

Summary of Mortality Differentials

Socioeconomic differences in mortality were evident no matter which indexes of socioeconomic level were employed. Highlights of the differentials follow.

Occupation Differentials

The data from the 1960 Matched Records Study for the United States are consistent with earlier findings in this country and abroad in revealing differences of considerable magnitude by broad occupation category (Chapter 3). Because of small frequencies, detailed specific occupational mortality differences could not be analyzed, and thus no information is available in this report on specific differential occupational risks except insofar as they are embodied in the broad occupational categories. In general, from the socioeconomic epidemiological perspective, improvement in the conditions of life of certain broad occupational groups might result in substantial mortality reduction for men; these are service workers, laborers (except farm and mine), and operatives. By reason of previously established correlations, such improvements should decrease not only the death rates of males for whom occupational data are available and analyzed but also those of their wives and other family members. At the extreme, mortality of white males 25 to 64 among service workers was 80 percent above that of the mortality of the occupational group with the lowest mortality, agricultural workers (mortality ratio of 1.37 compared with 0.76).

Education Differentials

Differentials in age-adjusted mortality ratios by education were greater for women than for men in the United States in 1960, and greater for persons below 65 than for those 65 and over (Chapter 2). White males 25 to 64 of lower education (less than five years of school) experienced mortality 64 percent above that of men with high education (four years of college). Among white females the comparable differential was 105 percent. The very large differential for women in this age group is mainly attributable to the high death rates of women with least education (less than five years of school) and may conceivably be, in part, associated with their relatively high fertility (see Chapter 6). White women 65 and over of lower education also experienced much higher mortality than women with high education, whereas among the older men the differentials were minor (67 percent higher for women compared with 4 percent for men). This suggests that improved socioeconomic conditions associated with education might have a marked effect on deaths of men 25 to 64 and on deaths to women of all ages 25 and over. Translation of these differences in mortality ratios into differences in expectation of life indicated that, at age 25, women with at least one year of college could expect to live almost 10 years longer, on the average, than women with less than five years of school; whereas the difference in the expectation of life at age 25 of males of high and low education, respectively, was only 3.2 years.

The sensitivity of age-adjusted death rates to education was evident within the nonwhite as well as the white population. Nonwhite males 25 to 64 years of age with less than five years of school experienced mortality 31 percent higher than that of nonwhite males who had completed at least one year of high school. Nonwhite females with less than five years of school experienced mortality at a level 70 percent above that of nonwhite women with at least one year of high school.

Income Differentials

Differentials in mortality by income were in general pattern similar to those by education. For example, mortality was inversely related to income level, and the income differentials were greater for persons 25 to 64 than for persons 65 and over. However, the income differentials were larger for white males than for white females, whereas education differentials were larger among females than among males. Moreover, among white females educational differences in mortality were as great as, or greater than, income differences whereas this was not the case for men. These findings, however, should not be interpreted to mean that among men income is more important as a factor in mortality than education. Income differentials, as has been indicated in Chapter 2, may be misleading because part of the income differential may be an artifact of a reverse causal path. That is, the basic presupposition in studies of socioeconomic differentials in mortality is that socioeconomic status has an effect on mortality. In the case of the income differentials, however, this causal path is complicated by a reverse path in which the approach of death itself is the cause of decreased income during the year preceding death. For this reason, it has been suggested that education differentials are probably more reliable indicators of socioeconomic differences in mortality than is income. Moreover, income differentials are subject to criticism not only because of a reverse causal path but also because income is subject to variation over time, as compared with education, which remains fixed after young adulthood.

Independent Influence of Education and Income

It was possible, for whites 25 to 64, to study the influence of education and income on mortality, with each, in turn, held constant. The educational differential in mortality of 40 percent for white males—between those with less than 8 years of school and those with at least one year of college—was reduced to 21 percent when income was controlled; and for white females it was reduced from 51 percent to 36 percent. Similarly for white males, the income differential of 77 percent was reduced to 56 percent when education was controlled; and for white females from 41 percent to 19 percent. These findings indicate that from the standpoint of socioeconomic epidemiology life conditions are different for persons with both high education and income status than for those with high education and low income or those with high income and low education. Apart from similar general impact, then, education and income, respectively, have important independent relationships with mortality.

Marital Status

Differences in mortality by marital status indicate that married persons of each sex, white and nonwhite, had lower age-adjusted death rates than the single, divorced, or widowed (Chapter 6).[2] Among both whites and nonwhites the men who were single, widowed, or divorced experienced relatively higher mortality compared with the married than did corresponding women. For example, age-adjusted death rates for the United States, 1959-1961, indicate that white males 35 to 64 years of age who were divorced experienced mortality more than twice that of their counterpart married (130 percent higher); the widowed more than three-fourths higher (78 percent), and the single three-fourths higher (75 percent). Among white females 35 to 64 the divorced experienced mortality 37 percent above the level of the married, the widowed 30 percent above, and the single 34 percent above.

Whereas among the whites the divorced of each sex experienced the highest mortality, among nonwhites it was the widowed of each sex who had the highest mortality. Among nonwhite males 35 to 64 who were widowed, age-adjusted death rates were 89 percent above the level of the married, the divorced 87 percent above, and the single 67 percent above. Among the nonwhite females 35 to 64 mortality for the widowed was 65 percent above that of the married, that of the divorced 6 percent above and that of the single 42 percent above.

The greater influence of unmarried status in generating high mortality for men compared with women may be attributable in part to the greater constraints hitherto placed on the behavior of unmarried women than of men. Apparently men, freed from the conventions imposed by marriage, undergo transformations in way of life disposing to higher mortality more than is the case for women. In assigning the reason for marital differences in mortality, however, it must be borne in mind that biological as well as socioeconomic factors may generate selection forces affecting marital status.

Parity

The mortality of ever-married white women with completed fertility (aged 45 to 64) standardized for age and education definitely varied with the number of children they have borne (Chapter 6). Mortality was greater for women with no children and with only one child (by 7 percent and 4 percent respectively above the average), and for women with 5 or 6 children (5 percent above average) and women with 7 or more children (14 percent above average). Women with 7 or more children experienced mortality 39 percent higher than women with 3 children. It is possible that women with one or no children were subfecund by reason of health problems which also led to their higher mortality. However, the positive association of high socioeconomic status and mammary cancer, with other evidence about the mortality of women who do not bear and nurse children, suggests that perhaps no or limited childbearing may also lead to higher mortality. The evidence is clear that women who bear relatively large numbers of children, five or more, may definitely be subject to higher mortality, independent of socioeconomic status, than those who bear two to four children. It would seem then that fertility control may, in addition to other reasons, be justified as a practice diminishing female mortality. This finding calls for additional and more intensive investigation of the relation of high levels of childbearing and mortality.

Nonwhite-white Differentials

Analyses of nonwhite-white differences in mortality based on uncorrected census and death registration data tend to overstate the excess mortality of nonwhites. With what appears to be the best correction possible with available data (correction for net census undercount), age-adjusted death rates of nonwhites in 1960 were 34 percent greater than white for females and 20 percent greater for males (Chapter 6). Uncorrected rates were 48 percent higher for females and 25 percent higher for males. The greater mortality of nonwhites was much higher at the younger than the older ages; and the mortality of older nonwhites, although distorted by problems of age reporting, may be below the level of white elders, especially after age 75. One theory—that higher death rates in the younger ages allow only the more hardy to survive to the older ages—would be consistent with such a pattern of nonwhite mortality.

Race Differentials

"Nonwhites" in the United States, although predominantly Negro, include other racial groups that can be identified in the official census and death registration data. The 1960 Matched Records Study provided comparison of response tabulations that permitted the correction of the official death statistics for the three-year period 1959-61 for differences in the reporting of race on the death certificate and in the census. The corrections had little effect on the mortality indexes of whites, all nonwhites, Negroes, and Japanese but did significantly change the indexes of Indians and Chinese. The corrected data indicate that the age-adjusted mortality indexes of Japanese 5 years of age and older of each sex were about one-third lower than white and only half as large as those of Negroes. (The Japanese also had infant and child mortality rates one-third below whites and two-thirds below Negroes.)

Negroes 5 years of age and older had the highest mortality of any of the identifiable racial groups, with corrected mortality indexes 47 percent above white for females and 28 percent above white for males. Indians had the next highest mortality with corrected mortality indexes 37 percent above white for females and 24 percent higher for males. Chinese male mortality was 10 percent higher than white but Chinese female mortality was 9 percent below that of white.

Although data on the effect of socioeconomic level on the mortality of the various racial groups were not available, analysis of median family income suggested that the racial differences were at least in part socioeconomic; that is, there was an inverse relationship between the mortality indexes by race and their average family income.

Racial differences in mortality were also summarized in terms of differences in expectation of life. Taking into account the quality of the available data, this analysis was limited to whites, all nonwhites, Japanese, and Negroes. Japanese in the United States had the highest expectation of life at birth, at age 25 and at age 55. Japanese men at birth, with a life expectancy of 74.4 years, could look forward to 6.8 more years of life, on the average, than white men and 13.1 more years of life than Negro men. Japanese women with a life expectancy at birth of 80.4 years could enjoy 5.7 more years of life than white women and 13.2 more years of life than Negro women.

Nativity Differences

Mortality rates by nativity and country of birth derived from reported death and population statistics can be very misleading, as indicated in Chapter 6. For the categories "native white" and "foreign-born white," correction of the reported 1959-61 death statistics for discrepancies in the reporting of nativity on death and census records actually reversed the relationship between native and foreign-born males 35 and over and also affected substantially the mortality differences between native and foreign-born females (see Table 6.7). The direction of the nativity differential also varied by age. For example, using the direct method of standardization for age and correcting the data for discrepancies in reporting of nativity on the death certificate and the census schedule, in the age group 35-64 the death rate for foreign-born white men was 13 percent below that of native white men, but in the age group 65 and over the foreign-born rate was 1 percent above the native. Similarly, the rate for foreign-born white women was 2 percent below that of native white women at ages 35-64 but 8 percent above for ages 65 and over.

Unfortunately the data needed to make adequate corrections of 1959-61 data to reach reliable conclusions about country of birth differences in mortality among the foreign born were not available. The data, partially corrected for discrepancies in reporting of country of birth on death certificates and census records, reveal broad patterns of lower mortality for foreign born originating in the Scandian countries and higher mortality for those originating in Eastern Europe; but obviously distorted data for other areas in Europe make the generalization above also suspect.

Infant Mortality

Only limited national data on infant mortality are presented in this report for two reasons: first, another monograph in this series has delved more deeply into differentials in infant mortality (Shapiro et al., 1968), and second, for reasons elaborated in Appendix A, results from the 1960 Matched Records Study were restricted to adult deaths. It may be noted, however, that in the nation in 1964-66 infant mortality was inversely related to family income and to the educational level of parents (Chapter 2). For mothers with only an elementary school education the infant mortality rate was 77 percent higher than for mothers who had graduated from college. Differentials of similar size obtained by the educational attainment of the father and, to a lesser degree, by family income.

Socioeconomic Differentials in a Metropolis

Prior to the 1960 Matched Records Study for the United States, information on socioeconomic differentials in mortality on a nation-wide basis was based on occupation, the only socioeconomic characteristic reported on the official death record. However, for several decades prior to 1960, data on socioeconomic differentials in death rates within a number of large cities were compiled on the basis of socioeconomic indexes for census tracts where persons (decedents and the base population for death rates) resided. A time series of comparable socioeconomic differentials in age-adjusted death rates, life expectancies, and infant mortality rates within the Chicago metropolitan area throughout the 30-year period from 1930 to 1960 was analyzed in Chapter 4.

Briefly the results showed very marked socioeconomic differentials in age-adjusted death rates and life expectancies in the Chicago area with very little convergence during the 30-year period. There was, however, very substantial convergence in socioeconomic differences in infant mortality during the period. More details on the patterns of these differentials within a large metropolis, and some implications on nationwide mortality patterns, are elaborated later in this chapter in the section on "excess mortality."

Socioeconomic Differentials by Cause of Death

Socioeconomic differences in mortality for selected general causes of death were analyzed for the United States in 1960 and for Chicago in 1950. No attempt will be made here to summarize the analysis that appears in Chapter 5, which is based on mortality indexes by four levels of education for the United States, and by five socioeconomic groups for Chicago. However, the overall impact of the differentials presented in Chapter 5 for the nation as a whole is summarized in the measures of "excess mortality" by cause of death which are analyzed later in this chapter.

Geographic Differentials

Previous studies have demonstrated that there are significant geographic variations in mortality, by region, division, economic subregions, urban-rural and metropolitan residence, and by community within a metropolitan area or central city. In general the findings reported in this study are consistent with previous findings (see Chapter 7). Geographic variations in mortality are presented by sex, color, and race, and an effort is made to determine the extent to which geographic mortality differences are associated with variations in average socioeconomic level of the geographic areas. A summary of these findings follows.

Divisions. Analyses of age-adjusted mortality by geographic division revealed that divisional mortality patterns tended to persist in each of three categories by type of metropolitan residence: metropolitan counties containing a central city of an SMSA (Standard Metropolitan Statistical Area), metropolitan counties without a central city (that is, suburban metropolitan counties), and nonmetropolitan counties.

For the white population mortality was 2 to 9 percent above the national level in the New England and Middle Atlantic divisions; at (for males) or above (for females) the national level in the East North Central division; at (for males) or below (for females) the national level in the South Atlantic division; and 2 to 11 percent below the national level in the West North Central, East and West South Central, Mountain and Pacific divisions. Among nonwhites mortality was above the national level by 1 to 10 percent in the South Atlantic, East South Central, West North Central and Middle Atlantic states; at about the national level in the East North Central states; and below the national level in the other divisions. Nonwhite mortality was exceptionally low—one-fourth below the national level—in the Pacific states, partly because a substantial proportion of the nonwhites in this division were Japanese or Chinese, two nonwhite groups with relatively low mortality rates. These divisional patterns tended to persist—with a few exceptions—for metropolitan counties with and without central cities and for the nonmetropolitan counties.

Types of metropolitan residence. Mortality in metropolitan counties was 5 percent above that in nonmetropolitan counties for white males and females. The greatest difference by type of metropolitan residence was in the West North Central division, where white male mortality in the metropolitan counties was 12 percent above the nonmetropolitan level and that for white females 9 percent above. Metropolitan mortality for white females in the East North Central division was also 9 percent above the nonmetropolitan level.

White mortality in metropolitan counties with a central city was higher than in nonmetropolitan counties for each sex in each geographic division (with two minor exceptions). For each sex in only three divisions (ENC, WNC, and ESC) white mortality in metropolitan counties without a central city was above or equal to that in nonmetropolitan counties. For each sex, in all but one division (ESC), white mortality in metropolitan counties with a central city was above that in metropolitan counties without a central city. Furthermore, for each sex the largest metropolitan-non-metropolitan differences in mortality were in the Middle West (ENC and WNC), where the central city-metropolitan age-adjusted death rates ranged from 7 to 13 percent above the nonmetropolitan level.

Mortality differentials by metropolitan residence varied for whites and nonwhites. Whereas mortality in metropolitan counties with a central city was for whites of each sex 7 percent above that in nonmetropolitan counties, that for nonwhites in central city-metro-politan counties was about the same as that in nonmetropolitan counties. Moreover, whereas for whites mortality in metropolitan counties without a central city was equal to or slightly above that in nonmetropolitan areas, for nonwhites mortality in the former was below that in the latter. Although there was considerable variation in these patterns by division, the evidence indicates that life conditions in suburbia and exurbia (metropolitan counties without a central city) are relatively favorable to nonwhites as shown by mortality, although nonwhite mortality is still above that of white. The highest level of metropolitan mortality for nonwhite males relative to that in nonmetropolitan areas was in the East North Central division, where mortality in metropolitan counties with a central city was 15 percent higher. For nonwhite females the highest mortality level relative to that in nonmetropolitan counties was in metropolitan counties with a central city in the Northeast division, 16 percent higher.

For the nation as a whole, then, and in almost all divisions, age-adjusted death rates for the white population of each sex were higher in metropolitan counties with a central city than in nonmetropolitan counties. In six of the nine divisions for each sex mortality in metropolitan counties without a central city was below that in nonmetropolitan areas. For whites the areas of highest mortality were in the metropolitan counties with a central city in the East North Central and West North Central divisions and in metropolitan counties without a central city in the East South Central division.

For nonwhites, whose mortality level was well above that of whites, highest relative mortality was for males in metropolitan counties with central cities in the East North Central, West South Central, and Middle Atlantic divisions; and for females in the same types of areas in NE, ENC, and WSC divisions.

Color and race. Analyses of regional variations in mortality by color (white-nonwhite), and color differentials in mortality by region, are appreciably affected by geographic variations in the racial composition of nonwhites, especially in the West. (The four broad regions used in this analysis were the Northeast, North Central, South, and West, each representing a combination of two or more of the geographic divisions in the preceding section.)

White males in the nation as a whole experienced mortality 3 percent above that in the West, where mortality was lowest. Nonwhite male mortality was 26 percent above that in the West, Negro 10 percent above, and Japanese 1 percent lower. White females in the nation as a whole experienced mortality 6 percent above that in the West, nonwhite females 28 percent above, Negro females 16 percent above, and Japanese females 4 percent below. For males of each race the highest level of mortality relative to that in the West was in the Northeast. The Northeast also had the highest relative mortality for white females, but there was very little mortality variation by region for nonwhite or Negro women. Mortality of Japanese women in the North Central region was 40 percent below that in the West.

If the mortality of whites in each region is used as a standard then it becomes clear that Negro mortality for each sex was higher than all nonwhite as well as white and Japanese mortality. Japanese mortality was well below that of white in each region. For the nation as a whole Negro male mortality was 36 percent above white, and Negro female mortality 55 percent above. In contrast Japanese male mortality was 32 percent below white and Japanese female mortality 33 percent below.

The gap between white and Negro mortality was smallest in the West (Negro males 27 percent, and females 42 percent higher). In the regions other than the West Negro male mortality was more than one-third above white, and Negro female mortality from about one-half to two-thirds above the white level. In contrast Japanese mortality for each sex was well below the white level.

States and subregions. Considered by states and economic subregions (119 geographic areas into which the nation is divided, as indicated in Figure B.1, Appendix B), it is apparent that the distributions of white and nonwhite age-adjusted death rates barely overlap. The median death rate of whites, when ranked by state, was for males 9.05 (deaths per 1,000 males per year) compared with 11.83 for nonwhite males. For females the median death rates were 5.33 and 8.80 respectively. For whites of both sexes combined the median death rate when ranked by the 119 economic subregions was 7.07, compared with 10.14 for nonwhites.

The series of six maps showing age-adjusted death rates by economic subregions reveal significant clusters of high, intermediate, and low mortality levels (Figures 7.1 to 7.6, Chapter 7). The detailed mappings merit serious ecological and epidemiological consideration. In brief overview the mortality patterns indicate that white mortality was highest in well-defined clusters of subregions in the Northeast, the Appalachians, and the Blue Ridge Mountains; in the South Atlantic Coastal Plains and Flatwoods; in parts of the Gulf Coast; in the cutover regions in the Northern Woods across Northern Michigan, Wisconsin, and Minnesota; and in the Chicago metropolitan and adjoining area; and in large parts of the desert and mountain areas in western United States.

For nonwhites the pattern of subregion mortality differentials varied from that of whites. Highest mortality was concentrated in the industrial parts of the Northeast; the old South and border states; in the West and Northwest parts of the great plains; and in scattered pockets elsewhere. In the North and South nonwhites were predominantly Negro; in the West over one-half were Indian, Japanese, or members of other races, mainly of Hispanic origin. Nonwhite mortality in the North, although above the level of white, was below that in the old South. Significant variations in mortality by economic subregion were found by sex for whites and by metropolitan residence for whites. These differences merit attention for mortality reduction programs but are too detailed for summary here.

Socioeconomic correlates. Assessment of the relationship between geographical variations in mortality and average socioeconomic level of geographic areas was undertaken by means of multivariate analyses (see Chapter 7). The results of this analysis, it should be emphasized, should not be interpreted as indicating relationships between mortality and socioeconomic characteristics of individuals. The findings are presented as ecological correlations, significant in their own right, and not as measurement of the relationship between mortality and characteristics of individuals presented in other chapters of the study. The ecological correlations given measure only the extent to which mortality differences among areas can be explained by variations in the average levels of other variables among the areas.

As was to be expected correlations between mortality and indexes of socioeconomic level for persons 25 to 64 were very different from those for persons 65 and over. Among the 48 states the correlation between age-adjusted death rates for persons 25 to 64 and persons 65 and over was only 0.32 for males and 0.33 for females, so that only 10 percent of the variation by states in death rates for persons 25-64 was associated with variations in death rates for persons 65 and over. Similarly there was very little association between white and nonwhite death rates by states, only 3 percent of the variation in death rates for nonwhite males being accounted for by variations in death rates for white males, and less than 1 percent for nonwhite females.

Significantly, the proportion of the population that was nonwhite (or Negro) accounted for more of the geographic variations in mortality among states and economic subregions than any other variable considered (median years of school, median income or earnings of males, median family income, percent metropolitan or percent in central cities of urbanized areas, population per square mile, percent employed in manufacturing industries, and M.D.'s per 100,000 population). The proportion of the population that was Negro accounted for 56 to 69 percent of the variation in the death rates of all persons 25-64 ($r = 0.75$ for males, 0.83 for females).

Correlations of median education level and median family income with age-adjusted death rates for states varied greatly and, on occasion, in opposite direction to the relationship between mortality and education or between mortality and family income which were found among individuals. For males and females 25 to 64 years of age, median years of school completed was negatively related to death rates ($r = -0.48$ for males and $r = -0.52$ for females). For white males 25 to 64 the relationship virtually disappeared ($r = 0.03$) whereas for nonwhite males it was higher (-0.53). Similarly, for white females 25 to 64 the relationship was negligible (0.02) whereas for nonwhite females 25 to 64 it was higher (-0.59). Median family income had a weaker negative correlation with death rates of states than did median years of schooling. Moreover, when the proportion of population that was Negro was held constant, the correlations became positive; that is, the death rates of states tended to increase with increasing average income levels of states. Clearly these ecological correlations cannot be interpreted as in any way measuring the relationship between the same variables considered for individuals. Chapters 2 and 5 document strong inverse relationships between mortality and income and between mortality and level of education among individuals 25-64 years of age.

For persons 65 and over mortality by states was positively related to median family income ($r = 0.45$ for males and 0.31 for females), to population density ($r = 0.52$ for males and 0.62 for females), to percent of workers employed in manufacturing ($r = 0.64$ for males and 0.72 for females) and to per capita number of physicians ($r = 0.43$ for males and 0.40 for females). These relationships imply that death rates of older persons, especially, are high in densely populated industrial cities, which also have higher than average income.

Age-adjusted death rates for census tracts within the city of Chicago were also correlated with indexes of socioeconomic level for the tracts. A strong inverse relationship was found between death rates and median family income ($r = -0.64$), a strong positive relationship with the proportion of dwelling units in substandard condition (r = 0.72), and a positive relationship with percent of population that was Negro (r = 0.54).

The negative association between mortality and median family income was stronger for Negroes than for whites (r = -0.68 compared with -0.46); somewhat stronger for Negro than white males (r = -0.64 compared with -0.56); and considerably stronger for Negro than white females (r = -0.57 compared with -0.21). The positive correlations between death rates and proportion of substandard dwelling units were slightly higher but similar in pattern.

Partial correlations indicated that, of the three independent variables studied, the proportion of substandard dwelling units had the strongest *independent* relationship to mortality (r = 0.61 with percent Negro held constant and r = 0.48 with both percent Negro and family income held constant). Of the variation in death rates by census tract, 56 percent was accounted for by the three variables combined (R = 0.75), about 55 percent by the income and substandard housing variables (R = 0.74), about 41 percent by median income alone (r = -0.64), and 52 percent by percent substandard dwelling units alone (r = 0.72). Among white females, however, the correlations were considerably weaker than among white males, nonwhite males and nonwhite females.

Noteworthy is the fact that the correlations between mortality and the indexes of socioeconomic level by census tracts in Chicago were similar in direction and intensity to the relationships between mortality and the socioeconomic characteristics of individuals; this did not hold for the correlations between mortality and socioeconomic indexes of states and economic subregions, which were quite different in pattern from the relationships between mortality and socioeconomic characteristics of individuals. The reason, of course, lies in the greater heterogeneity of the much larger state and subregion geographic areas.

Finally, analysis was made of the relationship between mortality and 23 independent variables for 201 Standard Metropolitan Statistical Areas (SMSA's) in the United States in 1960 (Chapter 7). A positive association was found between age-adjusted death rates and proportion of population that was Negro (r = 0.55 for males and 0.56 for females), a weaker negative association with education level (-0.33 to -0.36 for males, -0.48 to -0.49 for females, depending on the particular measure of education used), and a relatively low positive association with percent of dwelling units in substandard condition (r = 0.28 for males and 0.32 for females). Correlations with the other variables were too low to be substantively important.

The highest multiple correlation coefficient for all males was 0.76 and for all females 0.85. Thus about 58 percent of the variation in male death rates among the SMSA's and about 72 percent of the variation in female death rates were accounted for by the independent variables considered. Four of the variables together accounted for most of the explained variation: percent Negro, percent of persons 25 and over with 1 year or more of college, total population of SMSA (log), and median family income; multiple R with these variables was 0.65 for males and 0.77 for females.

For white females the highest multiple R was 0.73 but for white males only 0.43. Thus, although 53 percent of the variation in white female mortality was accounted for, only 18 percent of the variation in white male mortality was accounted for. The most important independent variable for these correlations was education level.

For nonwhites the patterns of relationship were different. Two of the socioeconomic indexes, family income and education level, were negatively associated with nonwhite mortality, and the housing index (substandard housing) was positively associated. The highest multiple R's were 0.67 for nonwhite males and 0.65 for nonwhite females, indicating that 42 to 45 percent of the variation in nonwhite mortality by SMSA was accounted for.

From the evidence gleaned from the analysis of mortality by geographic area the following conclusions may be drawn. First, significant variations in mortality were found which pinpoint the pockets of high death rates by region, division, state, economic subregions, SMSA's and for Chicago by census tracts. These are the areas which call for more intensive ecological and epidemiological investigation and mortality reduction programs—socioeconomic as well as biomedical. Second, areas of relatively low mortality were also identified which merit further investigation for clues to the factors associated with their relatively low mortality.

Excess Mortality

The analyses in Chapters 2 to 7 and the summary of differential mortality in the United States in the preceding section of this chapter have largely been based on relative differences in age-adjusted death rates or mortality ratios for different social-economic subgroups of the population.[3] To assess the impact of these socio-

Table 8.1. Index of excess mortality by color, sex, age and years of
school completed: United States, 1960

Sex, color and years of school completed	25 years & over	25-64 years	65 years & over
NUMBER OF EXCESS DEATHS			
Total population..........	291,838	139,528	152,310
All males...........................	92,049	84,139	7,910
All females.........................	199,789	55,389	144,400
All whites..........................	231,695	92,984	138,711
All nonwhites.......................	60,143	46,544	13,599
INDEX OF EXCESS MORTALITY (PERCENT)			
Total population............	19	26	15
All males...........................	11	25	1
All females.........................	30	29	30
All whites..........................	17	21	15
All nonwhites.......................	36	52	18
White males........................	10	21	2
0-4 years........................	9	30	3
5-7 years........................	12	29	2
8 years..........................	10	25	1
High school, 1-3 years........... } 11		24 }	0.1
High school, 4 years.............		16	
College, 1 year or more..........	0	0	0
Nonwhite males.....................	25	45	0.5
0-4 years........................	25	51	5
5-8 years........................	23	43	-8
High school or college...........	28	39	-3
White females......................	27	21	30
0-4 years........................	42	53	40
5-7 years........................	33	36	32
8 years..........................	31	30	31
High school, 1-3 years........... } 18		12 }	26
High school, 4 years.............		4	
College, 1 year or more..........	0	0	0
Nonwhite females...................	49	60	39
0-4 years........................	51	70	41
5-8 years........................	50	63	34
High school or college...........	44	42	41

Source: Population Research Center, University of Chicago,
1960 Matched Records Study. See text for definition of "excess
deaths." Index of excess mortality is defined as the percent of
total actual deaths in 1960 that were "excess."

economic differentials on the general level of mortality, measures of
"excess mortality" have been calculated. For this purpose excess
mortality has been defined in terms of the deaths that would have
been saved if the mortality level of white men (or women) of high
socioeconomic status had prevailed among all men (or women).

Adult Mortality in the United States, 1960

For the nation as a whole in 1960, excess deaths have been defined as the deaths which would not have occurred if the estimated age-specific death rates of white men (or women) 25 years of age and over who had completed at least one year of college had prevailed in each color-education subgroup of men (or women). They were calculated by applying the estimated annual age-specific death rates of college-educated white males (females) to the age composition of white and nonwhite males (females) in each education category reported in Table 8.1, and then subtracting the expected number of deaths under this assumption from the estimated actual number of deaths that occurred (see Appendix A, Section 5, for procedures used to estimate actual deaths and death rates by age and education level from the 1960 Matched Records Study). The index of excess mortality indicates the percent of total actual deaths that were estimated to be "excess"; negative indexes indicate that actual deaths were lower than expected and measure the percent by which actual deaths would increase *if* the age-specific death rates of college-educated white men (or women) prevailed in each color-education subgroup.

In the United States in 1960, by this definition there were almost 292,000 deaths of persons 25 and over that were excess, about 92,000 male deaths and 200,000 female deaths (Table 8.1). Since there were a total of 1.5 million deaths of persons 25 and over in the nation, about one-fifth (19 percent) of all deaths were excess, over one-tenth of male deaths (11 percent) and three-tenths of female deaths (30 percent). Of all deaths of white adults 25 and over, 17 percent were excess; for nonwhites the proportion of excess deaths was twice as great, 36 percent. Hence, if the mortality levels associated with white men and women having one or more years of college education could obtain for all men and women, over one-sixth of white adult deaths and more than one-third of adult nonwhite deaths might have been prevented.

Among men, excess mortality was greater for those 25 to 64 years of age, both white and nonwhite, than for older men. All males 25 to 64 had an excess mortality of 25 percent compared with only 1 percent for males 65 and over. Nonwhite men 25 to 64 had an excess mortality of 45 percent; white men of the same age, 21 percent. In contrast, nonwhite men 65 and over had 0.5 percent excess deaths and the older white men, 2 percent.

The pattern of excess mortality by age was quite different among women. Approximately three-tenths of all female deaths for both age groups were excess, 29 percent for women 25-64 and 30 percent for women 65 and over. Among white women, excess mortality was less at ages 25-64 (21 percent) than at ages 65 and over (30 percent). In contrast, 60 percent of all deaths to nonwhite females 25 to 64 were excess; whereas 39 percent of the deaths to nonwhite females 65 and over were excess.

The proportionate distribution of excess adult deaths by age for men and women was quite different. Only 9 percent (7,910 out of 92,049) of the excess deaths to males 25 and over occurred at ages 65 and over, whereas 72 percent (144,400 out of 199,789) of the excess female deaths occurred at the older ages. There were also substantial differences between whites and nonwhites in the percentage of excess adult deaths occurring after age 65, 60 percent of the white deaths compared to 23 percent of the nonwhite deaths.

It is doubtful that any other data as dramatically reveal the disadvantaged position of nonwhites in the nation (predominantly Negro) as these data on excess mortality. To demonstrate that excess mortality of adult nonwhites in the nation is over twice as great as white (36 percent compared with 17 percent), almost three times as great for nonwhite females 25 to 64 (60 percent compared with 21 percent), and over twice as great for nonwhite males 25 to 64 (45 percent as compared with 21 percent) is to point to the great potential for decreasing mortality through improved social and economic conditions of nonwhites in the nation.

Adult White Mortality by Cause of Death

Calculations of excess adult deaths have also been made for whites by cause of death; that is, estimates have been made of the number and percentage of white deaths from each cause in the nation in 1960 that would not have occurred if the mortality indexes for the less educated subgroups had been equal to the indexes for the college educated. The resulting indexes of excess mortality (percentages) are summarized in Table 8.2. They were derived from the mortality ratios prepared for the analysis in Chapter 5 by an indirect approximation because estimates of annual age-specific death rates from each cause were not available for college-educated whites.[4] Comparison of the indirect estimates of excess adult mortality for all causes of death in Table 8.2 with corresponding direct estimates

Table 8.2. Index of excess mortality from each cause of death, by sex and age, for the white population 25 years and over: United States, 1960

Cause of death (ISC codes)	White males			White females		
	25 & over	25-64 years	65 & over	25 & over	25-64 years	65 & over
ALL CAUSES...	9	25	0.1	29	22	32
1. Tuberculosis, all forms (001-019).............................	57	82	--[a]	--[a]	--[a]	--[a]
2. Malignant neoplasms, incl. lymph. & hematop. tissues (140-205)..	-1	17	-14	10	10[a]	11[a]
2a. of stomach (151)..	47	48	47	63	--	--
2b. of intestine & rectum (152-154)............................	4	3	4	30	29	30[a]
2c. of lung, bronchus & trachea (162,163)......................	28[a]	43[a]	11[a]	1	12	--[a]
2d. of breast (170)...	--	--[a]	--	-21	-13	-32
2e. of uterus, ovary, fallopian tube & broad ligament (171-175).	...	...[a]	...	22	36	2
2f. of prostate (177)...	-103	--[a]	-105	...	...	...
2g. Other malignant neoplasms.................................	-4	8	-15[a]	4	-1	8
3. Diabetes mellitus (260)....................................	13	32	--[a]	60	54	63
4. Major cardiovascular-renal diseases (330-334,400-468,592-594)...	8	22	2	37	38	37
4a. Vascular lesions affecting central nervous system (330-334).	17	10	18[a]	32	32	31[a]
4b. Rheumatic fever & chronic rheumatic heart disease (400-416).	13	24	--[a]	-3	15	--
4c. Arteriosclerotic & degenerative heart disease (420,422).....	9	21	2	41	45	40
4d. Hypertensive disease, with & without heart (440-447)........	1	33	-10	53	45	54
4e. Other cardiovascular-renal diseases.......................	-7	34	-22	24	29[a]	23
5. Influenza & pneumonia, except pneumonia of newborn (480-493)....	24	42	17[a]	33	--[a]	36[a]
6. Cirrhosis of liver (581)...................................	-19	7	--[a]	6	13	--[a]
7. All accidents (800-962)...................................	45	41	52[a]	29	7	43[a]
7a. Motor-vehicle accidents (810-835).........................	41	35	--[a]	7	-10[a]	--[a]
7b. Accidents except motor vehicle (800-802,840-962)...........	48	47	49[a]	38[a]	--[a]	--[a]
8. Suicide (963,970-979)......................................	37	33	--	--	--	--
9. Other causes of death......................................	8	33	-10	10	8	11

Source: Population Research Center, University of Chicago, 1960 Matched Records Study (see Appendix A). See text for definition of index of excess mortality.

[a] Mortality index not computed because of small numbers of deaths; mortality from this cause included in "residual" category.

reported in Table 8.1 shows that quite similar results are obtained by the two calculations.[5] For the following specific causes of death, more than one-fourth of the deaths would not have occurred (were excess) among at least one of the sexes, as summarized below:

Cause of Death	Percent Excess Deaths	
	Males	Females
Tuberculosis	57	—
Malignant neoplasm of stomach	47	63
of intestine and rectum	4	30
of lung, etc.	28	1
Diabetes mellitus	13	60
Vascular lesions	17	32
Arteriosclerotic heart disease	9	41
Hypertensive disease	1	53
Influenza and pneumonia	24	33
Motor vehicle accidents	41	7
Other accidents	48	38
Suicide	37	—

There are interesting variations in excess mortality between the older and younger men and women, respectively, as shown in Table 8.2.

For both men and women causes of death which were positively related to education tended, of course, to diminish the excess mortality for all causes of death combined. For males, the number of deaths from cancer of the prostate would have been more than doubled if the mortality of the college educated had prevailed at all education levels. Among females, the proportion of deaths from breast cancer would have been increased by 21 percent.

The combined effect of sensitivity to education and relative importance in contributing to total adult mortality is given by the proportionate distribution of "net excess" deaths by cause as shown in Table 8.3. The number of excess deaths in the cardiovascular-renal diseases alone was 53.1 percent as large as the total net excess mortality from all causes of death combined for males, and 78.0 percent as large as the total net excess for females (Table 8.3). If these percentages were based on the sum of all "positive excess"

Table 8.3. Proportionate distribution of "excess mortality" by cause of death and sex, for the white population 25 years and over: United States, 1960

Cause of death	White males	White females
All causes, persons 25 & over..................	100.0	100.0
1. Tuberculosis, all forms.............................	4.6	--[a]
2. Malignant neoplasms, incl. lymph. & hematop. tissues.	-2.0	6.5
2a. of stomach..	7.3	2.5
2b. of intestine & rectum.............................	1.0	3.3
2c. of lung, bronchus, & trachea.....................	10.9[a]	0.0
2d. of breast..	--	-2.6
2e. of uterus, ovary, fallopian tube & broad ligament	...	2.4
2f. of prostate......................................	-17.7	...
2g. Other malignant neoplasms........................	-3.4	0.9
3. Diabetes mellitus..................................	1.8	5.3
4. Major cardiovascular-renal diseases................	53.1	78.0
4a. Vascular lesions affecting central nervous system	18.3	16.0
4b. Rheumatic fever & chronic rheumatic heart disease	1.4	-0.2
4c. Arteriosclerotic & degenerative heart disease....	37.5	46.1
4d. Hypertensive disease, with & without heart.......	0.2	10.6
4e. Other cardiovascular-renal diseases..............	-4.2	5.4
5. Influenza & pneumonia, except pneumonia of newborn...	8.3	3.8
6. Cirrhosis of liver.................................	-3.2	0.2
7. All accidents......................................	22.8	3.2
7a. Motor-vehicle accidents..........................	8.6	0.2
7b. Accidents except motor vehicle...................	14.2	2.9[a]
8. Suicide..	6.4	--[a]
9. Other causes of death..............................	8.1	3.2

Source: Population Research Center, University of Chicago, 1960 Matched Records Study (see Appendix A). See text for definition of excess mortality. See Table 8.2 for ISC codes for each cause of death.

[a] Mortality index not computed because of small numbers of deaths; mortality from this cause included in "residual" category.

deaths instead of the total "net excess"—a more valid base, perhaps, for comparing men and women—the percentages would be reduced to 41.3 percent for males and 75.8 percent for females.[6]

Among males, four specific causes of death accounted for 62.9 percent of the "positive excess" mortality. These causes are arteriosclerotic and degenerative heart disease (29.1 percent), vascular lesions (14.2 percent), accidents except motor vehicle (11.1 percent), and cancer of the lung (8.5 percent). Among females, three causes accounted for 70.8 percent of the "positive excess" mortality. These causes are arteriosclerotic and degenerative heart disease (44.9 percent), vascular lesions (15.6 percent), and hypertensive disease (10.3 percent).

Trends in a Metropolis, 1930-60

In order to assess the trends in excess mortality in the Chicago Standard Metropolitan Statistical Area (SMSA) between 1930 and 1960, the indexes reported in Tables 8.4 and 8.5 were calculated. These indexes indicate the percentage of deaths that would not have occurred on each date if the age-specific death rates of white males (or females) in the group with the lowest mortality on that date had prevailed in all socioeconomic groups. Death rates for the ring of the SMSA provided the base for the calculation of excess mortality in 1960; in 1950 and earlier years the rates for SE group 5, the highest socioeconomic group within the city of Chicago, provided the base. The age-adjusted death rates in Table 4.3, Chapter 4, show that between 1950 and 1960 the lowest white death rates in the SMSA shifted from the city's SE group 5 to the ring of the SMSA. This shift may well reflect the flight to the suburbs of some of the more affluent white population during the decade and the relative lowering of the socioeconomic level of whites in the city that resulted (de Vise, 1967, p. 40).

Adult mortality. The greatest excess mortality during the 30-year period examined (1930-1960) occurred among nonwhite females 25 to 64. For the city as a whole, nonwhite female excess mortality among those 25 to 64 years of age ranged from a high of 74 percent in 1930 (and also 1940) to 64 percent in 1960; that is, as recently as 1960, 64 percent of deaths of nonwhite women 25 to 64 years of age would not have occurred had they enjoyed the age-specific death rates of white women in the ring of the SMSA. Furthermore, among

Table 8.4. Index of excess mortality by color, sex and socioeconomic group: Chicago Standard
Metropolitan Statistical Area (SMSA) and City of Chicago, 1930-1960

Sex, color and socioeconomic group[a]	Index of excess mortality[b]											
	All ages				Ages 25-64				Ages 65 & over			
	1960	1950	1940	1929-1931	1960	1950	1940	1929-1931	1960	1950	1940	1929-1931
White males												
Chicago SMSA..........	15	19	---	---	22	27	---	---	12	10	---	---
City of Chicago.....	24	22	14	23	33	31	18	26	18	13	8	8
SE 1 (low).......	44	41	37	45	55	53	45	51	37	28	23	17
SE 2.............	25	26	20	29	35	36	25	32	19	15	10	12
SE 3.............	16	11	5	17	26	20	5	20	11	3	3	7
SE 4.............	8	8	-2	8	14	15	-9	7	5	2	1	3
SE 5 (high)......	11	0	0	0	18	0	0	0	7	0	0	0
Ring (outside City).	0	5	---	---	0	7	---	---	0	-0.0	---	---
Nonwhite males												
Chicago SMSA..........	39	49	---	---	50	59	---	---	14	17	---	---
City of Chicago.....	41	50	57	67	52	60	64	69	15	19	19	27
SE 1 (low).......	51	56	64	73	65	68	72	76	26	23	29	30
SE 2.............	41	49	56	69	53	58	65	72	14	15	5	30
SE 3 (high)......	21	37	50	59	27	41	52	60	-3	15	26	22
Ring (outside City).	21	--*	---	---	--*	--*	---	---	--*	--*	---	---
White females												
Chicago SMSA..........	10	16	---	---	17	24	---	---	7	12	---	---
City of Chicago.....	16	18	19	25	26	27	29	29	10	13	11	11
SE 1 (low).......	35	34	41	44	52	49	52	50	26	23	26	16
SE 2.............	19	23	26	32	35	35	36	37	12	17	16	15
SE 3.............	10	15	17	23	21	22	26	27	4	12	11	12
SE 4.............	4	9	8	15	5	13	14	17	4	8	5	9
SE 5 (high)......	5	0	0	0	2	0	0	0	5	0	0	0
Ring (outside City).	0	5	---	---	0	9	---	---	0	4	---	---
Nonwhite females												
Chicago SMSA..........	45	51	---	---	63	69	---	---	7	8	---	---
City of Chicago.....	46	51	60	69	64	69	74	74	9	10	6	16
SE 1 (low).......	53	58	66	75	73	74	80	80	12	15	21	18
SE 2.............	46	50	60	71	63	68	74	75	10	12	1	28
SE 3 (high)......	36	40	55	61	52	62	69	68	4	-2	0.0	3
Ring (outside City).	26	--*	---	---	--*	--*	---	---	--*	--*	---	---

Source: Derived from age-specific death rates used to calculate the age-adjusted death rates reported
in Table 4.3 (see Source, Table 4.3).

See Table 4.3 for notes a and --*.

[b] For all years except 1960, this index indicates the percent of the actual deaths that would have been
saved in each group if the age-specific death rates for white persons of the same sex in the highest socioeconomic group in the City had prevailed in that group; for 1960 the index indicates the percent of actual
deaths that would have been saved if the death rates for white persons of the same sex living in the Ring
of the SMSA had prevailed. Negative percents indicate that actual deaths were lower than expected under
the same assumption; that is, a negative index indicates the percent by which actual deaths would increase
if the age-specific death rates of "white person of the same sex in the highest socioeconomic group in the
City (or the Ring)" had prevailed.

nonwhite women 25 to 64 in the lowest socioeconomic group excess
mortality was at the level of 80 percent in 1930 (and 1940) and was
still 73 percent in 1960. Even in the highest socioeconomic class
excess mortality for nonwhite females 25 to 64 years old was 52
percent in 1960.

Nonwhite males 25 to 64 ranked second in excess mortality over
the entire period. For the city as a whole, excess mortality of
nonwhite males 25 to 64 ranged from 69 percent in 1930 to 52
percent in 1960. Their excess mortality in the lowest socioeconomic
class ranged from 76 percent in 1930 to 65 percent in 1960. Striking

Table 8.5. Index of excess infant mortality by color, sex and socioeconomic group: Chicago Standard Metropolitan Statistical
Area (SMSA) and City of Chicago, 1930-1960

Color and socioeconomic group[a]	Index of excess infant mortality[b]					
	Males			Females		
	1960	1940	1929-1931	1960	1940	1929-1931
White, Chicago SMSA........	6	---	---	9	---	---
City of Chicago.........	12	12	40	18	-4	40
SE 1 (low)..........	29	24	56	31	9	57
SE 2.................	18	15	47	21	5	45
SE 3.................	0.0	8	30	8	-12	33
SE 4.................	-2	4	25	5	-23	21
SE 5 (high)..........	6	0	0	16	0	0
Ring of SMSA...........	0	---	---	0	---	---
Nonwhite, Chicago SMSA.....	45	---	---	55	---	---
City of Chicago.........	45	45	61	55	20	62
SE 1 (low)..........	47	36	65	55	19	64
SE 2.................	46	52	64	57	19	64
SE 3 (high)..........	39	36	53	51	21	59
Ring of SMSA...........	--*	---	---	--*	---	---

Source: Table 4.5. Data for 1950 indexes not available (see
Source, Table 4.5).

See Table 4.3 for notes a and --*.

[b] For each year except 1960 this index indicates the percent of
actual infant deaths that would have been saved in each group if the
infant mortality rate for white infants of the same sex in the highest
socioeconomic group in the City had prevailed in the group; for 1960 the
index indicates the percent of infant deaths that would have been saved
if the rate for white infants of the same sex in the Ring of the SMSA
had prevailed. Negative percents indicate that actual deaths were lower
than expected under the same assumption.

improvement in excess mortality for nonwhite males 25-64 in the
highest socioeconomic group is manifest in the drop of their excess
mortality between 1930 and 1960 from 60 percent to 27 percent.

Among white males 25 to 64 in the city, excess deaths decreased
from 26 percent in 1930 to 18 percent in 1940 and then increased to
31 and 33 percent, respectively, in 1950 and 1960. In the lowest
socioeconomic group excess mortality was 51 percent at the beginning of the period and was 55 percent in 1960. In fact, in 1960
excess mortality for white males 25 to 64 in each socioeconomic
group was larger than in 1930.

White females 25 to 64, who enjoy relatively low mortality,
nevertheless evidenced high excess mortality, especially in the lower
socioeconomic classes. Moreover, excess white female mortality in

the lowest classes showed relatively little change over the 30 years studied. Mortality for white women 25-64 was 29 percent in excess in 1930 and was still at 26 percent in 1960. In the lowest socioeconomic group white female excess mortality in 1960 was 52 percent, a level that was almost constant throughout the 30-year period. In the second lowest socioeconomic class excess mortality in 1960 was 35 percent, very close to its earlier levels. In the intermediate socioeconomic class excess (SE 3) mortality was still relatively high in 1960, 21 percent, but the excess deaths in this class showed some decline during the period (from 27 percent in 1930). In the ring, white female mortality for women 25 to 64 was 9 percent in excess of SE group 5 in 1950, and only 2 percent below the level of the same group in 1960.

Excess mortality, on the whole, was lower for persons 65 and over both for whites and nonwhites. In the city, the greatest excess mortality among these senior citizens in 1960 was to be found among white males, 18 percent; next, among nonwhite males, 15 percent; then among white females, 10 percent; and lowest among nonwhite females 65 and over, 9 percent.

White older males in the lowest socioeconomic class had 37 percent excess mortality in 1960, a level well above that in 1930 (17 percent). Consistent with the data reported above, excess mortality for older white men in the lowest socioeconomic class increased consistently over the period. White older females in the lowest class had 26 percent excess mortality in 1960, a level also considerably above that in 1930 (16 percent). Nonwhite older males in the lowest class had 26 percent excess mortality in 1960, a level below that in 1930 (30 percent). Nonwhite older females in the lowest class had 12 percent excess deaths in 1960, a level also below that in 1930 (18 percent).

Infant mortality. As was to be expected, excess nonwhite infant mortality was well above that of white. For the city as a whole in 1930 almost two-thirds of the nonwhite infant deaths, 61 percent for males and 62 percent for females, would not have occurred if nonwhites had had the infant mortality rates of whites in SE group 5; and in 1960 the excess was still quite high, 45 percent for nonwhite males and 55 percent for nonwhite females (Table 8.5). Excess infant mortality for whites in the city decreased sharply between 1930 and 1960, from 40 to 12 percent for males and from 40 to 18 percent for females.

Virtually all of the decrease in excess infant mortality in the Chicago area occurred during the first decade of the 30-year period, both for whites and for nonwhites. The apparent very low excess mortality for white and nonwhite females in 1940 is entirely due to the fact that the base population for measuring their excess mortality (SE group 5) had a relatively high infant mortality rate. If the infant mortality rate for white females in SE group 4, which was 23 percent below that of SE group 5 (see Table 4.5), is used as the base, the excess infant mortality for all white females in the city in 1940 is 18 percent, and that for all nonwhite females in the city is 54 percent. These revised measures of excess mortality for females in 1940 thus fall in line with the trend in excess male infant mortality, that is, sharp decreases between 1930 and 1940 and very little change between 1940 and 1960.

It is also clear from the indexes in Table 8.5 and the rates in Table 4.5 that since 1940 there has been no consistent inverse relationship between infant mortality and socioeconomic status within the nonwhite population in the city and also among the 60 percent of the white population in SE groups 3 to 5. The reasons for this merit further exploration.

Quality of Mortality Data

Measures of differential mortality are subject to error as a result of errors in the basic death and population statistics from which they are derived. To the extent that there are compensating errors in the two sources of data, errors in death rates derived from them are diminished. For example, if for a given age there is a 5-percent underregistration of deaths and a 5-percent undercount of population, there will be no error in the death rate calculated for this age group from the reported data. Currently in the United States there is very little basis for assuming compensating errors in reported deaths and population counts, however. In general, the registration of deaths is believed to be virtually complete, except possibly for a few isolated areas (NCHS, 1964, page 7-14), and response error is therefore the main source of error in death statistics.

Errors in census statistics stem from two sources, incomplete coverage and response error, the net result of which is called "net census undercount" (Siegel, 1968). Net census undercounts tend to be larger among lower status, disadvantaged subgroups of the population, a factor which leads to overestimation of mortality levels for these subgroups. This was documented for nonwhites in Chapter 6, where it was shown, for example, that the uncorrected death rate for nonwhite males was 25 percent higher than that for white males, as compared with a 20-percent differential after correction of both rates for net census undercounts. Similarly, an uncorrected nonwhite-white differential of 48 percent for females was reduced to 34 percent after correction for net census undercount. Thus, despite considerably poorer quality of census data for nonwhites than whites, the corrected nonwhite-white mortality differential was four-fifths as large as the uncorrected differential for males, and three-fourths as large as the uncorrected differential for females. No estimates have been made of net census undercounts by socioeconomic level within the white or nonwhite population. However, it may not be unrealistic to assume that the overestimation of socioeconomic differentials in mortality as a result of differential census undercounts is roughly of the same magnitude as the overestimation of the nonwhite-white differential in mortality. If this is true, no more than one-fourth of the socioeconomic differentials in mortality documented in this report—including the measures of excess mortality described earlier in this chapter—should be attributable to errors in census data.

The 1960 mortality differentials by education, income, occupation, and parity presented in this report, which were based on the 1960 Matched Records Study, include a built-in correction for discrepant responses on census and other records, as both the death and population statistics used in their calculation were classified by estimated "census characteristics" (see Appendix A). That is, of the two potential sources of error mentioned at the beginning of this section—death certificate response error and net census undercounts—the latter clearly are the main source of error in the mortality ratios calculated from the 1960 Matched Records Study.

However, death rates calculated from uncorrected tabulations of deaths and population statistics are subject to error—as shown in Chapter 6 in the analysis of mortality differentials by color and race, nativity, ethnicity, and marital status—not only because of errors in census data but also because of response errors on death records. In Chapter 6, efforts were made to assess the effects of net census undercounts by color, sex, and age, using Siegel's estimates of net census undercounts for the United States in 1960. In the absence of direct information on death certificate response error, data from the 1960 Matched Records Study on discrepancies in the reporting of race, nativity and ethnicity, and marital status on the death and census records were used to determine the extent of error in death rates from this source. Death rates for one or more subgroups of the population were significantly distorted by both sources of error, as indicated in Chapter 6.

Significance of Findings

The analyses of socioeconomic differences in mortality for the nation as a whole are restricted to the cross-section examination of differentials in 1960. Longitudinal data for the analysis of changes in socioeconomic differentials over time were analyzed only for the Chicago area. The time series of socioeconomic differentials in mortality in Chicago from 1930 to 1960 have important implications with respect to mortality trends in the nation as a whole, however, as elaborated below.

First, the Chicago data confirm one of the most significant findings of earlier studies as summarized by Antonovsky, in that the lowest socioeconomic class has continued to experience a much higher level of mortality and has shown no relative gain in recent decades. Antonovsky's suggested explanation of the continued great disparity in mortality between the lowest and other economic classes may well be applicable. That is, whereas the lowest socioeconomic class was able to share reasonably well in the earlier decreases in mortality brought about by the conquest of the infectious causes of death, it has not been in as favorable position in respect of the degenerative causes of death accompanied by chronic diseases which have made adequate medical care on a continuous basis more important in recent decades (1967, p. 67).

Second, the Chicago data help to illuminate why at least 15 nations have a longer life expectancy at birth than the United States (U.S. Department of Health, Education and Welfare, 1969, p. 6). For example, the expectation of life of 69.0 years for white males in the ring of the Chicago Metropolitan Area in 1960 was well above that (66.6 years) for all males in the United States, 1959-61, and closer to that of 71.3 years for males in Norway, 1956-60 (United Nations, 1967). Morever, expectation of life for white males in the lowest socioeconomic class in Chicago in 1960 was only 60.0 and that for nonwhite males in the lowest class but 56.7 years. The relatively high mortality of the United States compared with other advanced nations is undoubtedly in large measure a reflection of the high mortality of the disadvantaged in the nation—the lower socioeconomic groups of whites and the even more disadvantaged minority groups. This conclusion is supported by the Chicago area findings, which not only show that "excess deaths" constituted a large proportion of actual deaths in 1960, especially among disadvantaged groups, but also indicate that there was no significant decrease in excess mortality among white adults throughout the 30-year period 1930 to 1960 and that although excess mortality among nonwhites did decrease significantly during the period it was still very high—41 to 46 percent of all deaths—in 1960.

Particularly significant, among the findings for the nation as a whole, are the great differences between the death rates of whites and nonwhites, especially Negroes and Indians. The very high mortality of these minority groups constitutes stark evidence of their underprivileged status in this nation. Moreover, the emergence of large mortality differentials by socioeconomic level within the nonwhite population suggests that much, if not all, of the excess mortality of Negroes and Indians can be reduced with increases in levels of living and life styles.

The variations in mortality by geographic locale (including census tracts within cities as well as the larger economic subregions and states) can serve as indicators of specific areas in which more epidemiological research—both biomedical and socioeconomic—should be mounted; and also as areas in which experimental activities can be launched to effect reductions in mortality.

The conclusion advanced in Chapter 2 that education is probably the single most important indicator of socioeconomic status for mortality analysis makes a strong case for the addition of "highest year of school completed" to the standard death certificate in the United States. It is unfortunate that in the last revision of the standard certificates, education was added to the birth certificate but not to the death certificate (NCHS, 1968). In fact, the most economic and reliable approach to the measurement of socioeconomic differentials in mortality in the future—taking into account the experience gained from the 1960 Matched Records Study—would appear to be the addition of education as one item on the death certificate and the calculation of death rates by education level utilizing death tabulations from the death records and population statistics from the decennial census or Current Population Survey, including an adjustment for discrepant responses on the two records based on a small-scale matching of death certificates and census or survey records. (The small-scale matching study need not involve more than roughly 10,000 deaths.)

The data for the nation in 1960 also confirm earlier findings summarized by Antonovsky (1967, p. 66) that class differences in mortality are greatest in the young adult and middle years (see Tables 2.8 and 2.9).

Also a significant finding meriting more attention in research, policy, and program is the relatively high mortality of women, independent of socioeconomic class, who bear large numbers of children. The reasons for restricting family size, it would seem, can be bolstered by a significant additional reason—reduction of female mortality.

The findings of this study also suggest that if programs of sufficient magnitude including public health and medical programs had been mounted during the 30 years from 1930 to 1960, designed to narrow differences in socioeconomic status in the population, the overall death rates for metropolitan areas—and the country as a whole—would have decreased much more than they did. Programs designed to decrease mortality in the United States can be based on the socioeconomic epidemiological evidence presented. There can be little doubt that further reductions in national death rates can be achieved through the reduction of differentials in socioeconomic status in the United States. Although some of these differences in socioeconomic level may have been diminished since 1960, it is clear that any decrease that occurred still leaves great disparities in level of living and life style within the nation. Perhaps the most important next gain in mortality reduction is to be achieved through improved social-economic conditions rather than through increments to and application of biomedical knowledge. Certainly the biomedical know-how now available is either not available to the lower socioeconomic classes in the United States, or its impact, at this stage in the reduction of mortality, is relatively small compared with what could be achieved through reduction of the gap in levels of living and life styles associated with education, income, occupation, and geographic locale. If the United States is to demonstrate that she is indeed a land of equal opportunity, she must do considerably more to increase equality of opportunity on all those fronts which affect the most significant index of effective egalitarianism—the ability to survive—duration of life itself.

APPENDICES
NOTES
REFERENCES
INDEX

APPENDIX A
THE 1960 STUDY OF DEATHS
MATCHED WITH CENSUS RECORDS:
OBJECTIVES, DESIGN, AND
ESTIMATION PROCEDURES

The limited information reported on the legal death record in the United States has greatly restricted analysis of social and economic differentials in mortality, at least by any direct method wherein deaths tabulated by characteristics reported on death certificates are related to exposed population tabulated by characteristics reported on censuses or surveys. For example, the only measure of socioeconomic status on the death certificate is occupation, but any attempt to utilize this information for analysis of mortality by occupation is limited at the outset by the great discrepancy between the "usual occupation" reported on the death certificate and the "current (or last) occupation" reported in the population census.[1] Even in respect to other items on the death certificate, such as age, race, marital status, and country of birth, death rates are subject to error because of the lack of correspondence in the information reported for the same person on his death certificate and census schedule.

In a study conducted through the Population Research Center of the University of Chicago, with the cooperation of the National Center for Health Statistics and the Bureau of the Census, some of these problems were circumvented by matching death certificates for a sample of persons who died soon after the 1960 census to their 1960 census schedules. The major objective was to obtain tabulations of decedents by various social and economic characteristics reported on their census schedules, which would provide numerators for mortality ratios by these characteristics. Denominators for the mortality ratios were based on tabulations of the 1960 census population by the same characteristics. This appendix describes the procedures followed in carrying out the study and in deriving mortality ratios by selected social and economic characteristics. In the preceding chapters—as well as in this appendix—this study is referred to simply as the "1960 Matched Records Study."

The feasibility of the general approach used in the present study was tested in a small pilot study conducted jointly by the Bureau of the Census and the National Office of Vital Statistics in Memphis, Tennessee, in 1958. The results of the Memphis study were reported by Guralnick and Nam (1959), who concluded that a large-scale matching study, in conjunction with the 1960 census, was feasible if provision for estimation of the characteristics of unmatched decedents were incorporated into the study design.

1. Design of the Study

The 1960 Matched Records Study was designed to provide nationwide statistics on mortality differentials in the United States by various social and economic characteristics collected in the 1960 census. The sample of deaths selected for the study was limited to persons who died during the four months May through August 1960. This was soon enough after the April 1960 census so that addresses reported on the death certificate could be used to locate decedents in the Enumeration District files of the 1960 census records. Although the inclusion of deaths for an entire year after the census would have avoided the possibility of a seasonal bias, it was felt that the potentially high "nonmatch" rates for later months might introduce even more difficult problems and distortions.[2] The high unit cost of the manual search for decedents in the 1960 census records, combined with the heavy concentration of deaths above age 65, led to further limitation of the size of the sample by exclusion of one-half of the white decedents 65-74 years old and four-fifths of the white decedents 75 years and older. The net result was that of the 534,623 deaths which occurred in the United States during the four months from May through August 1960, some 340,033 were included in the study and searched in the 1960 census records.[3]

The project was supported by a research grant (RG-7134) from the National Institutes of Health to the Population Research Center (PRC), University of Chicago. Collection of the basic data was subcontracted to the National Center for Health Statistics (NCHS), which selected the sample of decedents and prepared duplicate copies of their death certificates and punched mortality cards, and the Bureau of the Census, which undertook the arduous task of searching the 1960 census records and preparing computer tapes and tabulations summarizing death certificate and census information for the matched decedents. Without the counsel and cooperation of both agencies the study would not have been possible.

In the 1960 census, information on most social and economic characteristics was collected from a 25-percent sample of the population, in what was called Stage II of the census. Consequently it was necessary, after decedents had been searched in the Stage I complete enumeration, also to search the Stage II records for those matched Stage I decedents who were included in the Stage II, 25-percent sample. This reduced the number of deaths for which socioeconomic census data were obtained to approximately one-fourth the number originally matched with the Stage I, 100-percent census enumeration. Procedures for matching were pretested on a small sample of April deaths. In general, the match operation involved the following steps:

a. Xerox prints of the death certificates for the 340,033 decedents were made from the microfilm records of deaths forwarded by the states to the NCHS.

b. The regular NCHS punched mortality card for each decedent was reproduced and attached to the corresponding Xerox print.

c. Each decedent was searched in the 100-percent enumeration records of the 1960 census, using census Enumeration District (ED) codes assigned to addresses listed on the death certificates to guide the search. The results of this match operation—including, for the "matched" decedents, the characteristics reported for them on the 100-percent enumeration schedules—were added to the punched mortality card for each decedent.

d. Decedents located in the 100-percent enumeration records and coded as "in the 25-percent sample" were then searched in the 25-percent sample records. Microfilms of the 25-percent sample schedules for these decedents were duplicated and processed through the regular census "editing" programs, the end result being a magnetic tape identical in content to the regular census tape for the 25-percent sample of the United States population.

e. A second tape was then compiled for decedents matched with the 25-percent sample census reports, collating information from their punched mortality cards and information from the computer tape described above in step (d).

Steps (a) and (b) were carried out under a subcontract with the NCHS. Steps (c), (d), and (e) were subcontracted to the Bureau of the Census. Thus, the handling of individual death certificates and census records in the matching operation was done entirely by the staffs of the NCHS and the Census Bureau, and the confidentiality of the returns on both records was scrupulously maintained.

The end products of the matching operation were three sets of basic data which could be used to compile tabulations of deaths by characteristics of decedents: (1) a deck of 340,033 punched cards, covering all of the decedents included in the study; (2) a magnetic tape, identical in content and format to the 25-percent sample census tape of the United States population, covering decedents matched with the 25-percent sample census records; (3) a collated tape for the decedents matched with the 25-percent sample census records, summarizing selected information from the punched cards and the 25-percent sample magnetic tape.

Information coded on the deck of punched cards includes (1) most of the NCHS codes available from their regular set of mortality punched cards for 1960; (2) the results of the search for each decedent in the 100-percent enumeration records, and the census characteristics from this record when the decedent was "matched"; (3) a special geographic code for each unmatched decedent indicating whether the residence address reported on his death certificate was inside an urbanized area, other urban, or rural, according to the geographic classification used in the 1960 census; and (4) identification of each decedent included and matched in the 25-percent sample census enumeration. The "death" tape that is identical to the 25-percent sample "population" tape includes all of the characteristics reported on the 25-percent sample census schedule for each decedent, his family and household, and the housing unit in which he lived in April 1960.

Table A.1 reports the results of the two stages of the match operation. For example, 262,966, or 77 percent, of the 340,033 decedents were located in the Stage I census records, and 64,675 of these were designated (on their Stage I records) for inclusion in the Stage II sample. However, 2,188 of the latter could not be located in the Stage II census records for various reasons, including the fact that the census sample was selected on the basis of housing units rather than persons or families and some units had a change of occupants between the Stage I and Stage II enumeration; in addition, some 82 decedents were lost in the collation of Stage II census data with death certificate information.

The net result was that the basic tabulations of matched decedents by social and economic characteristics as reported in the 1960 census

Table A.1.   Results of matching 340,033 death records with 1960 Census
             records, by color and sex: United States, May-August, 1960
             [unweighted count]

Result of census match operation	Total	White		Nonwhite	
		Males	Females	Males	Females
Total deaths in match operation	340,033	170,353	106,777	35,012	27,891
Matched with Stage I Census..	262,966	133,921	85,484	23,836	19,725
In Stage II sample and found...	62,487	31,993	20,326	5,557	4,611
In Stage II sample, not found..	2,188	971	608	363	246
Not in Stage II sample.........	198,291	100,957	64,550	17,916	14,868
Not matched with Stage I					
Number.....................	77,067	36,432	21,293	11,176	8,166
Percent....................	22.7	21.4	19.9	31.9	29.3

Source: Tabulation III, U.S. Bureau of the Census (compiled from
deck of punched mortality cards after matching death records with 1960
Census records and coding result of match operation on mortality cards).
Matched deaths tabulated by sex and color as reported Stage I Census (100%
enumeration); unmatched deaths tabulated by sex and color as reported on
death certificate.

refer to 62,405 persons who died during the period from May
through August 1960, and whose Stage II census data were located
and collated with their death certificate information. Social and
economic differentials in mortality based on these tabulations alone,
of course, would be subject to two types of bias: (1) a "match bias"
resulting from social and economic differences between matched and
unmatched decedents, and (2) a "seasonal bias" resulting from the
measurement of social and economic differentials during the summer
months only. However, provision was made in the study design to
estimate the social and economic characteristics of unmatched
decedents by undertaking an independent, self-contained, mail survey of a random sample of 9,541 of the total 340,033 decedents
included in the large-scale match operation. This survey was conducted by NCHS using procedures developed in their program of
"follow-back surveys linked to vital records."[4] A questionnaire
requesting information about each decedent, his family, and the
household in which he lived on April 1, 1960, was mailed to the
informant listed on the decedent's death certificate. The items
included in the questionnaire covered most of the "population"
items listed in the 25-percent sample schedule in the 1960 census.
Every attempt was made to duplicate the concepts employed in the
1960 census and to obtain information as of April 1, 1960, the
census date. The original query to the informant was sent by regular

first class mail. Two follow-up queries, the first by certified mail and the second by a special nonresponse letter, were sent to nonrespondents of previous mailings. Follow-up personal interviews with selected nonrespondents to the mail survey were undertaken by the field staff of the Census Bureau.

The 9,541 decedents included in the special survey sample were a random selection from the current mortality sample received by the National Center for Health Statistics for the four months May-August 1960; the probability of a person 65 years or older being included in the sample was one-half the probability for a person under 65 years of age. The survey was started in the summer of 1960, as soon as the advance samples of May 1960 deaths were transmitted by the individual states to the NCHS, and followed up as quickly as possible to avoid losses in response due to the informant's moving to another address as well as other losses in information that might result from greater elapsed time after death. The survey was completed by the end of June 1961, except for the coding and punching operations. The response rate was 88 percent from the mail survey, and this was raised to 94 percent after the personal interview follow-up. This response rate refers to the total number of usable questionnaires obtained, without taking into account the adequacy of the reporting of all the social and economic characteristics on the questionnaire.

Although the primary function of the NCHS Sample Survey was to provide estimates of census characteristics for decedents not matched with 1960 census records, the fact that it had to be carried out before the census match operation[5] and, therefore, before unmatched decedents could be identified had two important implications: (1) the survey was a sample of *all* deaths in the study, and (2) in order to identify unmatched decedents in the survey it was necessary to collate the survey data with the census data after the match operation was completed by the Census Bureau. This collation not only permitted the classification of NCHS Survey decedents into matched and unmatched groups but it also combined for each decedent data from all three sources—his NCHS Survey questionnaire, his death certificate, and his 1960 census schedule. As a result, the data collected in the survey served two useful purposes in addition to their main function: (1) they provided information on "match bias," that is, on differences in social and economic characteristics of matched and unmatched decedents; and (2) when collated with census data for those matched decedents who were included in

Table A.2. Response to selected questions in NCHS Survey, for 8,121 decedents 25 years of age and over, by color, sex, age and whether or not matched on Stage I Census record

Color, sex, match status in Stage I Census, and response to NCHS Survey	Number (unweighted count)			Percent		
	25 & over	25-64 years	65 & over	25 & over	25-64 years	65 & over
White males						
Total decedents in Survey.....	4,199	2,330	1,869	100.0	100.0	100.0
Responded to Survey.........	3,936	2,176	1,760	93.7	93.4	94.2
Reported marital status....	3,796	2,108	1,688	90.4	90.5	90.3
Reported family status.....	3,786	2,106	1,680	90.2	90.4	89.9
Reported education........	3,369	1,963	1,406	80.2	84.2	75.2
Matched with Census..........	3,384	1,849	1,535	100.0	100.0	100.0
Responded to Survey.........	3,198	1,747	1,451	94.5	94.5	94.5
Reported marital status...	3,089	1,699	1,390	91.3	91.9	90.6
Reported family status....	3,106	1,713	1,393	91.8	92.6	90.7
Reported education........	2,762	1,589	1,173	81.6	85.9	76.4
Not matched with Census.......	815	481	334	100.0	100.0	100.0
Responded to Survey.........	738	429	309	90.6	89.2	92.5
Reported marital status...	707	409	298	86.7	85.0	89.2
Reported family status....	680	393	287	83.4	81.7	85.9
Reported education........	607	374	233	74.5	77.8	69.8
White females						
Total decedents in Survey.....	2,936	1,176	1,760	100.0	100.0	100.0
Responded to Survey.........	2,762	1,092	1,670	94.1	92.9	94.9
Reported marital status...	2,616	1,045	1,571	89.1	88.9	89.3
Reported family status....	2,566	1,034	1,532	87.4	87.9	87.0
Reported education........	2,277	984	1,293	77.6	83.7	73.5
Matched with Census..........	2,379	955	1,424	100.0	100.0	100.0
Responded to Survey.........	2,257	899	1,358	94.9	94.1	95.4
Reported marital status...	2,136	862	1,274	89.8	90.3	89.5
Reported family status....	2,122	861	1,261	89.2	90.2	88.6
Reported education........	1,874	814	1,060	78.8	85.2	74.4
Not matched with Census.......	557	221	336	100.0	100.0	100.0
Responded to Survey.........	505	193	312	90.7	87.3	92.9
Reported marital status...	480	183	297	86.2	82.8	88.4
Reported family status....	444	173	271	79.7	78.3	80.6
Reported education........	403	170	233	72.4	76.9	69.3
Nonwhite males						
Total decedents in Survey.....	542	397	145	100.0	100.0	100.0
Responded to Survey.........	483	357	126	89.1	89.9	86.9
Reported marital status...	452	333	119	83.4	83.9	82.1
Reported family status....	420	307	113	77.5	77.3	77.9
Reported education........	382	299	83	70.5	75.3	57.2

(continued)

Table A.2. Response to selected questions in NCHS Survey, for 8,121 decedents 25 years of age and over, by color, sex, age and whether or not matched on Stage I Census record--(continued)

Color, sex, match status in Stage I Census, and response to NCHS Survey	Number (unweighted count)			Percent		
	25 & over	25-64 years	65 & over	25 & over	25-64 years	65 & over
Matched with Census...........	392	277	115	100.0	100.0	100.0
Responded to Survey.........	355	253	102	90.6	91.3	88.7
Reported marital status...	333	237	96	84.9	85.6	83.5
Reported family status....	317	223	94	80.9	80.5	81.7
Reported education........	281	212	69	71.7	76.5	60.0
Not matched with Census.......	150	120	30	100.0	100.0	100.0
Responded to Survey.........	128	104	24	85.3	86.7	80.0
Reported marital status...	119	96	23	79.3	80.0	76.7
Reported family status....	103	84	19	68.7	70.0	63.3
Reported education........	101	87	14	67.3	72.5	46.7
Nonwhite females						
Total decedents in Survey.....	444	295	149	100.0	100.0	100.0
Responded to Survey.........	399	261	138	89.9	88.5	92.6
Reported marital status...	377	247	130	84.9	83.7	87.2
Reported family status....	329	215	114	74.1	72.9	76.5
Reported education........	302	209	93	68.0	70.8	62.4
Matched with Census...........	326	217	109	100.0	100.0	100.0
Responded to Survey.........	298	197	101	91.4	90.8	92.7
Reported marital status...	282	188	94	86.5	86.6	86.2
Reported family status....	249	167	82	76.4	77.0	75.2
Reported education........	226	158	68	69.3	72.8	62.4
Not matched with Census.......	118	78	40	100.0	100.0	100.0
Responded to Survey.........	101	64	37	85.6	82.1	92.5
Reported marital status...	95	59	36	80.5	75.6	90.0
Reported family status....	80	48	32	67.8	61.5	80.0
Reported education........	76	51	25	64.4	65.4	62.5

Source: Population Research Center, University of Chicago. Tabulation of NCHS Survey decedents by color, sex and age as reported on death certificate; by response to marital status, family status, and education as reported on Survey questionnaire.

the survey, they provided comparisons of response to the same questions on census and survey questionnaires, and thus provided the data needed to adjust the reported survey characteristics for unmatched decedents to "estimated census" characteristics.

Table A.2 gives some information on response rates and the completeness of reporting of selected items on the NCHS Sample Survey questionnaires. Questionnaires were returned for 93 to 95 percent of all white males and females in two broad age groups, 25-64 and 65 or over. Not all questions were answered adequately on the questionnaires that were returned, however. For example, the education question was answered for only 80 percent of the white males 25 years of age or over, although questionnaires were returned for 94 percent of the group and 90 percent reported marital status and family status questions. Marital status was reported on almost all the questionnaires returned. Marital status was equally well reported for both age groups of white men and women, but education was less often reported for men and women 65 and over than for those 25-64 years of age.

Response rates were not quite as high for nonwhites as whites, although the differences were not large. For example, the response rate was 89 percent for nonwhite males 25 and over, compared with 94 percent for white males the same age. However, in a number of groups, responses to the family status and education questions were substantially lower for nonwhites than for whites. For example, only 62 and 65 percent of the "unmatched" nonwhite females 25-64 years of age had responses for the family status and education questions, respectively, compared with 78 and 77 percent of the "unmatched" white females the same age.

Especially gratifying—from the standpoint of the design of the study—was the fact that the response rates for unmatched decedents were almost as high as those for matched decedents. For example, between 87 and 93 percent of the unmatched white decedents had questionnaires returned for them, as compared with 94 to 95 percent of the matched decedents. Education was adequately reported for 69 to 78 percent of the unmatched compared with 74 to 86 percent of the matched white decedents. In other words, there was very little relationship between the match status of a decedent and whether a survey questionnaire was returned for him, a fact which enhanced the usefulness of the survey responses for purposes of estimating the social and economic characteristics of unmatched decedents.

2. Match Bias

If the social and economic characteristics of matched decedents were representative of all decedents, it would not be necessary to estimate the characteristics of unmatched decedents. This was not the case, however, as was anticiapted in the design of the study. The extent of match bias, or differences between matched and un-matched decedents with respect to selected characteristics, is sum-marized in Tables A.3 to A.8. The first two tables are based on tabulations of all deaths included in the census match operation, and they report match bias differentials by age, sex, color, and cause of death, items that are reported on the death certificate and which were, therefore, available for all matched and unmatched deaths. The other tables are based on tabulations of NCHS Survey deaths because they rely on survey characteristics for unmatched decedents. Nonwhites had roughly one and one-half times as many unmatched decedents as whites, and males had slightly higher "nonmatch" rates than females (Table A.3). That is, 32 percent of the nonwhite males and 29 percent of the nonwhite females were not matched with census records, compared with 21 and 20 percent, respectively, of the white males and females. Proportions not matched also varied considerably by age, with high rates for young adults—especially men

Table A.3. Percent not matched with Stage I Census records, for all decedents in census match operation, by color, sex and age: United States, May-August, 1960

Age	Total	White		Nonwhite	
		Male	Female	Male	Female
WEIGHTED COUNT[a]					
All ages--total deaths.......	533,742	268,381	202,202	35,233	27,926
All ages--percent not matched	21.1	20.1	19.5	31.7	29.2
Under 1 year...............	34.3	32.5	32.3	40.1	40.9
1-4 years.................	26.3	23.6	24.6	33.1	33.9
5-14 years.................	20.3	19.2	18.3	28.1	23.4
15-24 years...............	35.1	35.2	30.4	40.2	39.9
25-34 years...............	34.4	33.9	25.1	48.0	39.3
35-44 years.....	26.3	25.0	19.7	43.1	31.1
45-54 years...............	21.5	20.6	17.3	33.3	28.3
55-64 years...............	19.1	18.7	16.9	27.0	25.0
65-74 years...............	17.9	17.1	17.2	24.6	25.5
75 years & over...........	19.2	18.1	19.5	24.5	24.8
UNWEIGHTED COUNT					
All ages--total deaths[b]......	340,033	169,833	107,041	35,233	27,926
All ages--percent not matched	22.7	21.5	19.9	31.7	29.2
65-74 years...............	18.5	17.1	17.2	24.6	25.5
75 years & over...........	20.2	18.1	19.5	24.5	24.8

Source: Tabulations I (Revised) and II, same source as Table A-1. Matched and unmatched deaths tabulated by age, sex and color as reported on death certificate.

[a] Weighted as follows: "one" for all nonwhites and for whites under 65 years of age, "two" for whites 65-74 years of age, and "five" for whites 75 years and over.

[b] Minor differences between corresponding totals in Tables A-1 and A-3 reflect differences in reporting of sex and color on Stage I Census records and death certificates.

Table A.4. Percent not matched with Stage I Census records, for all white décedents 25 years of age and over
in census match operation, by cause of death, sex and age: United States, May-August, 1960

Cause of death (ISC codes)	White male			White female		
	25 & over	25-64 years	65 & over	25 & over	25-64 years	65 & over
All causes--weighted count[a]............................	241,633	92,285	149,348	185,445	48,847	136,598
All causes--percent not matched......................	18.9	20.9	17.7	18.5	17.9	18.7
Tuberculosis, all forms (001-019)..........................	25.4	27.7	22.8	25.0	26.3	23.5[b]
Malignant neoplasms, incl. lymph.&hematop. tissues (140-205)..	18.2	18.9	17.7	17.8	17.1	18.4
of digestive organs & peritoneum (150-156A, 157-159).......	16.9	16.9	16.8	17.5	16.4	18.0
of respiratory system (160-164)..........................	19.6	20.9	18.0	17.7	17.1	18.3
of breast (170)...				17.7	15.9	20.1
of genital organs (171-179)...............................	17.7	17.3	17.8	17.9	19.7	15.6
Diabetes mellitus (260)....................................	17.7	19.0	17.0	17.8	18.8	17.5
Major cardiovascular-renal diseases (330-334,400-468,592-594)	17.2	17.8	17.0	18.2	16.4	18.6
Vascular lesions affecting central nervous system (330-334)	18.3	18.9	18.2	19.6	16.8	20.0
Rheumatic fever & chronic rheumatic heart disease (400-416)	17.0	18.0	14.3	15.8	17.5	12.9
Arteriosclerotic & degenerative heart disease (420,422)....	16.6	17.2	16.2	17.2	15.8	17.5
Hypertensive disease (with & without heart) (440-447)......	17.9	18.5	17.7	17.8	15.9	18.2
Influenza & pneumonia except pneumonia of new born (480-493).	22.7	26.2	21.4	18.9	18.3	19.0
Cirrhosis of liver (581)....................................	26.9	28.7	22.8	21.9	23.5	18.4
Motor-vehicle accidents (810-835)..........................	28.6	30.8	20.7	22.2	22.3	21.8
Other accidents (800-802,840-962)..........................	26.5	29.4	21.1	22.5	23.7	22.0
Suicide (963,970-979)..........	24.7	27.1	17.5	20.3	21.2	16.4

Source: Tabulations I-A (Revised) and II-A, same source as Table A.1. Matched and unmatched deaths tabulated by cause of death, color, sex and age of decedent as reported on death certificate.

[a] See note a, Table A.3, for weights.

[b] Percent based on 20-99 deaths (unweighted count).

15-44 years of age and women 15-34 years of age—and children
under 5 years.

Although it was not possible to ascertain directly why unmatched
decedents could not be located in the 1960 census records—that is,
whether they were missed in the census enumeration, whether they
moved between the census date and the date of death, or whether
different names might have been used for the same person on the
two records[6] —the proportions of matched deaths were similar to
those in previous studies, and the patterns of match bias in accord
with expectations. For example, the match bias differentials in Table
A.3 reflect, in part at least, the geographic mobility of young
adults—and their preschool children—reinforced by the disproportionate concentration of migrants in the "difficult to enumerate"
residential areas of cities; both of these factors are related to the high
net census undercounts for these ages.[7]

The proportion of white decedents not matched with census
records varied considerably by cause of death. Nonmatch rates were
especially high for tuberculosis, cirrhosis of the liver, accidents, and
suicide (Table A.4). High rates for these causes are due, in part at

Table A.5. Percent not matched with Stage I Census records, for 8,121 decedents 25 years of age and over in NCHS Survey, by marital status and family status, by color, sex and age: United States, May-August, 1960

Color, marital status and family status	Males			Females		
	25 & over	25-64 years	65 & over	25 & over	25-64 years	65 & over
Marital status						
White decedents.........	18.9	20.6	17.9	19.0	18.8	19.1
Married (or separated)......	14.1	15.9	12.6	16.5	16.6	16.5
Widowed....................	24.5	30.6	23.9	20.0	20.4	20.0
Divorced...................	37.3	40.3	31.7[a]	27.7[a]	35.3[a]	19.4[a]
Never married..............	29.9	33.0	27.0	20.1	21.7[a]	19.6
Unknown....................	43.5[a]	--[a]	--[a]	--[a]	--[a]	--[a]
Nonwhite decedents.....	26.2	30.2	20.7	26.6	26.4	26.8
Married (or separated)......	19.1	24.8	10.1[a]	24.7	24.5	25.0[a]
Widowed....................	29.7[a]	22.9[a]	32.7[a]	27.7	25.3[a]	28.8
Divorced...................	29.2[a]	35.0[a]	--[a]	45.2[a]	--[a]	--[a]
Never married..............	50.0[a]	54.7[a]	--[a]	13.9[a]	--[a]	--[a]
Unknown....................	--[a]	--[a]	--[a]	--[a]	--[a]	--[a]
Family status						
White decedents.........	18.9	20.6	17.9	19.0	18.8	19.1
Family members..............	14.5	15.6	13.7	15.8	15.9	15.8
Unrelated individuals.......	33.0	41.4	29.5	17.8	23.7	16.7
Inmates....................	22.4	22.5[a]	22.4	25.9	11.6[a]	27.2
Family status not reported..	34.8	51.4[a]	27.5[a]	30.5	34.5[a]	29.7
No questionnaire returned...	27.4	33.8	22.9	28.8	33.3[a]	26.7[a]
Nonwhite decedents......	26.2	30.2	20.7	26.6	26.4	26.8
Family members..............	17.8	19.3	15.7[a]	21.0	18.3	23.8[a]
Unrelated individuals.......	43.4[a]	55.9[a]	--[a]	38.0[a]	35.0[a]	40.0[a]
Inmates....................	--[a]	--[a]	--[a]	--[a]	--[a]	--[a]
Family status not reported..	39.5[a]	40.0[a]	--[a]	27.7[a]	34.8[a]	20.8[a]
No questionnaire returned...	35.9[a]	40.0[a]	--[a]	35.7[a]	41.2[a]	--[a]

Source: Population Research Center, University of Chicago. Tabulation of NCHS Survey deaths by color, sex, age and marital status as reported on death certificate; by family status as reported on NCHS Survey; by whether or not matched with Stage I Census record. Percents computed from weighted numbers (see note a, Table A.3, for weights).

[a] Percent based on less than 100 deaths (unweighted count); percent not reported if based on less than 20 deaths.

least, to the high nonmatch rates for young adults, because considerably higher percentages of the deaths from these causes occur among persons 25-44 years old than is the case for other causes of death.

Nonmatch rates were much lower for married persons than for those who were single (had never married), widowed, or divorced (Table A.5). For example, among white males 25 years and older who were included in the NCHS Sample Survey, the proportion not matched was only 14 percent for married decedents as compared with 24, 30, and 37 percent, respectively, for widowed, never married, and divorced decedents. Among white females 25 and older, only 16 percent of the married group were not matched with census records compared with 20, 20, and 28 percent, respectively, for widowed, never married, and divorced. The nonmatch rates by family status in Table A.5 show much lower rates for family members than for nonfamily members, as would be expected from the marital status differentials just described.

The proportion of white decedents not matched with census records also varied with level of educational attainment, based on data from the NCHS Survey. Nonmatch rates tended to be lower for decedents with a high school education than for elementary- or college-trained decedents, except among women 65 and over (Table A.6).[8] Among these older women there was a consistent, though small, decline in the unmatched proportion as educational attainment increased—from 19 percent for women with less than 8 years of

Table A.6. Percent not matched with Stage I Census records, for 8,121 decedents 25 years of age and over in NCHS Survey, by years of school completed, color, sex and age: United States, May-August, 1960

Years of school completed	Males			Females		
	25 & over	25-64 years	65 & over	25 & over	25-64 years	65 & over
White decedents..........	18.9	20.6	17.9	19.0	18.8	19.1
Less than 8 years school......	19.3	21.6	18.4	19.1	19.1	19.1
Elementary, 8 years...........	17.4	18.2	16.9	18.2	16.6	18.7
High School, 1-4 years........	15.0	17.7	11.2	16.5	16.3	16.6
College, 1 year or more.......	18.5	19.4	17.6	16.2	19.1	14.8
Education not reported........	22.5	25.8	21.5	21.0	21.3[a]	21.0[a]
No questionnaire returned.....	27.4	33.8	22.9	28.8	33.3[a]	26.7[a]
Nonwhite decedents.......	26.2	30.2	20.7	26.6	26.4	26.8
None or elementary...........	23.5	28.6	15.3[a]	26.1	23.5	28.2[a]
High School, 1-4 years........	27.4[a]	22.9[a]	--[a]	24.3[a]	24.2[a]	--[a]
College, 1 year or more.......	35.7[a]	50.0[a]	--[a]	--[a]	--[a]	--[a]
Education not reported........	25.7	29.3[a]	23.3[a]	26.1[a]	25.0[a]	26.7[a]
No questionnaire returned.....	35.9[a]	40.0[a]	--[a]	35.7[a]	41.2[a]	--[a]

Source: Population Research Center, University of Chicago. Tabulation of NCHS Survey deaths by color, sex and age as reported on death certificate; by education as reported on NCHS Survey; whether or not matched with Stage I Census record. Percents computed from weighted numbers (see note a, Table A.3).

[a] Percent based on less than 100 deaths (unweighted count); percent not reported if based on less than 20 deaths.

school to 15 percent for women with one or more years of college.

Among males, nonmatch rates varied markedly by occupation, although the pattern was not consistent in the several age-color groups shown in Table A.7. Nonmatch rates were low (from 13 to 15 percent) among white males 65-74 years of age in the following occupations: craftsmen and foremen, managers-officials-proprietors, service workers, and clerical and sales workers. Among white males 25-64 years of age, only clerical and sales, and professional and technical workers had nonmatch rates below 15 percent, and the rate

Table A.7. Percent not matched with Stage I Census records, for 4,741 male decedents 25 years of age and over in NCHS Survey, by major occupation, color and age: United States, May-August, 1960

Color and major occupation group	25 & over	25-64 years	65-74 years
All white males.........................	18.9	20.6	17.8
Worked 1950 or later[a]	18.1	19.8	17.7
1 Professional, technical & kindred workers......	17.3	14.8	18.9[b]
2 Managers, officials & proprietors, exc. farm...	15.9	17.7	13.5[b]
3 Clerical & sales workers......................	13.7	14.2	14.7[b]
4 Craftsmen, foremen & kindred workers...........	14.9	18.1	13.1
5 Operatives & kindred workers..................	19.2	18.9	18.1[b]
6 Service workers (incl. private household)......	16.9	24.2	14.1[b]
7 Laborers, except farm & mine...................	20.6	19.7	23.4[b]
8 Agricultural workers[c]	19.9	22.9	21.5[b]
9 Occupation not reported.......................	26.3	33.3	26.1[b]
Did not work after 1949......................	19.5	18.8	17.1
No questionnaire returned....................	27.4	33.8	20.7[b]
All nonwhite males......................	26.2	30.2	22.2[b]
Worked 1950 or later[a]	27.2	29.4	25.0[b]
White collar workers (groups 1,2,3)..............	33.3[b]	44.8[b]	--[b]
Craftsmen & operatives (groups 4,5).............	29.7	27.5[b]	--[b]
Service workers & laborers (groups 6,7)..........	21.7	22.4[b]	23.8[b]
Agricultural workers[c] (group 8)...............	23.0[b]	36.1[b]	--[b]
Occupation not reported (group 9)...............	31.6	30.6[b]	--[b]
Did not work after 1949.....................	14.7[b]	25.8[b]	--[b]
No questionnaire returned....................	35.9[b]	40.0[b]	--[b]

Source: Population Research Center, University of Chicago. Tabulation of NCHS Survey deaths by color, sex and age as reported on death certificate; by occupation as reported on NCHS Survey questionnaire. Percents computed from weighted numbers (see note a, Table A.3).

[a] Includes decedents for whom work status was not reported (6.0 percent of white males and 12.0 percent of nonwhite males 25 and over for whom questionnaires were returned).

[b] Percent based on less than 100 deaths (unweighted count); percent not reported if based on less than 20 deaths.

[c] Includes farmers and farm managers, farm laborers and foremen.

Table A.8. Percent not matched with Stage I Census records, for 2,228 ever-married white female decedents 45 years of age and over in NCHS Sample Survey, by number of children ever borne: United States, May-August, 1960

Number of children ever borne	45 & over	45-64 years	65 & over
Ever married white women[a]...........	18.0	16.7	18.7
No children.....................	13.8	13.4	14.2
1 child.........................	18.1	17.1	18.9
2 children.....................	17.0	13.9	19.1
3 children.....................	14.6	9.6	17.8
4 children.....................	19.3	24.1[b]	17.1
5 or 6 children................	19.2	20.3[b]	18.8
7 children or more.............	21.5	24.2[b]	20.7
Unknown number of children......	24.2	25.5[b]	23.8

Source: Population Research Center, University of Chicago. Tabulation of NCHS Survey deaths by color, sex and age as reported on death certificate; by marital status and number of children ever borne as reported on Survey questionnaire; by whether or not matched with Stage I Census record. Percents computed from weighted numbers (see note a, Table A.3).

[a] Refers to decedents reported as married, separated, widowed or divorced on NCHS Survey questionnaires; excludes decedents 45 and over for whom questionnaires were not returned or whose marital status was not reported on their questionnaire.

[b] Percent based on 20-99 deaths (unweighted count).

for service workers was highest of all the occupations (24 percent). Among nonwhite males 25-64 years of age, the nonmatch rate of white collar workers was highest, 45 percent. There was also considerable variation in match rates among women when classified by number of children ever borne. Those with large families—four or more children—had higher nonmatch rates, especially among women 25-64 years old (Table A.8).

The wide variations in nonmatch rates reported in Tables A.3 to A.8 indicate that mortality differentials based on matched deaths alone would be subject to significant distortion and demonstrate the need for estimates of the social and economic characteristics of unmatched decedents. Such estimates were made in the Matched Records Study, using data collated from three sources—the NCHS Sample Survey questionnaires, the death certificates, and the 1960 census records—as described in the following section.

3. Derivation of Mortality Ratios

The mortality differentials obtained from the 1960 Matched Records Study are limited to persons 25 years of age and over.

Although death records for persons under 25 years of age were also matched with the 1960 census records—and their match rates were not substantially lower than those of other age groups—two problems complicated the estimation of differential mortality for persons under 25. First was the fact that most of these refer to infants, and most of the infants who died between May and August 1960 were born after April 1, the census date; this greatly complicated the problem of computing "expected deaths" for the age group under one. Second, a socioeconomic index for persons under 25 would have to be something like family income or father's occupation, items that were not available for all persons under 25.

The social and economic differentials in mortality derived from the study are based on ratios of actual to expected deaths, in which (1) actual deaths were obtained as the *sum* of "matched deaths classified by social and economic characteristics as reported on their census schedules" *plus* "unmatched deaths classified by social and economic characteristics as estimated from NCHS Survey questionnaires for the sample of unmatched deaths included in the survey," and (2) expected deaths were obtained by multiplying 1960 age-specific death rates for the total population of the United States by the 1960 age composition of the subpopulation in each category of the social and economic characteristics for which mortality ratios were calculated. The calculation of expected deaths presented no problems except in those cases where the Bureau of the Census had not tabulated the 1960 population of the United States in sufficient detail; usually it was the cross classification of a particular social or economic characteristic by the 10-year age intervals required for the control of age that was lacking. As a result it was necessary to underwrite and obtain from the Bureau of the Census several special tabulations of the population of the United States. Most of the methodological issues in the analysis of data from the Matched Records Study concerned the procedures used to estimate the social and economic characteristics of decedents not matched with 1960 census records, which are described in the following paragraphs.

a. Control Totals

The first step in the procedure for estimating characteristics of unmatched decedents was the derivation of control totals by color, sex, and age, to which estimated distributions of unmatched decedents by social and economic characteristics could be inflated.

Because the tabulations of matched decedents by census characteristics referred to 62,405 decedents matched with Stage II (25-percent sample) census records, classified by color, sex, age, and various social and economic characteristics reported on the census records, the color-sex-age control totals derived for unmatched decedents were defined in terms of a "State II census equivalent" of unmatched decedents by estimated census color, sex, and age. These unmatched control totals were obtained by first computing color-sex-age-specific ratios of all *matched Stage II deaths* in the study (tabulated by color, sex, and age as reported in the Stage II census) to all *matched Stage I deaths* (tabulated by death certificate color, sex, and age), and then applying these ratios to the distribution of *unmatched Stage I deaths* (tabulated by death certificate color, sex, and age).[9] Control totals for unmatched Stage II deaths and all (matched plus unmatched) Stage II deaths are shown in Table A.9.

Table A.9. Control totals for unmatched Stage II Census deaths and all (matched and unmatched) Stage II Census deaths, by color, sex and age: United States, May-August, 1960

Color and age	Male deaths			Female deaths		
	Matched Stage II Census	Unmatched (Stage II) control totals[a]	Total Stage II Census	Matched Stage II Census	Unmatched (Stage II) control totals[a]	Total Stage II Census
White, 25 & over...	46,100	10,845	56,945	34,579	7,826	42,405
25-34 years.....	983	503	1,486	592	199	791
35-44 years.....	2,369	791	3,160	1,489	365	1,854
45-54 years.....	5,349	1,389	6,738	2,798	587	3,385
55-64 years.....	9,493	2,177	11,670	5,210	1,056	6,266
65-74 years.....	13,647	2,824	16,471	9,413	1,955	11,368
75 & over.......	1,259	3,161	17,420	15,077	3,664	18,741
Nonwhite, 25 & over	4,473	1,917	6,390	3,867	1,431	5,298
25-34 years.....	221	204	425	180	117	297
35-44 years.....	382	289	671	380	171	551
45-54 years.....	704	352	1,056	572	226	798
55-64 years.....	972	359	1,331	757	252	1,009
65-74 years.....	1,187	386	1,573	975	333	1,308
75 & over.......	1,007	327	1,334	1,003	332	1,335

Source: Matched deaths tabulated from collated tape (see text) by Bureau of the Census, using color, sex and age as reported (or allocated) in 1960 Stage II Census. All numbers are weighted (see note a, Table A.3).

[a] Computed by multiplying (1) color-sex-age-specific ratios of matched Stage II deaths (tabulated by color, sex and age as reported in Stage II Census) to matched Stage I deaths (tabulated by color, sex and age as reported on death certificate), by (2) the color-sex-age composition of unmatched Stage I deaths (tabulated by color, sex and age as reported on death certificate).

Proportions not matched computed from this table will differ slightly from the percentages reported in Table A.3 because the latter are based on tabulations of deaths by color, sex, and age as reported on the death certificate whereas the control totals in Table A.9 summarize deaths by "estimated" color, sex, and age as reported in the census.

It was also necessary to derive control totals for unmatched decedents by color, sex, and age within each of the family status subgroups for which education and income differentials in mortality were to be calculated. This was essential for the income analysis especially, because family income was judged to be a better index of socioeconomic status than personal income for family members, but it obviously could be applied only to family members. The unmatched control totals by family status, sex, and color for two broad age groups are shown in column 3 of Table A.10. They were derived as follows: First, the distribution of unmatched NCHS survey decedents by family status as reported on the survey questionnaire (column 1, Table A.10) was adjusted to "estimated family status as reported on their 1960 census records" (column 2), using the cross classification in Table A.11, which compares responses to the family status questions on the NCHS survey questionnaire with responses to the same questions on the census schedules for those NCHS survey decedents who were matched with Stage II census records. Second, the estimated census family status distribution of unmatched survey decedents was then inflated to the color-sex control totals for the two broad age groups to obtain the family status control totals shown in column 3 of Table A.10.

b. Ratios by Education Level

After testing several methods of utilizing the NCHS Sample Survey data to derive estimates of the characteristics of unmatched decedents, it was clear that better estimates could be obtained by using data for matched as well as unmatched decedents in the survey. For example, because the comparison of response to the education question on the NCHS survey questionnaire and 1960 census schedule for the same decedent revealed rather large discrepancies in the reporting of education on the two records, education level reported for unmatched decedents in the NCHS survey was first adjusted to "estimated Census education" using the cross classified distribution in Table A.13, and then inflated to the unmatched Stage II control totals reported in Table A.9. These estimates of unmatched Stage II

Table A.10. Control totals for unmatched Stage II Census deaths and total (matched and unmatched) Stage II Census deaths, by family status, color, sex and age: United States, May-August, 1960

Color, sex, age and family status	Unmatched deaths			Matched Stage II Census (weighted)	Total Stage II Census
	NCHS Survey[a] (weighted)		Stage II control totals		
	Reported family status	Adjusted to Census family status			
	(1)	(2)	(3)	(4)	(5)
White					
Males 25-64 years.......	481	481.0	4,860	18,194	23,054
Family members.......	279	347.1	3,507	15,857	19,364
Unrelated individuals	94	116.3	1,175	1,618	2,793
Inmates.............	20	17.6	178	719	897
Unknown family status	88[b]	-	-	-	-
Males 65 & over.........	668	668.0	5,985	27,906	33,891
Family members.......	340	386.5	3,463	21,164	24,627
Unrelated individuals	160	188.0	1,684	3,952	5,636
Inmates.............	74	93.5	838	2,790	3,628
Unknown family status	94[b]	-	-	-	-
Females 25-64 years.....	221	221.0	2,207	10,089	12,296
Family members.......	136	177.8	1,776	8,430	10,206
Unrelated individuals	32	38.2	381	1,208	1,589
Inmates.............	5	5.0	50	451	501
Unknown family status	48[b]	-	-	-	-
Females 65 & over.......	672	672.0	5,619	24,490	30,109
Family members.......	296	357.1	2,986	15,655	18,641
Unrelated individuals	122	159.8	1,336	5,296	6,632
Inmates.............	124	155.1	1,297	3,539	4,836
Unknown family status	130[b]	-	-	-	-
Nonwhite					
Males 25-64 years.......	120	120.0	1,204	2,279	3,483
Family members.......	45	80.6	809	1,745	2,554
Unrelated individuals	38	35.1	352	396	748
Inmates.............	1	4.3	43	138	181
Unknown family status	36[b]	-	-	-	-
Males 65 & over.........	60	60.0	713	2,194	2,907
Family members.......	28	28.0	333	1,636	1,969
Unrelated individuals	8	30.0	356	415	771
Inmates.............	2	2.0	24	143	167
Unknown family status	22[b]	-	-	-	-
Females 25-64 years.....	78	78.0	766	1,889	2,655
Family members.......	30	58.8	578	1,534	2,112
Unrelated individuals	14	14.2	139	280	419
Inmates.............	4	5.0	49	75	124
Unknown family status	30[b]	-	-	-	-
Females 65 & over.......	80	80.0	665	1,978	2,643
Family members.......	38	61.1	508	1,393	1,901
Unrelated individuals	24	14.2	118	411	529
Inmates.............	2	4.7	39	174	213
Unknown family status	16[b]	-	-	-	-

Source: Column (1) from Population Research Center, University of Chicago, tabulation of NCHS Survey deaths by color, sex and age as reported on death certificate; by family status as reported on Survey questionnaire. Column (4) from U.S. Bureau of the Census, tabulation of matched Stage II deaths by census characteristics of decedents (Tables 1, 8, 9 and 12, collated tape). See text for explanation of other columns.

[a] Weighted as follows: one for all decedents under 65; two for all decedents 65 and over.

[b] Includes decedents for whom no Survey questionnaire was returned as well as those for whom family status was not reported on the questionnaire.

Table A.11. Comparison of response to family status questions on NCHS Survey questionnaire and Stage II Census record, for decedents 25 years of age and over in NCHS Sample Survey who were matched with Stage II Census records, by color, sex and age

Color, sex, age, and family status (Stage II Census)	Family status (NCHS Survey)				
	Total	Family members	Unrelated individuals	Inmates	Unknown[a]
White					
Males 25-64 years........	436	367	30	17	22
Family members........	381	363	1	-	17
Unrelated individuals.	40	4	29	2	5
Inmates..............	15	-	-	15	-
Males 65 & over..........	323	240	36	26	21
Family members........	247	235	3	-	9
Unrelated individuals.	44	1	31	3	9
Inmates..............	32	4	2	23	3
Females 25-64 years......	249	194	25	14	16
Family members........	211	192	8	-	11
Unrelated individuals.	24	2	17	-	5
Inmates..............	14	-	-	14	-
Females 65 & over........	298	179	57	33	29
Family members........	186	166	3	-	17
Unrelated individuals.	69	9	53	-	7
Inmates..............	43	4	1	33	5
Nonwhite					
Males 25-64 years........	63	43	6	3	11
Family members........	52	43	2	-	7
Unrelated individuals.	7	-	4	-	3
Inmates..............	4	-	-	3	1
Males 65 & over..........	26	19	4	1	2
Family members........	19	19	-	-	-
Unrelated individuals.	6	-	4	-	2
Inmates..............	1	-	-	1	-
Females 25-64 years......	52	31	9	3	9
Family members........	40	30	2	-	8
Unrelated individuals.	8	-	7	-	1
Inmates..............	4	1	-	3	-
Females 65 & over........	31	20	5	-	6
Family members........	26	19	3	-	4
Unrelated individuals.	4	1	2	-	1
Inmates..............	1	-	-	-	1

Source: Population Research Center, University of Chicago. Tabulation of NCHS Survey deaths by color, sex and age as reported on death certificate; by family status as reported on NCHS Survey questionnaire and by family status as reported on Stage II Census record (unweighted count). See text for definitions of family status categories.

[a] Includes decedents for whom no questionnaire was returned as well as those for whom family status was not reported on the questionnaire.

Table A.12. Numbers of deaths on which education differentials in mortality are based, by family status, color, sex and age: United States, May-August, 1960

Family status, color, sex, age and years of school completed	Matched Stage II Census (unweighted)	Unmatched deaths		Stage II Census (weighted)	Matched Stage II Census (weighted)	Total Stage II Census or actual deaths
		NCHS Survey (unweighted)				
		Reported education	Adjusted to Census education			
	(1)	(2)	(3)	(4)	(5)	(6)=(4)+(5)
Total white decedents						
Males 25-64 years.............	18,194	481[a]	481.0	4,860	18,194	23,054
Less than 5 years..........	1,482	31	44.7	452	1,482	1,934
Elementary, 5-7 years.......	3,192	72	107.2	1,083	3,192	4,275
Elementary, 8 years........	4,403	93	108.1	1,092	4,403	5,495
High School, 1-3 years......	3,565	66	92.9	939	3,565	4,504
High School, 4 years........	3,100	57	73.2	740	3,100	3,840
College, 1-3 years.........	1,283	27	31.9	322	1,283	1,605
College, 4 years or more....	1,169	28	23.0	232	1,169	1,401
Unknown....................	-	107[b]	-	-	-	-
Males 65 & over..............	9,676	336[a,c]	336.0	5,985	27,906	33,891
Less than 5 years..........	2,005	48	85.5	1,523	6,029	7,552
Elementary, 5-7 years.......	2,291	57	74.0	1,318	6,579	7,897
Elementary, 8 years........	2,653	73	93.5	1,666	7,683	9,349
High School, 1-3 years......	1,038 }	28	52.0	926	2,845 }	5,990
High School, 4 years.......	782 }				2,219 }	
College, 1-3 years.........	529 }	28	31.0	552	1,447 }	3,103
College, 4 years or more....	378 }				1,104 }	
Unknown....................	-	102[b]	-	-	-	-
Females 25-64 years...........	10,089	221[a]	221.0	2,207	10,089	12,296
Less than 5 years..........	918	12	25.8	258	918	1,176
Elementary, 5-7 years.......	1,632	26	39.6	395	1,632	2,027
Elementary, 8 years........	2,365	42	43.9	439	2,365	2,804
High School, 1-3 years......	1,788	28	42.2	421	1,788	2,209
High School, 4 years........	2,148	40	41.9	418	2,148	2,566
College, 1-3 years.........	783	11	16.3	163	783	946
College, 4 years or more....	455	11	11.3	113	455	568
Unknown....................	-	51[b]	-	-	-	-
Females 65 & over.............	7,722	336[a]	336.0	5,619	24,490	30,109
Less than 5 years..........	1,427	51	66.6	1,114	4,557	5,671
Elementary, 5-7 years.......	1,597	41	80.7	1,350	5,031	6,381
Elementary, 8 years........	2,291	74	97.3	1,627	7,456	9,083
High School, 1-3 years......	875 }	50	76.9	1,286	2,602 }	7,032
High School, 4 years........	967 }				3,144 }	
College, 1-3 years.........	348 }	17	14.5	242	1,053 }	1,942
College, 4 years or more....	217 }				647 }	
Unknown....................	-	103[b]	-	-	-	-
Total nonwhite decedents						
Males 25-64 years.............	2,279	120	120.0	1,204	2,279	3,483
Less than 5 years..........	832	31	49.8	500	832	1,332
Elementary, 5-8 years.......	900	35	40.9	410	900	1,310
High School or College......	547	21	29.3	294	547	841
Unknown....................	-	33[b]	-	-	-	-
Males 65 & over..............	2,194	31[c]	31.0	713	2,194	2,907
Less than 5 years..........	1,284	9	21.9	503	1,284	1,787
Elementary, 5-8 years.......	679	2	5.5	127	679	806
High School or College......	231	3	3.6	83	231	314
Unknown....................	-	17[b]	-	-	-	-
Females 25-64 years...........	1,889	78	78.0	766	1,889	2,655
Less than 5 years..........	530	11	27.3	268	530	798
Elementary, 5-8 years.......	832	21	37.3	366	832	1,198
High School or College......	527	19	13.4	132	527	659
Unknown....................	-	27[b]	-	-	-	-
Females 65 & over.............	1,978	40	40.0	665	1,978	2,643
Less than 5 years..........	1,074	14	20.5	341	1,074	1,415
Elementary, 5-8 years.......	670	10	12.6	209	670	879
High School or College......	234	1	6.9	115	234	349
Unknown....................	-	15[b]	-	-	-	-
White family members						
Males 25-64 years.............	15,857	279[d]	279.0	3,507	15,857	19,364
Less than 8 years..........	3,941	75	82.4	1,036	3,941	4,977
Elementary, 8 years........	3,810	56	57.9	728	3,810	4,538
High School, 1-3 years......	3,139	49	56.3	708	3,139	3,847
High School, 4 years.......	2,761	41	44.9	564	2,761	3,325
College, 1 year or more.....	2,206	42	37.5	471	2,206	2,677
Unknown....................	-	16	-	-	-	-

(continued)

Table A.12. Numbers of deaths on which education differentials in mortality are based, by family status, color, sex and age: United States, May-August, 1960--(continued)

Family status, color, sex, age and years of school completed	Matched Stage II Census (unweighted)	NCHS Survey (unweighted)		Stage II Census (weighted)	Matched Stage II Census (weighted)	Total Stage II Census or actual deaths
		Reported education	Adjusted to Census education			
	(1)	(2)	(3)	(4)	(5)	(6)=(4)+(5)
Males 65 & over...............	7,523	170[d]	170.0	3,463	21,164	25,627
Less than 8 years..........	3,302	64	80.7	1,644	9,535	11,179
Elementary, 8 years.........	2,092	40	44.1	898	5,847	6,745
High School, 1-4 years......	1,423	16	29.0	591	3,830	4,421
College, 1 year or more.....	706	17	16.2	330	1,952	2,282
Unknown....................	-	33	-	-	-	-
Females 25-64 years...........	8,430	136	136.0	1,776	8,430	10,206
Less than 8 years..........	2,062	29	37.7	493	2,062	2,555
Elementary, 8 years.........	1,964	31	24.9	325	1,964	2,289
High School, 1-3 years......	1,543	19	26.5	346	1,543	1,889
High School, 4 years.......	1,849	27	28.5	372	1,849	2,221
College, 1 year or more.....	1,012	17	18.4	240	1,012	1,252
Unknown....................	-	13	-	-	-	-
Females 65 & over.............	5,121	148[d]	148.0	2,986	15,655	18,641
Less than 8 years..........	2,166	54	69.8	1,408	6,612	8,020
Elementary, 8 years.........	1,522	37	42.9	866	4,795	5,661
High School, 1-4 years......	1,119	24	28.9	583	3,349	3,932
College, 1 year or more.....	314	9	6.4	129	899	1,028
Unknown....................	-	24	-	-	-	-
White unrelated individuals						
Males 25-64 years.............	1,618	94[d]	94.0	1,175	1,618	2,793
0-8 years..................	840	42	58.9	736	840	1,576
High School, 1-4 years......	567	25	24.9	311	567	878
College, 1 year or more.....	211	12	10.2	128	211	339
Unknown....................	-	15	-	-	-	-
Males 65 & over...............	1,332	80[d]	80.0	1,684	3,952	5,636
0-8 years..................	950	43	62.1	1,307	2,822	4,129
High School or College......	382	16	17.9	377	1,130	1,507
Unknown....................	-	21	-	-	-	-
Females 25-64 years...........	1,208	32[d]	32.0	381	1,208	1,589
0-8 years..................	596	13	18.1	215	596	811
High School, 1-4 years......	423	11	7.6	90	423	513
College, 1 year or more.....	189	4	6.4	76	189	265
Unknown....................	-	4	-	-	-	-
Females 65 & over.............	1,657	61[d]	61.0	1,336	5,296	6,632
0-8 years..................	1,003	29	40.1	878	3,261	4,139
High School or College......	654	16	20.9	458	2,035	2,493
Unknown....................	-	16	-	-	-	-
White inmates of institutions						
Males 25-64 years.............	719	20[d]	20.0	178	719	897
0-8 years..................	486	7	14.9	132	486	618
High School or College......	233	3	5.1	46	233	279
Unknown....................	-	10	-	-	-	-
Males 65 & over...............	821	37[d]	37.0	838	2,790	3,628
0-8 years..................	605	22	31.7	718	2,087	2,805
High School or College......	216	3	5.3	120	703	823
Unknown....................	-	12	-	-	-	-
Females 25-64 years...........	451	5[d]	5.0	50	451	501
0-8 years..................	293	5	4.6	46	293	339
High School or College......	158	0	0.4	4	158	162
Unknown....................	-	2	-	-	-	-
Females 65 & over.............	944	62[d]	62.0	1,297	3,539	4,836
0-8 years..................	624	29	45.0	942	2,376	3,318
High School or College......	320	10	17.0	355	1,163	1,518
Unknown....................	-	23	-	-	-	-

Source: Column (2) from Population Research Center, University of Chicago, tabulation of NCHS Survey deaths by color, sex and age as reported on death certificate; by family status and education as reported on Survey questionnaire. Column (5) from U.S. Bureau of the Census, tabulation of matched Stage II deaths by Census characteristics of decedents (Tables 1, 8, 12, collated tape). Other columns explained in text.

[a] Numbers of white family members, unrelated individuals, and inmates do not sum to total white decedents because the latter include persons for whom family status was not reported in the NCHS Survey, as follows: 88 males 25-64, 49 males 65 & over, 48 females 25-64, 65 females 65 & over.

[b] Includes decedents for whom no Survey questionnaire was returned as well as those for whom education or family status was not reported on the questionnaire.

[c] Includes decedents of unknown age (2 white males, 1 nonwhite male).

[d] Excludes decedents for whom no Survey questionnaire was returned and those for whom family status was not reported on the questionnaire.

deaths by color, sex, age, and educational attainment were then added to the Census Bureau's tabulations of matched Stage II deaths by census education, color, sex, and age in order to obtain final estimates of "matched plus unmatched deaths" by education level. (It should be noted that some of the discrepancies in response reported in Table A.13 may be due to the fact the NCHS survey questionnaires for some decedents did not report whether the highest grade attended had been completed, and these decedents were coded and tabulated by highest grade attended.)

Table A.12 reports the numbers of matched and unmatched deaths from which the estimates of education differentials in mortality presented in Chapter 2 were derived. The numbers of deaths involved in each step of the estimation procedure can be followed in this table. Column 2 gives the (unweighted) number of NCHS survey deaths which could not be matched with Stage I census records, distributed by education as reported on the survey questionnaires. This distribution of unmatched survey decedents was "adjusted" to the distribution by estimated census education shown in column 3 by allocating unmatched decedents reported in each survey education category in column 2 according to the census education distribution in Table A.13 for the same survey education category, and summing the results over all the survey education categories (including the "unknown" survey category). The estimated distributions by census education in column 3 of Table A.12 were next inflated to the color-sex-age control totals for unmatched Stage II deaths, as shown in column 4, and then added to tabulations of matched Stage II deaths by census education (column 5) to obtain the estimated census education distribution of total Stage II deaths shown in column 6. The unweighted count of matched Stage II deaths in column 1 is an estimate of the actual number of decedents matched with Stage II census records.[10] Thus, columns 1 and 2 represent the numbers of matched and unmatched deaths, respectively, for which education information was collected in the Matched Records Study.

Two aspects of the estimation procedure may require clarification: (1) We have already noted that the unmatched Stage II control totals may be defined as the "Stage II census equivalent" of unmatched deaths, classified by estimated census color, sex, and age. As a result, the sum of matched Stage II deaths (tabulated by census color, sex, and age) plus the unmatched Stage II control totals yields an estimated total (matched and unmatched) decedents for the Stage II census, classified by estimated census color, sex, and age. (2) The

Table A.13. Comparison of response to education question on NCHS Survey questionnaire and Stage II Census record, for decedents 25 years of age and over in NCHS Sample Survey who were matched with Stage II Census records, by color, sex and age: United States, May-August, 1960

Color, sex, age and years of school completed (Stage II Census)	Total[a]	Less than 5 years	Elementary		High School		College		Un-known[b]
			5-7 years	8 years	1-3 years	4 years	1-3 years	4 years or more	
White males 25-64 years..........	410[a]	28	62	91	58	68	27	28	48
Less than 5 years.............	34	21	6	1	-	-	-	-	6
Elementary, 5-7 years.........	82	4	41	15	7	1	-	-	14
Elementary, 8 years...........	91	3	11	58	5	3	-	-	11
High School, 1-3 years........	78	-	2	13	39	13	-	2	9
High School, 4 years..........	74	-	1	4	5	49	9	1	5
College, 1-3 years............	28	-	1	-	2	2	16	4	3
College, 4 years or more......	23	-	-	-	-	-	2	21	-
White males 65 & over............	289[a]	38	44	80	23	19	19	8	58
Less than 5 years.............	61	29	10	2	-	1	-	-	19
Elementary, 5-7 years.........	61	5	16	25	1	1	-	-	13
Elementary, 8 years...........	84	2	17	43	5	2	2	-	13
High School, 1-3 years........	29	-	1	5	13	3	3	-	4
High School, 4 years..........	26	2	-	4	3	9	3	1	4
College, 1 year or more.......	28	-	-	1	1	3	11	7	5
White females 25-64 years........	233[a]	19	24	46	35	54	18	8	29
Less than 5 years.............	27	15	3	3	-	-	-	-	6
Elementary, 5-7 years.........	36	2	15	10	2	1	-	-	6
Elementary, 8 years...........	44	2	3	24	4	4	1	-	6
High School, 1-3 years........	46	-	3	7	24	6	1	1	4
High School, 4 years..........	49	-	-	2	4	37	1	-	5
College, 1-3 years............	22	-	-	-	1	5	14	1	1
College, 4 years or more......	9	-	-	-	-	1	1	6	1
White females 65 & over..........	265[a]	42	45	57	14	31	8	11	57
Less than 5 years.............	51	35	3	1	-	1	-	1	10
Elementary, 5-7 years.........	67	4	30	14	5	1	-	-	13
Elementary, 8 years...........	72	2	8	37	3	5	-	-	17
High School, 1-3 years........	34	1	2	3	6	8	2	2	10
High School, 4 years..........	26	-	2	2	-	15	-	1	6
College, 1 year or more.......	15	-	-	-	-	1	6	7	1
Nonwhite males 25-64 years.......	53[a]	11	25		7		1		9
Less than 5 years.............	19	8	6		-		-		5
Elementary, 5-8 years.........	21	3	15		1		-		2
High School, 1-4 years........	10	-	3		5		-		2
College, 1 year or more.......	3	-	1		1		1		-
Nonwhite males 65 & over.........	25[a]	9	7		-		-		9
Less than 5 years.............	17	6	3		-		-		8
Elementary, 5-8 years.........	6	3	2		-		-		1
High School, 1-4 years........	2	-	2		-		-		-
College, 1 year or more.......	-	-	-		-		-		-
Nonwhite females 25-64 years.....	41[a]	9	15		9		1		7
Less than 5 years.............	14	7	2		2		-		3
Elementary, 5-8 years.........	19	2	10		3		-		4
High School, 1-4 years........	7	-	2		4		1		-
College, 1 year or more.......	1	-	1		-		-		-
Nonwhite females 65 & over.......	28[a]	9	7		1		2		9
Less than 5 years.............	13	7	2		-		-		4
Elementary, 5-8 years.........	9	2	3		-		1		3
High School, 1-4 years........	6	-	2		1		1		2
College, 1 year or more.......	-	-	-		-		-		-

Source: Population Research Center, University of Chicago. Tabulation of NCHS Survey deaths by color, sex and age as reported on death certificate; by years of school completed as reported on NCHS Survey questionnaire, and by years of school completed as reported (or as allocated, if not reported) on Stage II Census record (unweighted count). Some of the discrepancies in response summarized in this table may be due to the fact that the NCHS Survey questionnaires for some decedents did not report whether or not the highest grade of school attended had been completed, and these decedents were tabulated by highest grade attended.

[a] Excludes 133 decedents (26 white males, 25-64, 34 white males 65 and over, 15 white females 25-64, 33 white females 65 and over, 10 nonwhite males 25-64, 1 nonwhite male 65 and over, 11 nonwhite females 25-64, 3 nonwhite females 65 and over) for whom years of school was "allocated" by computer in edit of Stage II Census tape.

[b] Includes decedents for whom no questionnaire was returned as well as those for whom education was not reported on the questionnaire.

procedure for estimating the educational attainment of all unmatched Stage II decedents from the education reported for the
subsample in the NCHS survey also incorporates an adjustment to
estimate their census "level of education." Consequently, our final
estimates of "matched plus unmatched" deaths were designed to
yield the best possible distribution of total (Stage II) deaths by
estimated *census* characteristics of decedents. Use of these estimates
for deaths in conjunction with tabulations of population data by
census characteristics yields mortality indexes designed to measure
the relative incidence of death in subgroups of the population as
classified in the 1960 census records.[11] In this connection it may be
worth mentioning a rather obvious alternative estimation procedure
in which: (1) distributions of matched Stage II deaths by census
education could be inflated to matched Stage I deaths, with controls
by color, sex, and age; (2) distributions of unmatched NCHS survey
deaths by estimated census education could be inflated to unmatched Stage I deaths, with controls by color, sex, and age; and
(3) these two inflated Stage I estimates summed to obtain estimates
representing all deaths in the study. Such a procedure had two
shortcomings relative to the one used: (1) it involved more computations because tabulations of the matched Stage II decedents would
also have had to be inflated before being combined with estimates
for unmatched decedents, and (2) the resulting numbers would have
been further removed from the actual numbers of deaths for which
data were collected. In any case, the education differentials obtained
by the two procedures would be identical because our procedure for
deriving Stage II control totals for unmatched deaths preserved the
Stage I weights for summing matched and unmatched deaths by
color, sex, and age.

The estimates of total Stage II deaths in column 6 of Table A.12
provided the numerators (actual deaths) for mortality indexes by
level of educational attainment derived from the study. These
indexes were calculated as ratios of actual deaths (column 6, Table
A.12) to expected deaths in which the number of expected deaths
for each education group was computed by *multiplying* 1960
age-specific death rates for the total United States population *by* the
age composition of each sex, color, and education subgroup of the
population as tabulated from the 1960 United States census of
population. (Age categories used in the calculation of expected
deaths were as follows: 25-34, 35-44, 45-54, 55-64, 65-74, 75 and

over.) The mortality ratios by years of school completed which are reported in the tables in Chapter 2 are not the ratios of actual to expected deaths just described. Rather they are "relatives" which express the ratios of actual to expected deaths for the various education levels to the corresponding ratio for the color-sex-age subtotal to which the education subgroups belong (see note 3, Chapter 2, for further elaboration of this point).

Mortality ratios by education level within each of the three family status groups (family members, unrelated individuals, and inmates) reported in Chapter 2 were calculated by procedures identical to those described above for all persons 25 and over, except that broader categories of educational attainment were used. For each family status group, estimates of the education distribution for total Stage II decedents—which provided the "actual deaths" for the numerators of mortality ratios—were obtained in three steps. The steps for family members, for example, were as follows: First, the education level reported on the NCHS survey questionnaires for unmatched decedents reported as family members on the question-naires was adjusted to "estimated census education" using a cross classification comparing responses to the education question on the survey questionnaire with responses to the same question on the 1960 census schedule for those family members in the NCHS survey who were matched with Stage II census records (this cross classifi-cation is not included in the Appendix tables). Second, the estimated census education distribution of these unmatched NCHS survey family members was then inflated to the unmatched Stage II control totals for family members taken from column 3 of Table A.10. Third, these estimates of unmatched Stage II family members by education level were then added to the Census Bureau's tabulation of matched Stage II decedent family members to obtain the estimates of total Stage II deaths by education level, which provided the actual deaths for the numerators of the mortality indexes for family members. The mortality indexes by education level from which the mortality ratios for family members in Chapter 2 were derived are age-adjusted ratios of actual deaths to expected deaths, in which the number of expected deaths for each education level was obtained by *multiplying* 1960 age-specific death rates for the total United States population by the age composition of family members in that education level in the 1960 census enumeration.

c. Ratios by Education Level and Cause of Death

Estimates of actual deaths (total Stage II deaths) by education level were made for each of the 23 selected causes of death listed in Table A.14. The 23 categories include 19 unduplicated cause-of-death groups (causes 1, 2a-2g, 3, 4a-4e, 5, 6, 7a-7b, 8), 3 major causes (causes 2, 4, 7) and a residual (cause 9).[1][2]

The procedures followed in deriving estimates of the education distribution of total Stage II deaths from each cause of death were identical to those described, for all causes combined, in the preceding section of this appendix, *except that:* (1) it was first necessary to derive color-sex-age control totals for unmatched Stage II deaths from each cause, and (2) estimates were made only for 4 levels of educational attainment. The "unmatched Stage II" control totals for each cause of death were obtained by first computing color-sex-age-specific ratios of all *matched Stage II deaths from each cause* (tabulated by cause as reported on the death certificate, by color, sex, and age as reported in the Stage II census) to all *matched Stage I deaths for the same cause*[13] (tabulated by cause, color, sex, and age as reported on the death certificate), and then applying these ratios to the color-sex-age distribution of *unmatched Stage I deaths for that cause* (tabulated by cause, color, sex, and age as reported on the death certificate).

Estimates of the education distribution of total Stage II deaths from each cause were derived in three steps. First, the reported education of unmatched NCHS survey deaths from each cause was "adjusted" to estimated census education, using the cross classification in Table A.13. Second, the estimated census education distribution of unmatched survey deaths from each cause was inflated to the unmatched Stage II control totals for that cause. Third, the inflated education distribution for unmatched Stage II deaths from each cause was added to the education tabulation of matched Stage II deaths from that cause.

Table A.14 reports the numbers of matched Stage II deaths and unmatched NCHS survey deaths, as well as several other relevant categories of 1960 deaths, for each of the 23 causes of death included in the analysis. The number of deaths involved in each step of our estimation procedure can be followed in this table. Column 1 gives the (unweighted) number of NCHS survey deaths from each

Table A.14. Numbers of deaths on which education differentials in mortality for selected causes of death are based, compared with total 1960 deaths, by sex and age: white decedents in Stage II Census and NCHS Sample Survey

Cause of death (ISC codes), sex and age	Deaths, May-August, 1960				Total deaths, 1960		Seasonal index	Matched Stage II deaths (unweighted)
	Unmatched		Matched Stage II Census (weighted)	Total Stage II Census (weighted)			Percent Stage II Census of total deaths, 1960	
	NCHS Survey (unweighted)	Stage II Census (weighted)			Number	Percent by cause a		
	(1)	(2)	(3)	(4)	(5)	(6)	(7)	(8)
ALL CAUSES								
White males 25 & over.....	817	10,845	46,100	56,945	781,800	100.0	7.3	27,869
25-64...................	481	4,860	18,194	23,054	288,753	100.0	8.0	18,194
65 & over..............	336	5,985	27,906	33,891	493,047	100.0	6.9	9,675
White females 25 & over...	557	7,826	34,579	42,405	593,051	100.0	7.2	17,810
25-64...................	221	2,207	10,089	12,296	151,706	100.0	8.1	10,089
65 & over..............	336	5,619	24,490	30,109	441,345	100.0	6.8	7,721
1. Tuberculosis,all forms (001-019)								
White males 25 & over.....	8	113	325	438	5,977	0.8	7.3	231
25-64...................	7	67	172	239	3,172	1.1	7.5	172
65 & over..............	1	46	153	199	2,805	0.6	7.1	59
2. Malignant neoplasms,incl. lymph. & hematop. tissues (140-205)								
White males 25 & over.....	159	1,798	8,063	9,861	126,761	16.2	7.8	5,080
25-64...................	98	791	3,377	4,168	52,609	18.2	7.9	3,377
65 & over..............	61	1,007	4,686	5,693	74,152	15.0	7.7	1,703
White females 25 & over...	122	1,491	6,910	8,401	110,116	18.6	7.6	4,664
25-64.....:............	73	701	3,377	4,078	49,801	32.8	8.2	3,377
65 & over..............	49	790	3,533	4,323	60,315	13.7	7.2	1,287
2a. of stomach (151)								
White males 25 & over.....	13	160	787	947	11,309	1.4	8.4	437
25-64...................	6	52	252	304	3,681	1.3	8.3	252
65 & over..............	7	108	535	643	7,628	1.5	8.4	185
White females 25 & over...	6	87	406	493	6,903	1.2	7.1	221
25-64...................	2	25	125	150	1,903	1.3	7.9	125
65 & over..............	4	62	281	343	5,000	1.1	6.9	96
2b. of intestine and rectum (152-154)								
White males 25 & over.....	11	242	1,193	1,435	18,187	2.3	7.9	679
25-64...................	6	82	400	482	6,252	2.2	7.7	400
65 & over.....	5	160	793	953	11,935	2.4	8.0	279
White females 25 & over...	19	247	1,184	1,431	19,171	3.2	7.5	723
25-64...................	10	90	458	548	6,456	4.3	8.5	458
65 & over..............	9	157	726	883	12,715	2.9	6.9	265
2c. of lung, bronchus, & trachea (162,163)								
White males 25 & over.....	43	429	1,753	2,182	28,494	3.6	7.7	1,286
25-64...................	30	254	954	1,208	15,177	5.3	8.0	954
65 & over..............	13	175	799	974	13,317	2.7	7.3	332
White females 25 & over...	6	68	318	386	4,702	0.8	8.2	225
25-64...................	3	36	172	208	2,353	1.6	8.8	172
65 & over..............	3	32	146	178	2,349	0.5	7.6	53
2d. of breast (170)								
White females 25 & over...	23	286	1,365	1,651	21,854	3.7	7.6	1,052
25-64...................	17	164	865	1,029	12,585	8.3	8.2	865
65 & over..............	6	122	500	622	9,269	2.1	6.7	187
2e. of uterus, ovary, fallopian tube & broad ligament (171-175)								
White females 25 & over...	25	278	1,268	1,546	19,317	3.3	8.0	929
25-64...................	16	177	720	897	11,052	7.3	8.1	720
65 & over..............	9	101	548	649	8,265	1.9	7.9	209
2f. of prostate (177)								
White males 25 & over.....	12	159	758	917	12,624	1.6	7.3	327
25-64...................	1	22	119	141	1,510	0.5	9.3	119
65 & over..............	11	137	639	776	11,114	2.3	7.0	208
2g. Other malignant neoplasms[b]								
White males 25 & over.....	80	808	3,572	4,380	56,147	7.2	7.8	2,351
25-64...................	55	381	1,652	2,033	25,989	9.0	7.8	1,652
65 & over..............	25	427	1,920	2,347	30,158	6.1	7.8	699
White females 25 & over...	43	525	2,369	2,894	38,169	6.4	7.6	1,514
25-64...................	25	209	1,037	1,246	15,452	10.2	8.1	1,037
65 & over..............	18	316	1,332	1,648	22,717	5.1	7.3	477

(continued)

Table A.14. Numbers of deaths on which education differentials in mortality for selected causes of death are based, compared with total 1960 deaths, by sex and age: white decedents in Stage II Census and NCHS Sample Survey-- (continued)

Cause of death (ISC codes), sex and age	Deaths, May-August, 1960				Total deaths, 1960		Seasonal index	Matched Stage II deaths (un-weight-ed)
	Unmatched		Matched Stage II Census (weight-ed)	Total Stage II Census (weight-ed)	Number	Percent by cause[a]	Percent Stage II Census of total deaths, 1960	
	NCHS Survey (un-weight-ed)	Stage II Census (weight-ed)						
	(1)	(2)	(3)	(4)	(5)	(6)	(7)	(8)
3. Diabetes mellitus (260)								
White males 25 & over.....	15	145	671	816	10,626	1.4	7.7	391
25-64.................	7	57	242	299	3,762	1.3	7.9	242
65 & over.............	8	88	429	517	6,864	1.4	7.5	149
White females 25 & over...	15	205	940	1,145	15,162	2.6	7.6	492
25-64.................	5	56	238	294	4,049	2.7	7.3	238
65 & over.............	10	149	702	851	11,113	2.5	7.7	254
4. Major cardiovascular-renal diseases (330-334,400-468,592-594)								
White males 25 & over.....	406	5,882	28,170	34,052	471,932	60.4	7.2	15,976
25-64.................	206	2,119	9,732	11,851	146,309	50.7	8.1	9,732
65 & over.............	200	3,763	18,438	22,201	325,623	66.0	6.8	6,244
White females 25 & over...	301	4,696	21,232	25,928	367,290	61.9	7.1	9,248
25-64.................	73	797	4,055	4,852	58,796	38.8	8.3	4,055
65 & over.............	228	3,899	17,177	21,076	308,494	69.9	6.8	5,193
4a. Vascular lesions affecting central nervous system (330-334)								
White males 25 & over.....	68	1,048	4,680	5,728	80,050	10.2	7.2	2,172
25-64.................	24	237	1,016	1,253	14,799	5.1	8.5	1,016
65 & over.............	44	811	3,664	4,475	65,251	13.2	6.9	1,156
White females 25 & over...	78	1,190	4,913	6,103	88,232	14.9	6.9	2,004
25-64.................	20	168	825	993	12,163	8.0	8.2	825
65 & over.............	58	1,022	4,088	5,110	76,069	17.2	6.7	1,179
4b. Rheumatic fever & chronic rheumatic heart disease(400-416)								
White males 25 & over.....	11	110	534	644	7,786	1.0	8.3	440
25-64.................	10	83	377	460	5,479	1.9	8.4	377
65 & over.............	1	27	157	184	2,307	0.5	8.0	63
White females 25 & over...	11	101	541	642	8,594	1.4	7.5	413
25-64.................	9	71	336	407	5,579	3.7	7.3	336
65 & over.............	2	30	205	235	3,015	0.7	7.8	77
4c. Arteriosclerotic & degenerative heart disease(420,422)								
White males 25 & over.....	246	3,731	18,749	22,480	310,798	39.8	7.2	11,176
25-64.................	139	1,485	7,129	8,614	107,154	37.1	8.0	7,129
65 & over...	107	2,246	11,620	13,866	203,644	41.3	6.8	4,047
White females 25 & over...	153	2,401	11,606	14,007	197,023	33.2	7.1	5,041
25-64.................	27	398	2,119	2,517	29,393	19.4	8.6	2,119
65 & over.............	126	2,003	9,487	11,490	167,630	38.0	6.9	2,922
4d. Hypertensive disease,with & without heart (440-447)								
White males 25 & over.....	24	341	1,572	1,913	27,188	3.5	7.0	817
25-64.................	11	95	422	517	6,551	2.3	7.9	422
65 & over.............	13	246	1,150	1,396	20,637	4.2	6.8	395
White females 25 & over...	23	450	2,092	2,542	34,828	5.9	7.3	912
25-64.................	10	70	370	440	5,401	3.6	8.1	370
65 & over.............	13	380	1,722	2,102	29,427	6.7	7.1	542
4e. Other cardiovascular-renal diseases								
White males 25 & over.....	57	652	2,635	3,287	46,110	5.9	7.1	1,371
25-64.................	22	219	788	1,007	12,326	4.3	8.2	788
65 & over.............	35	433	1,847	2,280	33,784	6.9	6.7	583
White females 25 & over...	36	554	2,080	2,634	38,613	6.5	6.8	878
25-64.................	7	90	405	495	6,260	4.1	7.9	405
65 & over.............	29	464	1,675	2,139	32,353	7.3	6.6	473
5. Influenza & pneumonia, except pneumonia of newborn (480-493)								
White males 25 & over.....	24	253	860	1,113	25,714	3.3	4.3	450
25-64.................	10	84	238	322	6,821	2.4	4.7	238
65 & over.............	14	169	622	791	18,893	3.8	4.2	212
White females 25 & over...	8	169	731	900	19,533	3.3	4.6	307
25-64.................	3	32	139	171	3,454	2.3	5.0	139
65 & over.............	5	137	592	729	16,079	3.6	4.5	168

(continued)

Table A.14. Numbers of deaths on which education differentials in mortality for selected causes of death are based, compared with total 1960 deaths, by sex and age: white decedents in Stage II Census and NCHS Sample Survey--(continued)

Cause of death (ISC codes), sex and age	Deaths, May-August, 1960				Total deaths, 1960		Seasonal index	Matched Stage II deaths (unweighted)
	Unmatched		Matched Stage II Census (weighted)	Total Stage II Census (weighted)	Number	Percent by cause[a]	Percent Stage II Census of total deaths, 1960	
	NCHS Survey (unweighted)	Stage II Census (weighted)						
	(1)	(2)	(3)	(4)	(5)	(6)	(7)	(8)
6. Cirrhosis of liver (581)								
White males 25 & over.....	18	229	618	847	12,167	1.6	7.0	503
25-64.................	14	171	421	592	8,344	2.9	7.1	421
65 & over..............	4	58	197	255	3,823	0.8	6.7	82
White females 25 & over...	9	113	412	525	5,906	1.0	8.9	318
25-64.................	7	78	259	337	4,106	2.7	8.2	259
65 & over..............	2	35	153	188	1,800	0.4	10.4	59
7. All accidents (800-962)								
White males 25 & over.....	76	822	2,164	2,986	37,504	4.8	8.0	1,744
25-64.................	62	643	1,497	2,140	25,505	8.8	8.4	1,497
65 & over..............	14	179	667	846	11,999	2.4	7.1	247
White females 25 & over...	21	301	1,051	1,352	19,018	3.2	7.1	665
25-64.................	8	144	493	637	7,332	4.8	8.7	493
65 & over..............	13	157	558	715	11,686	2.6	6.1	172
7a. Motor-vehicle accidents(810-835)								
White males 25 & over.....	33	353	873	1,226	15,503	2.0	7.9	754
25-64.................	27	300	675	975	11,906	4.1	8.2	675
65 & over..............	6	53	198	251	3,597	0.7	7.0	79
White females 25 & over...	9	109	384	493	5,836	1.0	8.4	330
25-64.................	7	83	295	378	4,087	2.7	9.2	295
65 & over..............	2	26	89	115	1,749	0.4	6.6	35
7b. Accidents except motor vehicle (800-802,840-962)								
White males 25 & over.....	43	469	1,291	1,760	22,001	2.8	8.0	990
25-64.................	35	343	822	1,165	13,599	4.7	8.6	822
65 & over..............	8	126	469	595	8,402	1.7	7.1	168
White females 25 & over...	12	192	667	859	13,182	2.2	6.5	335
25-64.................	1	61	198	259	3,245	2.1	8.0	198
65 & over..............	11	131	469	600	9,937	2.3	6.0	137
8. Suicide (963,970-979)								
White males 25 & over.....	28	271	828	1,099	12,840	1.6	8.6	679
25-64.................	26	225	604	829	9,616	3.3	8.6	604
65 & over..............	2	46	224	270	3,224	0.7	8.4	75
9. Other causes of death[d]								
White males 25 & over.....	83	1,332	4,401	5,733	78,279	10.0	7.3	2,815
25-64.................	51	703	1,911	2,614	32,615	11.3	8.0	1,911
65 & over..............	32	629	2,490	3,119	45,664	9.3	6.8	904
White females 25 & over...	81	851	3,303	4,154	56,026	9.4	7.4	2,116
25-64.................	52	399	1,528	1,927	24,168	15.9	8.0	1,528
65 & over..............	29	452	1,775	2,227	31,858	7.2	7.0	588

Source: Column (2) from Population Research Center, University of Chicago, tabulation of NCHS Survey deaths by color, sex, age and cause of death as reported on death certificate. Column (3) from U.S. Bureau of the Census, tabulation of matched Stage II deaths by color, sex and age as reported on Census record; by cause of death as reported on death certificate (Table 15, collated tape). Columns (5) and (6) from National Center for Health Statistics, Vital Statistics of United States, 1960, Vol. II, Part A, Tables 3-5, 5-7, and 5-9. Column (8) unweighted numbers estimated by applying sampling proportions (one for ages 25-64, one-half for ages 65-74, and one-fifth for ages 75 and over) to weighted counts of matched Stage II deaths in column (3). Other columns explained in text.

[a] Deaths from each cause are expressed as percents of corresponding sex-age subtotals.

[b] For males, cause 2g includes cause 2d as well as cancer sites not listed in this table.

[c] For females, cause 9 includes causes 1 and 8, in addition to causes not listed in this table.

cause which were not matched with census records; distributions of these deaths by survey education were converted to estimated distributions by census education, using the cross classification of survey education by census education reported in Table A.13, and then inflated to the unmatched Stage II control totals shown for each cause of death in column 2.[14] The resulting estimates of unmatched Stage II deaths by education, sex, and age for each cause of death were then added to tabulations of matched Stage II deaths by education, sex, and age for each cause, to derive the estimates of total Stage II deaths by education, sex, and age which provided the numerators (actual deaths) of mortality indexes by education and cause of death. Column 8 of Table A.14 reports the unweighted counts of matched Stage II deaths, and indicates for each cause of death the actual number of decedents matched with Stage II census records. Thus, columns 1 and 8 represent the numbers of unmatched and matched deaths, respectively, for which education information by cause of death was collected in the Matched Records Study.

Column 5 of Table A.14 reports the total number of 1960 deaths from each cause; column 6 the percentages of all 1960 deaths, separately for each sex-age subgroup, that were in each cause of death category; and column 7, the percentages of all 1960 deaths covered in our total Stage II (matched plus unmatched) census estimates. Column 7, therefore, is a measure of seasonal selectivity by cause of death. If deaths from each cause had been equally distributed throughout the year *and* if the Stage II census had been an exact 25-percent sample, all the percentages in column 7 should be 8.3, or one-twelfth of all 1960 deaths (because May through August is one-third of the year, and Stage II would be exactly one-fourth of the Stage I census enumeration). Actually, however, the ratio of matched Stage II to matched Stage I deaths was slightly less than 25 percent—23.7 percent to be exact.[15]

The mortality ratios by education level reported for the United States in Table 5.2 of Chapter 5 were derived from ratios of actual deaths (total Stage II census deaths in column 4, Table A.14) to expected death from each cause, in which the number of expected deaths for each education group was computed by *multiplying* 1960 age-specific death rates from each cause for the total United States population *by* the age composition of white males and females in each education group as tabulated in the 1960 census of population.

d. Ratios by Family Income and Personal Income

Mortality ratios by family income for family members, and by personal income for unrelated individuals, are reported in Chapter 2. These mortality ratios were calculated by procedures identical to those described above for family members by level of education attainment. For example, estimates of the family income distribution for total Stage II family members—which provided the "actual deaths" for the numerators of the mortality ratios—were obtained in three steps, and the numbers of deaths involved in each step can be followed in Table A.15. First, the family income reported on the NCHS survey questionnaire for unmatched decedents reported as family members on the questionnaire (column 2) was adjusted to "estimated census income" (column 3) using the cross classified distribution in Table A.16, which compares responses to the income questions on the survey questionnaire with responses to the same questions on the 1960 census schedules for those family members in the NCHS survey who were matched with Stage II census records. Second, the estimated census income distribution of unmatched NCHS survey family members was then inflated to the unmatched Stage II control totals for family members (from column 3, Table A.10) to obtain the estimates of unmatched Stage II family members by family income which are reported in column 4 of Table A.15. Third, these estimates of unmatched Stage II family members by family income level were then added to the Census Bureau's tabulation of matched Stage II family members by family income (column 5) to obtain the estimates of total Stage II family members (column 6).

e. Ratios by Occupation for Men

For several reasons occupation differentials in mortality were estimated only for white males 25-74 years of age. Most important was the fact that the 1960 census collected information on the "current" occupation of persons classified as "employed" during the last week of March 1960 and the last occupation held by other persons who had worked at any time since 1949. It was decided to combine these two groups for analysis of mortality by occupation because a substantial proportion of those who died between May and August 1960 were ill or incapacitated at the time of the 1960 census and therefore were excluded from the employed group. Combination

Table A.15. Numbers of deaths on which income differentials in mortality of the white population are based, by family status, sex and age: United States, May-August, 1960

Family status, sex, age, and income	Matched Stage II Census (unweighted)	Unmatched deaths			Matched Stage II Census (weighted)	Total Stage II Census or actual deaths
		NCHS Survey (unweighted)		Stage II Census (weighted)		
		Reported income	Adjusted to Census income			
	(1)	(2)	(3)	(4)	(5)	(6)=(4)+(5)
Family members by family income						
White males 25-64 years...................	15,857	279[a]	279.0	3,507	15,857	19,364
Under $2,000...........................	1,954	31	41.1	517	1,954	2,471
$2,000-3,999...........................	2,664	29	42.8	538	2,664	3,202
$4,000-5,999...........................	3,442	33	60.9	765	3,442	4,207
$6,000-7,999...........................	2,852	16	46.4	583	2,852	3,435
$8,000-9,999...........................	1,947	18	39.7	499	1,947	2,446
$10,000 or more.......................	2,998	16	48.1	605	2,998	3,603
Inadequately reported..................	-	136[b]	-	-	-	-
White males 65 & over.....................	7,523	170[a]	170.0	3,463	21,164	24,627
Under $2,000...........................	2,355	39	63.7	1,298	7,007	8,305
$2,000-3,999...........................	2,036	19	41.0	835	5,527	6,362
$4,000-7,999...........................	1,865	18	38.2	778	5,026	5,804
$8,000 or more.........................	1,267	8	27.1	552	3,604	4,156
Inadequately reported..................	-	86[b]	-	-	-	-
White females 25-64 years................	8,430	136[a]	136.0	1,776	8,430	10,206
Under $2,000...........................	1,170	14	18.4	240	1,170	1,410
$2,000-3,999...........................	1,485	16	26.8	350	1,485	1,835
$4,000-5,999...........................	1,857	15	24.6	321	1,857	2,178
$6,000-7,999...........................	1,531	14	25.7	336	1,531	1,867
$8,000-9,999...........................	952	7	16.9	221	952	1,173
$10,000 or more.......................	1,435	11	23.6	308	1,435	1,743
Inadequately reported..................	-	59[b]	-	-	-	-
White females 65 & over..................	5,121	148[a]	148.0	2,986	15,655	18,641
Under $2,000...........................	1,282	22	40.0	807	3,941	4,748
$2,000-3,999...........................	1,215	15	30.2	609	3,541	4,150
$4,000-7,999...........................	1,582	21	43.8	884	4,836	5,720
$8,000 or more.........................	1,042	10	34.0	686	3,337	4,023
Inadequately reported..................	-	80[b]	-	-	-	-
Unrelated individuals by personal income						
White males 25-64 years...................	1,618	94[a]	94.0	1,175	1,618	2,793
Under $2,000...........................	738	13	37.3	466	738	1,204
$2,000-3,999...........................	366	7	26.4	330	366	696
$4,000 or more.........................	514	11	30.3	379	514	893
Inadequately reported..................	-	63[b]	-	-	-	-
White males 65 & over.....................	1,332	80[a]	80.0	1,684	3,952	5,636
Under $2,000...........................	977	38	51.5	1,084	3,002	4,086
$2,000 or more.........................	355	15	28.5	600	950	1,550
Inadequately reported..................	-	27[b]	-	-	-	-
White females 25-64 years................	1,208	32[a]	32.0	381	1,208	1,589
Under $2,000...........................	751	11	17.5	208	751	959
$2,000-3,999...........................	261	5	5.0	60	261	321
$4,000 or more.........................	196	3	9.5	113	196	309
Inadequately reported..................	-	13[b]	-	-	-	-
White females 65 & over..................	1,657	61[a]	61.0	1,336	5,296	6,632
Under $2,000...........................	1,418	36	49.1	1,075	4,585	5,660
$2,000 or more.........................	239	7	11.9	261	711	972
Inadequately reported..................	-	18[b]	-	-	-	-

Source: Column (2) from Population Research Center, University of Chicago, tabulation of NCHS Survey deaths by age, sex and color as reported on death certificate; by family status and income as reported on Survey questionnaire. Column (5) from U.S. Bureau of the Census, tabulation of matched Stage II deaths by Census characteristics of decedents (Tables 8 and 9, collated tape). See text for explanation of other columns.

[a] Includes only those decedents for whom Survey questionnaires were returned and family status reported.

[b] Includes decedents for whom the income questions were not answered at all, or were incompletely or otherwise inadequately answered.

Table A.16. Comparison of response to income questions on NCHS Survey questionnaire and Stage II Census record, for white decedents 25 years of age and over in NCHS Sample Survey who were matched with Stage II Census records, by sex and age: United States, May-August, 1960

Color, sex, age and 1959 income (Stage II Census)	Total	1959 income of decedent or family (NCHS Survey)						Income not adequately reported[a]
		With income adequately reported						
		Under $2,000	$2,000-3,999	$4,000-5,999	$6,000-7,999	$8,000-9,000	$10,000 or more	
Family members by family income								
White males 25-64 years	335[b]	24	39	43	37	28	34	130
Under $2,000	40	15	5	4	0	0	0	16
$2,000-3,999	49	5	23	3	1	0	1	16
$4,000-5,999	71	1	6	27	3	1	1	32
$6,000-7,999	59	1	4	6	20	3	2	23
$8,000-9,999	54	0	0	3	10	19	6	16
$10,000 or more	62	2	1	0	3	5	24	27
White females 25-64 years	187[b]	17	27	35	17	7	18	66
Under $2,000	19	9	0	2	0	0	0	9
$2,000-3,999	41	5	18	5	0	0	0	12
$4,000-5,999	40	0	6	18	4	0	0	12
$6,000-7,999	34	2	1	8	11	1	0	11
$8,000-9,999	22	1	2	2	2	4	4	8
$10,000 or more	30	0	0	0	0	2	14	14
White males 65 & over	213[b]	47	36	23		9		98
Under $2,000	78	38	10	1		0		29
$2,000-3,999	55	4	18	3		1		29
$4,000-7,999	48	3	8	16		1		20
$8,000 or more	32	2	0	3		7		20
White females 65 & over	163[b]	38	15	22		12		76
Under $2,000	50	26	0	1		0		23
$2,000-3,999	31	4	8	2		0		17
$4,000-7,999	46	5	6	13		2		20
$8,000 or more	36	3	1	6		10		16
Unrelated individuals by personal income								
White males 25-64 years	23[c]	-	3		7			13
Under $2,000	7	-	-		2			5
$2,000-3,999	6	-	2		-			4
$4,000 or more	10	-	1		5			4
White females 25-64 years	22[c]	10	4		4			4
Under $2,000	15	10	3		-			2
$2,000-3,999	-	-	-		-			-
$4,000 or more	7	-	1		4			2
White males 65 & over	31[c]	21		8				2
Under $2,000	19	14		4				1
$2,000 or more	12	7		4				1
White females 65 & over	54[c]	35		8				11
Under $2,000	45	33		4				8
$2,000 or more	9	2		4				3

Source: Population Research Center, University of Chicago. Tabulation of NCHS Survey deaths by color, sex and age as reported on death certificate; by family status and income as reported on NCHS Survey questionnaire; by income as reported on Stage II Census record (unweighted count).

[a] Includes persons for whom the income questions were not answered at all, or were incompletely or otherwise inadequately answered.

[b] Excludes two groups of decedents reported as family members in NCHS Survey: (1) those who were not reported as family members in Stage II Census; (2) those for whom family income was "allocated" by computer in edit of Stage II Census tape.

[c] Excludes decedents reported as unrelated individuals in NCHS Survey whose personal income was "allocated" by computer in edit of Stage II Census tape.

of the two groups, employed persons classified by current occupation *plus* "other persons with civilian work experience since 1950" classified by last occupation held, made it possible to assign to an occupation all persons with work experience since 1950, a combination which covered 94 percent of the white males 25-74 years old in the United States in 1960 (see Table 3.2, Chapter 3). As might be expected, the coverage was considerably less for those 65-74 years of age (82 percent) than for those 25-64 years old (96 percent). Less than one-half (48 percent) of the white males 75 years or older had worked at some time since 1950, and this age group was excluded from the analysis.

The mortality ratios by occupation for the United States in 1960 reported in Chapter 3 were derived by procedures comparable to those for educational attainment, which are described above in this appendix. As in the case of educational attainment, estimates of the occupation distribution for total (Stage II) decedents were obtained

Table A.17. Numbers of deaths on which occupation differentials in mortality of males are based, by color and age: United States, May-August, 1960

Color, age and major occupation group	Matched Stage II Census (unweighted)	Unmatched deaths		Stage II Census (weighted)	Matched Stage II Census (weighted)	Total Stage II Census or actual deaths
		NCHS Survey (unweighted)				
		Reported occupation	Adjusted to Census occup.			
	(1)	(2)	(3)	(4)	(5)	(6)=(4)+(5)
White males 25-64 years............	18,194	481	481.0	4,860	18,194	23,054
Did not work 1950 or later..............	1,656	24	28.2	285	1,656	1,941
Worked 1950 or later a	16,538	405	452.8	4,575	16,538	21,113
1 Professional & technical workers....	1,235	23	25.3	256	1,235	1,491
2 Managers, officials, proprietors....	2,059	50	52.7	532	2,059	2,591
3 Clerical & sales workers...........	2,289	32	47.6	481	2,289	2,770
4 Craftsmen & foremen................	3,607	78	96.9	979	3,607	4,586
5 Operatives & kindred workers........	3,158	67	90.8	917	3,158	4,075
6 Service workers (incl. pvt. hh.)....	1,276	40	47.2	477	1,276	1,753
7 Laborers, except farm & mine........	986	23	40.5	409	986	1,395
8 Agricultural workers b	1,112	30	27.7	280	1,112	1,392
9 Occupation not reported.............	816	62	24.1	244	816	1,060
No NCHS Survey questionnaire returned...	...	52	...	...	...	...
White males 65-74 years............	6,824	154	154.0	2,824	13,647	16,471
Did not work 1950 or later..............	1,879	19	29.9	548	3,757	4,305
Worked 1950 or later a	4,945	123	124.1	2,276	9,890	12,166
1 Professional & technical workers....	314	7	8.9	163	627	790
2 Managers, officials, proprietors....	595	12	8.5	156	1,190	1,346
3 Clerical & sales workers...........	685	11	12.7	233	1,370	1,603
4 Craftsmen & foremen................	1,032	16	20.7	380	2,065	2,445
5 Operatives & kindred workers........	782	17	20.3	372	1,565	1,937
6 Service workers (incl. pvt. hh.)....	485	9	9.5	174	970	1,144
7 Laborers, except farm & mine........	346	11	13.8	253	691	944
8 Agricultural workers b	521	17	22.5	413	1,042	1,455
9 Occupation not reported.............	185	23	7.2	132	370	502
No NCHS Survey questionnaire returned...	...	12	...	...	...	...
Nonwhite males 25-64 years.........	2,279	120	120.0	1,204	2,279	3,483
Did not work 1950 or later..............	397	8	10.2	102	397	499
Worked 1950 or later....................	1,882	96	109.8	1,102	1,882	2,984
White collar workers (groups 1,2,3)...	161	13	13.3	133	161	294
Craftmen & operatives (groups 4,5)....	584	25	27.9	280	584	864
Other workers (groups 6,7,8)..........	967	32	48.0	482	967	1,449
Occupation not reported (group 9).....	170	26	20.6	207	170	377
No NCHS Survey questionnaire returned...	...	16	...	...	...	...

Source: Column (2) from Population Research Center, University of Chicago, tabulation of NCHS Survey deaths by age, sex and color as reported on death certificate; by occupation as reported on Survey questionnaire. Column (5) from U.S. Bureau of the Census, tabulation of matched Stage II deaths by Census characteristics of decedents (Table 5, collated tape). See text for explanation of other columns.

ᵃ Includes decedents for whom "year last worked" was not reported (following procedures used in 1960 Census of Population). Persons not employed at time of 1960 Census are classified by last occupation.

ᵇ Includes farmers and farm managers, farm laborers and foremen.

in three steps, and the numbers of deaths involved in each step can be followed in the columns of Table A.17. First, the work experience and major occupation reported on the NCHS survey questionnaires[16] for unmatched decedents included in the NCHS survey (column 2) were adjusted to "estimated census work experience and census occupation" (column 3) using the cross classified distribution in Table A.18, which compares responses to the occupation question on the survey questionnaire with responses to the same question on the 1960 census schedule for those decedents in the NCHS survey who were matched with Stage II census records. Second, the estimated census occupational composition of unmatched NCHS

Table A.18. Comparison of response to work experience and occupation questions on NCHS Survey questionnaire and Stage II Census record, for male decedents 25-74 years of age in NCHS Sample Survey who were matched with Stage II Census records, by color and age: United States, May-August, 1960

Color, age, work experience since 1950 and major occupation group (Stage II Census)	Total	Did not work 1950 or later	Worked 1950 or later, last occupation was in group:										No questionnaire returned
			Total[a]	1	2	3	4	5	6	7	8	9	
White males 25-64 years	434[b]	22	396	35	51	47	87	74	27	18	24	33	16
Did not work 1950 or later	22	11	10	-	-	2	1	1	1	1	1	3	1
Has worked 1950 or later[c]	412	11	386	35	51	45	86	73	26	17	23	30	15
1 Professional & technical workers	33	-	32	27	-	1	2	2	-	-	-	-	1
2 Managers, officials, proprietors	52	-	52	2	36	3	4	2	-	-	1	4	-
3 Clerical & sales workers	57	1	56	4	2	37	5	2	2	-	-	4	-
4 Craftsmen & foremen	88	-	84	1	6	1	57	9	-	2	-	8	4
5 Operatives & kindred workers	80	2	74	-	2	1	8	52	1	3	-	7	4
6 Service workers (incl. pvt. hh.)	31	3	26	-	1	-	-	1	21	2	-	1	2
7 Laborers, except farm & mine	26	-	22	-	1	-	4	3	-	10	-	4	4
8 Agricultural workers[d]	23	-	23	-	-	1	-	1	-	-	21	-	-
9 Occupation not reported	22	5	17	1	3	1	6	1	2	-	1	2	-
White males 65-74 years	144	28	113	5	22	12	20	16	7	6	10	15	3
Did not work 1950 or later	38	24	14	-	4	1	2	4	1	1	-	1	-
Has worked 1950 or later[c]	106	4	99	5	18	11	18	12	6	5	10	14	3
1 Professional & technical workers	8	-	8	4	-	1	3	-	-	-	-	-	-
2 Managers, officials, proprietors	14	-	14	-	12	-	1	1	-	-	-	-	-
3 Clerical & sales workers	13	-	13	1	1	8	1	1	-	-	-	1	-
4 Craftsmen & foremen	22	2	20	-	2	-	13	-	-	-	-	5	-
5 Operatives & kindred workers	14	-	13	-	-	-	-	8	-	1	-	4	1
6 Service workers (incl. pvt. hh.)	7	-	7	-	-	-	-	-	6	1	-	-	-
7 Laborers, except farm & mine	8	-	7	-	2	-	-	-	-	3	-	2	1
8 Agricultural workers[d]	12	-	11	-	-	-	-	-	-	-	10	1	1
9 Occupation not reported	8	2	6	-	1	2	-	2	-	-	-	1	-
Nonwhite males 25-64 years	63	5	54	4			16		19			15	4
Did not work 1950 or later	5	-	5	1			-		1			3	-
Worked 1950 or later[d]	58	5	49	3			16		18			12	4
White collar workers (groups 1,2,3)	6	-	6	2			-		1			3	-
Craftsmen & operatives (groups 4,5)	16	1	14	-			11		2			1	1
Other workers (groups 6,7,8)	26	3	21	-			3		12			6	2
Occupation not reported (group 9)	10	1	8	1			2		3			2	1

Source: Population Research Center, University of Chicago. Tabulation of NCHS Survey deaths by color, sex and age as reported on death certificate; by work experience and occupation as reported on NCHS Survey questionnaire; and by work experience and occupation as reported on Stage II Census record (unweighted count).

[a] Includes decedents for whom work experience was not reported on Survey questionnaire.

[b] Excludes 2 males for whom occupation was allocated by computer in edit of Stage II Census tape.

[c] Includes decedents for whom work experience was not reported on the 1960 Census schedule; excludes decedents for whom occupation was allocated by the computer in the edit of Stage II Census tape.

[d] Includes farmers and farm managers, farm laborers and foremen.

survey decedents was inflated to the unmatched Stage II control totals for males 25-64 and 65-74 years of age (column 4, Table A.17). Third, these estimates of unmatched Stage II male decedents, by age and occupation, were then added to the Census Bureau's tabulation of matched Stage II male decedents by age and occupation (column 5), to obtain estimates of total Stage II deaths (column 6).

The mortality indexes by occupation computed from the Matched Records Study were age-adjusted ratios of actual deaths to expected deaths, in which the number of expected deaths for each occupation was obtained by *multiplying* 1960 age-specific death rates for the total United States population by the age composition of white or nonwhite males in that occupation in the 1960 census enumeration, and the number of actual deaths was the estimated number of total Stage II deaths obtained for that occupation in column 6 of Table A.17. Columns 1 and 2 of the same table report the unweighted numbers of matched Stage II deaths and unmatched NCHS survey deaths on which the estimates of actual deaths by occupation are based.

f. Ratios by Marital Status

Mortality ratios by marital status were derived from the 1960 Matched Records Study following procedures essentially comparable to those described above for education level but with some minor differences because marital status—unlike education and income—was reported on the death certificate as well as on the NCHS survey questionnaire. In this case, estimates of the marital composition for total Stage II decedents were obtained in the following three steps, and the numbers of deaths involved in each step are indicated in Table A.19. First, the marital status reported on the death certificate[17] for unmatched decedents included in the NCHS Sample Survey (column 2) was adjusted to "estimated census marital status" (column 3), using the cross classification in Table A.20, which compares responses to the marital status question on the death certificate and Stage I census record for all decedents in the Matched Records Study who were matched with Stage I census records and had age coded in the same 10-year age interval on the death certificate and census record. Second, the estimated census marital composition of unmatched NCHS survey decedents was then inflated to the unmatched Stage II control totals for each of the three age

Table A.19. Numbers of deaths on which marital status differentials in mortality of white population are based, by sex and age: United States, May-August, 1960

Sex, age and marital status	Matched Stage II Census (unweighted)	Unmatched deaths			Matched Stage II Census (weighted)	Total Stage II Census or actual deaths
		NCHS Survey (unweighted)		Stage II Census (weighted)		
		By death certificate marital status	Adjusted to Census marital status			
	(1)	(2)	(3)	(4)	(5)	(6)=(4)+(5)
White males 25-44 years..........	3,352	123	123.0	1,294	3,352	4,646
Married (or separated)........	2,608	79	82.4	866	2,608	3,474
Widowed......................	33	1	1.1	12	33	45
Divorced.....................	123	14	10.6	112	123	235
Never married................	588	27	28.9	304	588	892
Unknown......................	-	2[a]	-	-	-	-
White males 45-64 years..........	14,842	358	358.0	3,566	14,842	18,408
Married (or separated)........	12,185	201	213.0	2,122	12,185	14,307
Widowed......................	711	32	32.0	319	711	1,030
Divorced.....................	628	50	40.1	399	628	1,027
Never married................	1,318	69	72.9	726	1,318	2,044
Unknown......................	-	6[a]	-	-	-	-
White males 65 & over............	9,676	334	334.0	5,985	27,906	33,891
Married (or separated)........	6,630	138	146.0	2,616	17,866	20,482
Widowed......................	2,091	134	130.8	2,344	7,380	9,724
Divorced.....................	192	13	10.7	192	500	692
Never married................	763	43	46.5	833	2,160	2,993
Unknown......................	-	6[a]	-	-	-	-
White females 25-44 years........	2,081	45	45.0	564	2,081	2,645
Married (or separated)........	1,655	30	31.4	394	1,655	2,049
Widowed......................	95	1	1.1	14	95	109
Divorced.....................	103	9	7.3	91	103	194
Never married................	228	5	5.2	65	228	293
Unknown......................	-	-[a]	-	-	-	-
White females 45-64 years........	8,008	176	176.0	1,643	8,008	9,651
Married (or separated)........	5,412	101	104.8	978	5,412	6,390
Widowed......................	1,616	44	42.7	399	1,616	2,015
Divorced.....................	301	15	12.7	119	301	420
Never married................	679	15	15.8	147	679	826
Unknown......................	-	1[a]	-	-	-	-
White females 65 & over..........	7,722	336	336.0	5,619	24,490	30,109
Married (or separated)........	2,606	72	76.7	1,283	6,758	8,041
Widowed......................	4,313	227	223.0	3,729	15,180	18,909
Divorced.....................	122	6	5.4	90	318	408
Never married...	681	30	30.9	517	2,234	2,751
Unknown......................	-	1[a]	-	-	-	-

Source: Column (2) from Population Research Center, University of Chicago, tabulation of NCHS Survey deaths by age, sex, color and marital status as reported on death certificate. Column (5) from U.S. Bureau of the Census, tabulation of matched Stage II deaths by Census characteristics of decedents (Table 11, collated tape).

[a] Refers to decedents for whom marital status was not reported on the death certificate.

groups, as shown in column 4 of Table A.19. Third, the estimates for unmatched Stage II decedents were then added to the Census Bureau's tabulation of matched Stage II deaths (column 5) by age and marital status, to obtain the estimates of total Stage II deaths (column 6) which provided the numerators of the mortality indexes from which the mortality ratios by marital status were derived.

Because marital status is an item reported on the death certificate it was not necessary to rely only on data from the 1960 Matched Records Study to measure differences in mortality by marital status. The uncorrected marital status differentials reported in Chapter 7 were based on tabulations of 1959-61 deaths provided by the National Center for Health Statistics; the corrected rates incorporate an adjustment for discrepancies in responses to the marital status question on death certificates and census records derived from the Matched Records Study. This procedure provided much more stable estimates of differences in mortality by marital status than could be obtained from the Matched Records Study alone because of the much larger numbers of deaths for the three-year period.

Table A.20. Comparison of response to marital status question on Stage I Census record and death certificate, for white decedents 25 years and over who were matched with Stage I Census records and had age coded in same 10-year interval on death certificate and census record, by sex and age: United States, May-August, 1960

Sex, age and marital status (Stage I Census, unedited)	Total	Marital status (death certificate)				
		Married (or separated)	Widowed	Divorced	Never married	Not stated
White males 25-44 years...........	11,396	8,787	113	581	1,877	38
Married (or separated).........	8,849	8,642	39	103	45	20
Widowed.......................	96	16	64	9	6	1
Divorced......................	480	48	4	397	28	3
Never married.................	1,940	60	6	69	1,791	14
Not stated....................	31	21	-	3	7	-
White males 45-64 years...........	55,649	45,168	2,578	2,742	4,912	249
Married (or separated).........	45,458	44,580	304	319	166	89
Widowed.......................	2,506	140	2,020	215	108	23
Divorced......................	2,350	169	115	1,898	122	46
Never married.................	5,121	170	117	274	4,479	81
Not stated....................	214	109	22	36	37	10
White males 65 & over..............	111,336	69,066	30,186	2,772	8,739	573
Married (or separated).........	69,824	67,705	1,596	229	190	104
Widowed.......................	29,296	740	27,267	648	467	174
Divorced......................	2,290	116	420	1,618	92	44
Never married.................	9,295	264	677	254	7,873	227
Not stated....................	631	241	226	23	117	24
White females 25-44 years.........	7,008	5,637	210	385	761	15
Married (or separated).........	5,671	5,551	34	54	23	9
Widowed.......................	200	23	161	11	3	2
Divorced......................	353	25	12	301	14	1
Never married.................	757	21	-	17	716	3
Not stated....................	27	17	3	2	5	-
White females 45-64 years.........	28,702	19,731	5,348	1,197	2,355	71
Married (or separated).........	19,938	19,391	358	108	53	28
Widowed.......................	5,115	131	4,768	164	31	21
Divorced......................	1,128	68	136	876	38	10
Never married.................	2,393	54	65	43	2,220	11
Not stated....................	128	87	21	6	13	1
White females 65 & over............	96,065	25,432	60,256	1,528	8,575	274
Married (or separated).........	26,370	24,483	1,666	85	61	75
Widowed.......................	58,870	706	56,971	673	373	147
Divorced......................	1,419	57	580	723	48	11
Never married.................	8,720	82	561	41	7,998	38
Not stated....................	686	104	478	6	95	3

Source: Table 7, matrix numbers 135-141 and 213-219, special tabulations (weighted counts) comparing responses on death certificates and Stage I Census record prepared by the Bureau of the Census for the National Center for Health Statistics, compiled from matched deaths in the deck of 340,033 punched mortality cards (see Source, Table A.1). Exclude decedents under 1 year of age according to death certificate age and persons 100 years or over according to Census age; decedents with sex, race or age not reported on the Stage I Census schedule (unedited); decedents with age reported in different 10-year age intervals on the death certificate and Stage I Census record; and a few decedents with "not valid" codes for marital status. Although marital status was allocated in the computer edit of the 1960 Stage I Census tape, the marital status coded on the punched mortality cards and used in this crossclassification was an unedited independent code assigned during the match operation. Similar comparison of response data for 10-year age intervals is published in National Center for Health Statistics, Series 2, Number 34, Comparability of Marital Status, Race, Nativity and Country of Origin on the Death Certificate and Matching Census Record, May, 1969, Table 1; minor discrepancies between Table 1 and this table reflect differences in handling "not valid" and "not stated" codes.

However, because it was necessary to estimate "unmatched Stage II" deaths by marital status in order to obtain the control totals for ever-married women that were needed to compute mortality ratios by parity for these women, it was decided to carry out the computations of marital status differentials from the Matched Records Study as well, and to compare them with the results reported in Chapter 7, which were derived from deaths for the three-year period 1959-61.

Mortality ratios by marital status computed from the 1960 Matched Records Study are summarized below for white males and females (the numbers of deaths were too small for nonwhite widowed and divorced persons to warrant publication), with ratios for married persons set equal to 1.00.

	White Males 25-64	White Females 25-64	White Males 65 & Over	White Females 65 & Over
Single	1.76	1.30	1.21	1.08
Married	1.00	1.00	1.00	1.00
Widowed	1.73	1.30	1.17	1.13
Divorced	2.12	1.47	1.04	—[a]

[a]Not calculated because less than 10 unmatched NCHS survey deaths reported in this category.

These ratios compare reasonably well with those reported in Chapter 7 for the three-year period 1959-61, except for males 65 and over, who have larger differentials than those reported here.

g. Ratios by Parity for Married Women

Mortality differentials by number of children ever borne were estimated for all white women 45 years or older who had ever been married, that is, for those women who were classified as married, separated, widowed, or divorced in the 1960 census enumeration. Estimates of the parity distribution of ever-married female decedents for the numerators of the mortality indexes by parity were calculated in three steps, and the number of deaths involved in each step is summarized in Table A.21. First, the parity reported on the NCHS survey questionnaire for ever-married white women in the survey who were not matched with census records (column 2) was adjusted to "estimated census parity" (column 3), using the cross classifi-

Table A.21. Numbers of deaths on which mortality differentials by parity of women are based: United States, May-August, 1960

Age of woman and number of children ever borne (parity)	Matched Stage II Census (unweighted)	NCHS Survey (unweighted)		Stage II Census (weighted)	Matched Stage II Census (weighted)	Total Stage II Census or actual deaths
		Reported parity	Adjusted to Census parity			
	(1)	(2)	(3)	(4)	(5)	(6)=(4)+(5)
Ever married white women 45-64 years...	7,329	131	131.0	1,496	7,329	8,825
No children......................	1,501	19	22.1	252	1,501	1,753
1 child.........................	1,417	22	26.0	297	1,417	1,714
2 children......................	1,558	21	26.4	301	1,558	1,859
3 children......................	1,018	11	13.2	151	1,018	1,169
4 children......................	620	13	14.5	166	620	786
5 or 6 children.................	641	15	18.1	207	641	848
7 children or more..............	574	16	10.7	122	574	696
Unknown.........................	-	14[a]	-	-	-	-
Ever married white women 65 & over.....	7,041	270	270.0	5,102	22,256	27,358
No children......................	1,127	30	45.9	867	3,526	4,393
1 child.........................	1,022	33	33.2	627	3,177	3,804
2 children......................	1,257	43	56.4	1,066	3,848	4,914
3 children......................	975	31	42.1	796	2,967	3,763
4 children......................	761	20	21.1	399	2,525	2,924
5 or 6 children.................	900	31	31.0	586	2,904	3,490
7 children or more..............	999	48	40.3	761	3,309	4,070
Unknown.........................	-	34[a]	-	-	-	-

Source: Column (2) from Population Research Center, University of Chicago, tabulation of NCHS Survey deaths by age, sex and color as reported on death certificate; by marital status and number of children ever borne as reported on Survey questionnaire. Column (5) from U.S. Bureau of the Census, tabulation of matched Stage II deaths by Census characteristics of decedents (Table 13, collated tape).

[a] Includes only those women for whom NCHS Survey questionnaires were returned and marital status was reported as married, separated, widowed or divorced.

cation in Table A.22, which compares responses to the parity question on the survey questionnaires with responses to the same question on the 1960 census schedules for those ever-married women in the NCHS survey who were matched with Stage II census records. Second, the estimated census parity distribution of unmatched NCHS survey decedents was then inflated to unmatched Stage II control totals for ever-married white female decedents in two age groups, 25-64 years and 65 years or over; control totals for this purpose were obtained from column 4 of Table A.19, by summing married, widowed, and divorced females in the two age groups. Third, these estimates of unmatched Stage II ever-married white female decedents by age and parity were then added to the Census Bureau's tabulation of matched Stage II ever-married white female decedents by age and parity (column 5, Table A.21) to obtain the estimates of total Stage II white female decedents by age and parity (column 6).

Two sets of mortality indexes by parity were computed for ever-married white females from the Matched Records study, one standardized for age and the second for age and education level simultaneously. Both indexes may be defined as ratios of actual to

Table A.22. Comparison of response to question on number of children ever borne, NCHS Survey questionnaire and Stage II Census record, for white female decedents 45 years of age and over in NCHS Sample Survey who were matched with Stage II Census records and were reported as "ever married" on both records: United States, May-August, 1960

Number of children ever borne (Stage II Census)	Number of children ever born (NCHS Survey)									
	Total	None	1	2	3	4	5 or 6	7 or 8	9 or more	Un-known
Ever married white women										
45-64 years, total.......	150	24	31	26	26	10	14	6	6	7
No children..........	27	24	1	-	1	-	-	-	-	1
1 child..............	32	-	28	1	-	-	-	1	-	2
2 children...........	29	-	2	23	1	-	-	-	-	3
3 children...........	26	-	-	1	23	1	-	1	-	-
4 children...........	11	-	-	1	-	9	-	-	-	1
5 or 6 children.......	17	-	-	-	1	-	14	2	-	-
7 or 8 children.......	2	-	-	-	-	-	-	2	-	-
9 children or more....	6	-	-	-	-	-	-	-	6	-
65 years & over, total...	216	32	24	32	24	24	24	21	16	19
No children..........	41	30	1	-	2	-	1	-	-	7
1 child..............	23	-	18	-	1	-	-	-	-	4
2 children...........	42	1	4	28	1	2	1	1	1	3
3 children...........	32	-	1	3	20	2	2	1	-	3
4 children...........	23	-	-	1	-	20	-	-	1	1
5 or 6 children.......	24	1	-	-	-	-	18	3	1	1
7 or 8 children.......	15	-	-	-	-	-	-	15	-	-
9 children or more....	16	-	-	-	-	-	2	1	13	-

Source: Population Research Center, University of Chicago. Tabulation of NCHS Survey deaths by color, sex and age as reported on death certificate; by marital status and number of children ever borne as reported on Survey questionnaire and Stage II Census record (unweighted count). Excludes women for whom Survey questionnaires were not returned, women whose marital status was not reported on their Survey questionnaire, and women whose marital status or parity was allocated by computer edit in the Stage II Census.

expected deaths, in which the numbers of actual deaths (the numerators) were the estimated numbers of total Stage II deaths obtained in column 6 of Table A.21. Expected deaths for the age-adjusted ratios were computed by *multiplying* 1960 age-specific death rates for the total United States population *by* the age composition of ever-married white females of each parity in the 1960 census enumeration. Expected deaths for the age-education-adjusted ratios were computed by *multiplying* estimated age-education-specific death rates for the total United States population *by* the age-education composition of ever-married white females of each parity in the 1960 census enumeration.

4. Reliability of Mortality Ratios

Several aspects of our estimation procedure made it difficult to measure the sampling error of the mortality ratios used in our analysis. First, the limitation of deaths to those occurring during the four-month period May-August introduces a potential seasonal bias. Second, the estimation and inflation procedures for unmatched Stage II deaths, which are described above in this appendix, present more complications because the procedures include adjustments for discrepancies in responses to the same questions on death certificates, 1960 census records, and the special NCHS survey questionnaires. Although this adjustment has the advantage of correcting the mortality indexes for one kind of response error common to conventional death rates, namely, response errors resulting from discrepancies in the reporting of the same characteristic on death certificates and census records, it has an undetermined effect on sampling error. Lastly, even if random sampling theory could reasonably be applied to our mortality indexes, the formulas for sampling errors of age-adjusted ratios are very complicated and difficult to compute[18] and, still more important, do not apply to our measures of differential mortality, which themselves are ratios of two age-adjusted mortality ratios. Given this situation, we have selected rather arbitrary minimum reliability requirements, in terms of the numbers of deaths matched with Stage II census records and the numbers of unmatched deaths in the NCHS survey, the latter because the NCHS survey provided our only data on social and economic characteristics of unmatched decedents. The minimum reliability requirements appear in notes to each table summarizing results from the study.

5. Derivation of 1960 Life Tables by Education Level

Selected life table functions for the adult white population within six levels of educational attainment are reported in Table 2.4, Chapter 2. Life tables for these six education levels were derived from the Matched Records Study following the procedures outlined below.

Step 1. First, education level as reported on the survey questionnaire for unmatched decedents 25 and over (classified by 10-year age intervals up to ages 75 and over) who were included in the NCHS survey was adjusted to "estimated census education level" using the cross classification of "NCHS survey education by 1960 census education" summarized in Table A.13, except that the cross classification was specific for three age categories rather than two (25-44, 45-64, 65 and over). In these calculations, the cross classification for matched NCHS survey decedents 25-44 years old was used to adjust the reported survey education of persons 25-34 years old and persons 35-44 years old. Similarly the cross classification for matched survey decedents 45-64 years old was used to adjust the reported survey education of unmatched decedents 45-54 and 55-64 years old; and the cross classification for matched decedents 65 and over was used to adjust the reported education of unmatched decedents 65-74 years old and those 75 and over. The net result was an "estimated census education" distribution of NCHS unmatched survey decedents by 10-year age intervals from age 25 to ages 75 and over.

Step 2. The "estimated census education distributions" of unmatched decedents (by 10-year age intervals) obtained in Step 1 were next inflated to the control totals for white males and females by 10-year age intervals (shown in Table A.9), to obtain estimates of unmatched Stage II decedents by estimated census education level for each 10-year age group. The latter estimates were then added to a special tabulation of matched Stage II white decedents by census education and age to obtain estimates of total Stage II white deaths by census education and age.

Step 3. The distributions of total Stage II deaths obtained in Step 2 represent all the deaths that occurred in the United States during the four months May-August. These distributions were next inflated to total deaths for the entire year, 1960, by multiplying the education distribution obtained in Step 2 for each 10-year age interval to the total number of 1960 deaths for that age interval. The age classification of 1960 deaths selected for this purpose was corrected for discrepancies in the reporting of age on the death certificate and 1960 census records (NCHS, 1968).

Step 4. The net result of Step 3 was an estimated distribution of all 1960 white deaths by "estimated census" age (in 10-year age intervals), by "estimated census" education level. This distribution provided the numerators of age-specific annual death rates for the United States in 1960 by level of education. Denominators for the rates were obtained from a comparable classification of the United States population by age and education level (Bureau of the Census, 1963).

Step 5. The age-specific annual death rates obtained in Step 4 were used to calculate abridged life tables beginning at age 25, as follows:

(a) $_nq_x$ values were calculated from the age-specific death rates using the Reed-Merrell tables.[19] (b) ℓ_{25} was assumed to be 95,097 for white males in each education level, and 96,386 for white females in each education level (the values of ℓ_{25} reported in the official abridged life tables for the United States in 1960).[20] (c) ℓ_x and $_nd_x$ were calculated from their basic definitions. (d) $_nL_x$ was calculated from the formulas below.[21]

ages 25-34: $_{10}L_{25} = 5\,(\ell_{25} + \ell_{35})$

ages 35-64: $_{10}L_x = 5\,(\ell_x + \ell_{x+10}) + 0.41667\,(_{10}d_{x+10} - _{10}d_{x-10})$

ages 65-74: $_{10}L_{65} = 0.8333\,(-\ell_{55} + 8\ell_{65} + 5\ell_{75})$

ages 75 & over: $_\infty L_{75} = \ell_{75} \div {_\infty}M_{75}$

(e) T_x and $\overset{\circ}{e}_x$ were calculated from their basic definitions.

This procedure does not allow for any education differentials in mortality before age 25. This assumption, however, affects only the life table functions ℓ_x and $_nL_x$ which are not used in the Chapter 2 analysis. The $_nq_x$ probabilities of death and the $\overset{\circ}{e}_x$ expectations of remaining years of life are affected only by the death rates above age x.

APPENDIX B

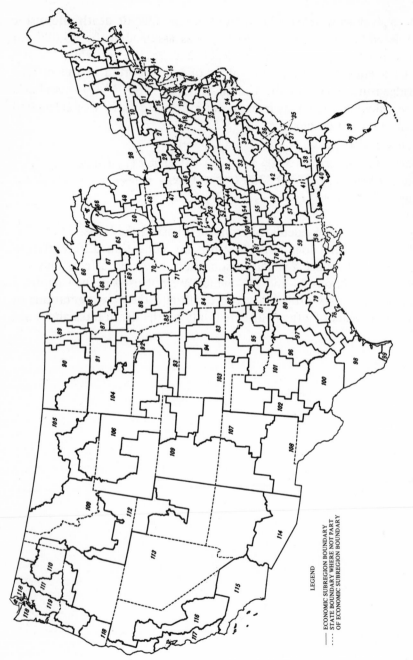

Figure B.1. Outline map of economic subregions, United States, 1960.

Table B.1. Age-adjusted death rates (per 1,000 population), by color, sex, and metropolitan or nonmetropolitan county of residence, for economic subregions (direct method, 1940 total population as standard): United States, 1959-61

Economic subregion	Total non-white	Total white population			White metropolitan population			White nonmetro-politan population		
		Total	Male	Female	Total	Male	Female	Total	Male	Female
United States, total.................	10.26	7.19	9.06	5.50	7.30	9.23	5.62	7.01	8.83	5.28
1. Northern New England.....................	--[a]	7.48	9.41	5.69	--[a]	--[a]	--[a]	7.48	9.41	5.69
2. New England Secondary Industrial..........	--[a]	7.42	9.49	5.67	7.56	9.77	5.75	7.30	9.27	5.61
3. Eastern Massachusetts-Rhode Island.......	9.54	7.40	9.33	5.82	7.41	9.36	5.83	7.04	8.84	5.54
4. Southern New England.....................	9.60	7.07	8.89	5.51	7.10	8.91	5.55	6.92	8.83	5.24
5. New York City and Environs...............	10.46	7.56	9.30	6.04	7.58	9.32	6.07	7.27	9.06	5.68
6. Hudson Valley.............................	9.31[a]	7.64	9.65	5.88	7.91[a]	10.05[a]	6.08[a]	7.42	9.32	5.70
7. St. Lawrence-Champlain....................	--[a]	7.99	9.99	6.15	--[a]	--[a]	--[a]	7.99	9.99	6.15
8. Eastern Lake Plains-Mohawk Adirondack.....	9.58	7.49	9.32	5.87	7.41	9.22	5.79	7.79	9.68	6.12
9. Western Lake Plains-Ontario Shore.........	9.83	7.46	9.30	5.84	7.54	9.40	5.91	7.07	8.79	5.50
10. Pennsylvania-New York Border..............	9.59	7.45	9.38	5.72	7.12	8.84	5.64	7.53	9.49	5.74
11. Pennsylvania Anthracite....................	--[a]	8.90	11.24	6.90	9.04	11.49	6.99	8.71[a]	10.91[a]	6.78[a]
12. Lehigh Valley.............................	--[a]	7.54	9.30	5.98	7.54	9.30	5.98	--[a]	--[a]	--[a]
13. Philadelphia (part in Pennsylvania).......	10.30	7.82	9.78	6.18	7.82	9.78	6.18	--[a]	--[a]	--[a]
14. Philadelphia (part in New Jersey).........	9.78	7.63	9.37	6.10	7.63	9.37	6.10	--[a]	--[a]	--[a]
15. S. Jersey Coast, Delmarva & Va. Peninsulas	11.53	7.53	9.47	5.78	7.59	9.57	5.85	7.51	9.45	5.73
16. Southeastern Pennsylvania-North. Maryland.	11.02	7.21	9.03	5.64	7.06	8.88	5.51	7.53	9.34	5.91
17. Northern Allegheny Mountains..............	8.43	7.59	9.37	5.98	7.66[a]	9.66[a]	5.95[a]	7.56	9.27	5.99
18. Shenandoah Valley-Blue Ridge..............	11.13	7.36	9.51	5.45	--[a]	--[a]	--[a]	7.36	9.51	5.45
19. Northern Piedmont.........................	11.14	7.46	9.62	5.71	7.47	9.63	5.74	7.35	9.47	5.36
20. Central Virginia Piedmont.................	10.91	7.22	9.50	5.34	7.28	9.76	5.37	7.08	8.99	5.27
21. Virginia-North Carolina Coastal Plain.....	10.71	7.59	10.24	5.27	--[a]	--[a]	--[a]	7.59	10.24	5.27
22. North Carolina Tidewater..................	11.59	7.78	10.26	5.46	--[a]	--[a]	--[a]	7.78	10.26	5.46
23. Pee Dee & Lumber River....................	11.81	8.02	10.59	5.75	--[a]	--[a]	--[a]	8.02	10.59	5.75
24. North Carolina Upper Coastal Plain.......	11.07	7.74	10.21	5.60	6.73	8.91	4.92	8.06	10.62	5.83
25. Old Belt Brightleaf Tobacco...............	11.16	6.84	8.95	5.02	6.90	9.18	5.07	6.81	8.84	4.98
26. Central Appalachian Ridge & Valley........	11.32	7.40	9.30	5.65	6.96	8.84	5.35	7.59	9.49	5.78
27. Pittsburgh Steel & Bituminous Fuel........	10.98	7.70	9.45	6.07	7.72	9.47	6.11	7.63	9.43	5.93
28. N.E. Ohio - N.W. Pennsylvania.............	9.88	7.40	9.18	5.78	7.47	9.27	5.84	7.25	8.96	5.65
29. E. Central Ohio - N.W. West Virginia......	10.29	7.36	9.00	5.82	7.70	9.49	6.01	7.17	8.73	5.72
30. Central Allegheny Plateau.................	9.73	7.17	8.83	5.59	7.37	9.33	5.62	7.10	8.66	5.58
31. Southern Appalachian Coal Mining..........	10.31	7.66	9.68	5.68	7.60	9.74	5.65	7.68	9.69	5.69
32. Southern Appalachian Ridge & Valley.......	11.82	7.22	9.03	5.59	7.13	9.14	5.42	7.29	8.97	5.71
33. Southern Blue Ridge Mountains.............	11.41	6.66	8.42	5.04	7.00	8.97	5.26	6.57	8.27	4.97
34. Central Piedmont.........................	11.61	7.14	9.38	5.23	7.19	9.82	5.11	7.13	9.28	5.26
35. South Carolina-Ga. Fall Line Sand Hills...	11.62	7.35	9.81	5.32	7.28	9.78	5.25	7.89	10.22	5.82
36. South Carolina-Georgia Upper Coastal Plain	11.77	8.08	10.80	5.69	--[a]	--[a]	--[a]	8.08	10.80	5.69
37. South Carolina-Georgia Atlantic Flatwoods.	12.81	7.77	10.25	5.63	7.84[a]	10.52[a]	5.69[a]	7.68	9.98	5.54
38. Georgia-Florida Lower Coastal Plain.......	10.73	7.08	9.21	5.12	--[a]	--[a]	--[a]	7.08	9.21	5.12
39. Florida Peninsula.........................	10.72	6.36	8.28	4.58	6.39	8.35	4.60	6.28	8.13	4.53
40. Florida Flatwoods.........................	11.60	7.32	9.45	5.33	7.44	9.77	5.38	7.11	9.00	5.24
41. Georgia-Alabama Central Coastal Plain.....	10.96	7.26	9.55	5.22	6.84	9.09	4.89	7.34	9.67	5.27
42. Southern Piedmont.........................	11.38	6.84	9.13	4.94	6.96	9.34	5.11	6.79	9.07	4.80
43. Georgia-Alabama Appalachian Ridge & Valley	11.24	7.20	9.40	5.28	7.09[a]	9.31[a]	5.23[a]	7.31	9.49	5.35
44. Eastern & Western Highland Rim............	11.35	7.10	8.69	5.56	--[a]	--[a]	--[a]	7.10	8.69	5.56
45. Kentucky Bluegrass........................	11.04	7.10	8.78	5.53	6.63	8.47	5.09	7.22	8.89	5.64
46. Ohio-Indiana Flatlands....................	11.32	7.35	9.33	5.67	7.44	9.56	5.72	6.96	8.50	5.45
47. West Central Ohio-Central Indiana.........	10.17	7.16	9.05	5.51	7.26	9.27	5.56	7.02	8.77	5.43
48. Michigan-Ohio-Indiana Tri-State..........	8.97	7.03	8.80	5.44	6.81	8.57	5.30	7.10	8.87	5.49
49. Southeastern Michigan.....................	9.21	7.36	9.18	5.66	7.36	9.19	5.66	7.35	9.05	5.69
50. Western Michigan Lakeshore................	9.35	6.98	8.72	5.39	6.96	8.76	5.37	7.02	8.71	5.41
51. Lower Wabash & Ohio Valley................	11.54	7.26	9.16	5.56	7.42[a]	9.45[a]	5.69[a]	7.17	9.01	5.49
52. S. Central Indiana & W. Central Ky. Hills.	9.65	6.83	8.38	5.30	--[a]	--[a]	--[a]	6.83	8.38	5.30
53. Pennyroyal & Jackson Purchase.............	10.95	6.84	8.54	5.25	--[a]	--[a]	--[a]	6.84	8.54	5.25
54. Nashville Basin...........................	11.69	6.93	8.99	5.18	6.89	9.13	5.09	6.99	8.83	5.31
55. Middle Tennessee Valley & Sand Mountain...	11.22	6.95	8.84	5.20	7.12	9.15	5.32	6.94	8.83	5.19
56. Alabama Upper Coastal Plain...............	9.88	6.51	8.33	4.81	5.44	6.93	4.04	6.97	8.93	5.15
57. Alabama-Mississippi Black Prairie.........	10.78	6.97	9.25	5.06	7.10	9.77	5.09	6.93	9.10	5.04
58. Central Gulf Coast........................	10.96	7.63	9.97	5.58	7.85	10.40	5.76	7.20	9.27	5.18
59. Miss.-Ala. Piney Woods & S. Brown Loam....	9.78	6.92	8.94	5.10	6.51[a]	9.05[a]	4.54[a]	7.02	8.98	5.22
60. Tenn.-Miss. Fall Line Slopes & Pine Hills.	9.71	6.45	7.98	5.02	--[a]	--[a]	--[a]	6.45	7.98	5.02
61. Tennessee-Mississippi River Hills.........	9.81	6.83	9.04	4.98	6.98[a]	9.37[a]	5.12[a]	6.73	8.84	4.88
62. Southern Illinois.........................	10.10	7.30	9.22	5.52	--[a]	--[a]	--[a]	7.30	9.22	5.52
63. East Central Illinois.....................	8.68	6.81	8.60	5.24	6.95	8.83	5.36	6.73	8.48	5.16
64. Southern Lake Mich. Industrial Conurbation	10.69	7.70	9.63	5.98	7.73	9.67	6.00	6.84	8.46	5.35
65. Eastern Wisconsin.........................	8.41	6.68	8.26	5.22	6.52	8.13	5.07	6.75	8.32	5.27
66. Northern Woods............................	9.83[a]	7.59	9.27	5.83	7.59[a]	9.39[a]	5.80[a]	7.59	9.23	5.85
67. Central Wisconsin.........................	--[a]	6.67	8.20	5.16	--[a]	--[a]	--[a]	6.67	8.20	5.16
68. Upper Mississippi River Hill Lands........	9.28	6.61	8.34	5.05	6.75	8.70	5.10	6.39	7.84	4.97
69. Corn Belt-Dairy Transition................	9.81	6.54	8.23	4.99	6.65	8.32	5.18	6.50	8.17	4.93
70. Eastern Iowa-Western Illinois.............	9.98	6.71	8.49	5.11	6.84	8.73	5.19	6.65	8.38	5.08

(continued)

Table B.1. Age-adjusted death rates (per 1,000 population), by color, sex, and metropolitan or nonmetropolitan county of residence, for economic subregions (direct method, 1940 total population as standard): United States, 1959-61--(continued)

Economic subregion	Total non-white	Total white population			White metropolitan population			White nonmetropolitan population		
		Total	Male	Female	Total	Male	Female	Total	Male	Female
71. S. Iowa - N. Missouri - W. Central Ill....	11.04	6.56	8.32	4.94	--a	--a	--a	6.56	8.32	4.94
72. Mo. - Ill. Ozark-Corn Belt Transition.....	10.73a	7.09	9.07	5.41	7.22	9.30	5.50	6.55	8.18	4.98
73. Ozark Plateau............................	--	6.56	8.24	4.91	6.68	8.93	4.82	6.54	8.12	4.94
74. Middle Arkansas Valley & Ozark Slopes.....	10.10	6.47	8.40	4.69	6.62a	8.90a	4.66a	6.32	7.99	4.72
75. Crowley's Ridge & Arkansas Prairies.......	8.96	6.78	8.68	4.93	--a	--a	--a	6.78	8.68	4.93
76. Mississippi Delta........................	10.03	7.16	9.25	5.22	6.95a	9.24a	4.98a	7.22	9.27	5.28
77. Louisiana Sugarcane......................	10.27	7.13	9.45	5.03	--	--	--	7.13	9.45	5.03
78. Louisiana-Texas Coast Prairies...........	9.91	7.07	9.18	5.15	7.15a	9.37a	5.20a	6.81	8.66	5.01
79. Texas-Louisiana Timbered.................	8.64	6.67	8.75	4.61	--	--	--	6.67	8.75	4.61
80. Arkansas-Louisiana-Texas Coastal Plain....	8.85	6.57	8.59	4.70	6.48	8.48	4.71	6.59	8.61	4.70
81. Ouachita Mountains.......................	8.10	6.76	8.81	4.79	--a	--a	--a	6.76	8.81	4.79
82. Springfield Upland.......................	10.34	6.94	8.75	5.26	--a	--a	--a	6.94	8.75	5.26
83. Flint Hills & Cherokee Plains............	8.93a	6.78	8.77	5.01	6.90a	9.09a	5.06a	6.73	8.67	4.97
84. Kansas-Missouri Corn Belt Border..........	--	6.37	7.96	4.88	--	--	--	6.37	7.96	4.88
85. Central Missouri River Valley............	10.50	6.72	8.57	5.08	6.91	8.97	5.17	6.39	7.93	4.93
86. North Central Iowa-Southwestern Minnesota.	9.16a	6.49	8.27	4.88	6.94a	9.09a	5.18a	6.32	7.98	4.75
87. Minnesota-South Dakota Corn Belt Margin...	--a	6.16	7.66	4.62	--a	--a	--a	6.16	7.66	4.62
88. Minnesota Forest Margin..................	--a	6.30	7.45	5.07	--a	--a	--a	6.30	7.45	5.07
89. Red River Valley........................	--a	6.38	7.99	4.71	6.11a	7.85a	4.44a	6.50	8.07	4.83
90. North Dakota Central Plateau.............	--	6.42	7.88	4.84	--a	--a	--a	6.42	7.88	4.84
91. Black Prairies..........................	--a	6.65	8.35	4.89	--a	--a	--a	6.65	8.35	4.89
92. Nebraska-South Dakota Corn Belt Margin...	--a	6.39	8.11	4.72	--a	--a	--a	6.39	8.11	4.72
93. Kans-Nebr.Corn Belt-Winter Wheat Transition	--a	6.08	7.50	4.75	--a	--a	--a	6.08	7.50	4.75
94. Wichita Prairies........................	9.25	6.32	8.12	4.75	6.42	8.37	4.77	6.29	8.01	4.75
95. Central Oklahoma........................	9.14	6.74	8.79	4.91	6.74	8.90	4.90	6.76	8.76	4.92
96. Grand Prairie & West Cross Timbers........	10.01	6.60	8.70	4.73	6.77	9.03	4.85	6.49	8.49	4.63
97. Texas Blackland.........................	9.78	6.38	8.44	4.61	6.42	8.52	4.68	6.32	8.37	4.48
98. Corpus Christi-San Antonio...............	9.55a	7.03	8.82	5.45	6.99	8.81	5.45	7.14	8.91	5.42
99. Lower Rio Grande Valley..................	--a	6.80	8.20	5.46	7.20	8.81	5.73	6.50	7.77	5.26
100. Edwards Plateau.........................	--	6.47	8.26	4.81	6.80	8.52	5.28	6.38	8.20	4.69
101. Texas-Oklahoma Rolling Plains............	9.84	6.33	8.30	4.53	6.10	8.03	4.40	6.54	8.61	4.64
102. Southern High Plains....................	9.86	6.52	8.58	4.57	6.46	8.76	4.41	6.64	8.51	4.78
103. South Central Plains....................	8.71	6.71	8.53	5.06	6.91	8.84	5.26	6.44	8.17	4.75
104. W. S.Dak., N.W. Nebr., & S.E. Mont.......	13.80	6.88	8.75	4.84	--a	--a	--	6.88	8.75	4.84
105. S.W. North Dakota & North. Montana Plains.	11.69	7.18	8.77	5.43	8.03	10.00	6.01	6.95	8.46	5.27
106. Upper Platte River Yellowstone Valley & Big Horn Basin...	11.26	6.71	8.45	5.00	6.45	8.22	4.87	6.80	8.54	5.05
107. Southeast Colorado & Northeast New Mexico.	--a	6.83	8.25	5.40	6.26	7.65	4.92	7.10	8.52	5.65
108. Trans Pecos & Southern New Mexico........	8.95	7.26	8.94	5.65	7.44	9.01	6.09	7.13	8.93	5.30
109. The Rocky Mountain......................	9.00	7.58	9.43	5.65	7.26	9.11	5.57	7.64	9.51	5.67
110. Palouse-Columbia River Basin............	11.11	6.67	8.45	4.90	6.89	8.85	5.04	6.49	8.14	4.77
111. Yakima Valley-Okanogan Highlands.........	--a	6.87	8.72	4.97	--a	--a	--a	6.87	8.72	4.97
112. Snake River & Utah Valleys, & Wasatch Front	8.75	6.56	8.20	5.00	6.55	8.19	5.07	6.57	8.22	4.95
113. Western Desert, Semi-Desert, & Mountain...	9.28	7.70	9.68	5.49	8.45	10.75	5.90	7.52	9.45	5.39
114. Southern Arizona........................	10.46	7.32	9.51	5.19	7.23	9.39	5.17	7.73	10.06	5.29
115. Southern California.....................	7.66	6.79	8.69	5.20	6.81	8.72	5.21	6.26	7.65	4.84
116. California Central Valley...............	8.85	7.32	9.39	5.23	7.47	9.58	5.35	7.11	9.11	5.07
117. Central Pacific Coast & San Francisco Bay.	7.50	7.07	8.96	5.38	7.12	9.07	5.43	6.85	8.58	5.16
118. North. Pacific Coast & North. Puget Sound..	10.44	7.18	9.00	5.27	6.99	8.66	5.34	7.22	9.08	5.26
119. Southern Puget Sound-Willamette Valley....	8.26	6.98	8.93	5.19	7.07a	9.08a	5.25a	6.62	8.34	4.95
120. Alaska.	9.62	7.85	9.32	5.49	--a	--a	--a	7.85	9.32	5.49
121. Hawaii..................................	6.15	8.09	9.92	6.38	7.74	9.46	6.14	9.77	11.91	7.63

a Rate not reported because based on less than 10,000 population.

Table B.2. Death rates and independent variables for correlation analysis, total population, 48 states: United States, 1960

State	Age-adjusted death rates, 1959-61 (direct method, 1940 U.S. standard)						Infant mortality rate (total pop.)	Independent variables						
	All males			All females				Median years school, persons 25 & over	Median family income, all families	% of pop. in central cities of urbanized areas	% Negro (of total pop.)	Physicians per 100,000 civilian pop.	Pop. per sq. mile of land area	% of workers employed in mfg.
	All ages	65 & over	25-64 years	All ages	65 & over	25-64 years								
	X_A	X_B	X_C	X_A	X_B	X_C	X_D	X_1	X_3	X_5	X_7	X_{11}	X_{12}	X_{13}
UNITED STATES.	9.37	68.0	7.60	5.84	46.8	4.10	26.0	10.6	$5,660	32.3	10.5	...	50.5	27.1
Alabama.......	10.04	66.0	8.85	6.44	45.9	5.06	32.4	9.1	3,937	26.7	30.0	73.9	64.0	26.5
Arizona.......	9.76	63.8	8.40	5.45	39.4	3.99	31.9	11.3	5,568	50.1	3.3	87.6	11.5	12.8
Arkansas......	8.86	60.3	7.38	5.47	41.1	3.95	27.4	8.9	3,184	13.4	21.8	88.1	34.0	20.1
California....	8.92	65.5	7.19	5.35	42.5	3.79	23.3	12.1	6,726	35.2	5.6	152.4	100.4	24.1
Colorado......	8.64	62.3	6.81	5.30	42.5	3.55	27.5	12.1	5,780	37.4	2.3	144.7	16.9	15.8
Connecticut...	8.87	69.7	6.74	5.62	48.6	3.67	21.1	11.0	6,887	34.4	4.2	161.7	517.5	40.3
Delaware......	9.83	72.7	7.95	6.26	51.3	4.48	23.8	11.1	6,197	21.5	13.6	112.1	225.6	32.7
Florida.......	9.09	56.0	8.38	5.39	37.1	4.34	29.7	10.9	4,722	25.6	17.8	100.0	91.3	13.1
Georgia.......	10.47	66.6	9.62	6.41	43.7	5.41	33.0	9.0	4,208	24.1	28.5	89.5	67.7	26.3
Idaho.........	8.51	62.8	6.47	5.05	41.0	3.31	22.9	11.8	5,259	0.0	0.2	82.7	8.1	13.5
Illinois......	9.64	71.9	7.73	6.06	49.2	4.25	25.0	10.5	6,566	42.1	10.3	118.6	180.3	31.8
Indiana.......	9.19	69.2	7.17	5.70	47.5	3.82	23.9	10.8	5,798	30.0	5.8	92.8	128.9	35.4
Iowa..........	8.35	64.1	6.30	5.00	42.9	3.13	21.9	11.3	5,069	22.0	0.9	92.9	49.2	18.6
Kansas........	8.23	61.7	6.30	4.98	41.7	3.22	22.1	11.7	5,295	17.2	4.2	101.6	26.6	16.6
Kentucky......	9.33	65.0	7.81	5.85	47.0	3.97	27.9	8.7	4,051	16.0	7.1	82.4	76.2	21.2
Louisiana.....	10.23	68.8	8.82	6.43	47.3	4.92	32.0	8.8	4,272	32.5	31.9	108.0	72.2	15.6
Maine.........	9.52	71.9	7.31	5.80	48.4	3.82	25.5	11.0	4,873	14.2	0.3	95.6	31.3	33.2
Maryland......	10.26	75.2	8.45	6.48	51.8	4.67	27.3	11.4	6,309	30.3	16.7	127.8	314.0	24.5
Massachusetts.	9.35	71.7	7.40	5.79	49.5	3.87	21.6	11.6	6,272	34.7	2.2	173.9	654.5	35.5
Michigan......	9.22	70.6	7.09	5.86	48.3	4.02	24.1	10.8	6,256	32.9	9.2	103.7	137.2	38.0
Minnesota.....	8.27	63.6	6.18	5.04	43.2	3.18	21.6	10.8	5,573	27.1	0.7	126.2	42.7	19.5
Mississippi...	9.94	65.2	8.36	6.58	46.6	4.96	41.6	8.9	2,884	6.6	42.0	71.9	46.1	19.2
Missouri......	9.17	67.0	7.39	5.60	45.3	3.85	24.7	9.6	5,127	32.4	9.0	109.6	62.5	24.7
Montana.......	9.59	67.9	7.68	5.61	44.7	3.87	25.0	11.6	5,403	16.0	0.2	87.8	4.6	10.1
Nebraska......	8.24	62.9	6.18	4.93	41.8	3.12	21.9	11.6	4,862	30.5	2.1	101.5	18.4	12.2
Nevada........	10.90	75.1	9.20	6.19	44.9	4.64	30.1	12.1	6,736	40.6	4.7	97.1	2.6	6.3
New Hampshire.	9.48	73.0	7.20	5.61	48.2	3.52	23.6	10.9	5,636	14.5	0.3	122.7	51.3	39.7
New Jersey....	9.54	72.9	7.52	6.20	51.4	4.27	24.6	10.6	6,786	18.7	8.5	116.5	806.7	36.1
New Mexico....	8.95	60.3	7.18	5.65	42.9	3.85	33.2	11.2	5,371	21.2	1.8	74.6	7.8	7.5
New York......	9.69	72.9	7.71	6.26	52.3	4.28	24.1	10.7	6,371	55.8	8.4	186.7	350.1	28.6
North Carolina	10.18	67.0	9.02	6.13	46.6	4.47	31.7	8.9	3,956	16.0	24.5	89.7	92.9	31.7
North Dakota..	8.05	61.3	5.92	5.03	43.3	3.06	24.8	9.3	4,530	7.4	0.1	75.1	9.1	3.7
Ohio..........	9.28	69.9	7.35	5.92	49.1	4.06	24.0	10.9	6,171	35.2	8.1	112.0	236.9	37.0
Oklahoma......	8.86	62.9	7.24	5.12	40.0	3.54	25.5	10.4	4,620	27.8	6.6	93.5	33.8	13.2
Oregon........	8.89	64.9	7.02	5.17	42.2	3.45	23.2	11.8	5,892	24.0	1.0	119.9	18.4	23.4
Pennsylvania..	9.83	74.3	7.87	6.33	52.8	4.37	24.5	10.2	5,719	31.1	7.5	126.7	251.5	36.4
Rhode Island..	9.21	72.1	7.20	5.87	50.8	3.82	23.3	10.0	5,589	33.6	2.1	118.2	812.4	39.3
South Carolina	11.29	68.7	10.89	7.07	45.5	6.29	34.3	8.7	3,821	9.6	34.8	72.7	78.7	32.0
South Dakota..	8.65	62.4	6.65	5.09	42.4	3.18	28.1	10.4	4,251	9.6	0.2	67.8	8.9	6.6
Tennessee.....	9.40	65.8	7.82	5.99	46.6	4.23	29.4	8.8	3,949	25.5	16.5	98.7	85.4	26.0
Texas.........	8.94	62.9	7.29	5.32	40.4	3.78	28.9	10.4	4,884	46.3	12.4	94.7	36.5	16.3
Utah..........	8.30	62.1	6.44	5.13	43.0	3.31	19.6	12.2	5,899	35.3	0.5	118.7	10.8	16.0
Vermont.......	9.48	72.6	7.21	5.63	47.9	3.61	24.1	10.9	4,890	0.0	0.1	140.7	42.0	25.0
Virginia......	10.01	70.1	8.47	6.23	48.5	4.53	29.8	9.9	4,964	25.1	20.6	95.8	99.6	22.4
Washington....	8.90	66.2	7.05	5.24	43.5	3.47	23.4	12.1	6,225	31.1	1.7	107.1	42.8	24.6
West Virginia.	9.57	66.3	8.07	5.89	47.9	3.99	25.5	8.8	4,572	13.5	4.8	80.1	77.3	23.4
Wisconsin.....	8.58	66.1	6.39	5.42	46.9	3.39	21.8	10.4	5,926	28.4	1.9	97.8	72.2	32.9
Wyoming.......	9.15	64.8	7.00	5.36	43.3	3.52	28.2	12.1	5,877	0.0	0.7	80.5	3.4	7.7

Source: National Center for Health Statistics, special tabulations of deaths for 1959-61 and Vital Statistics of United States, 1960, Vol. II, Pt. A, Table 3E. Bureau of the Census, 1960 Census of Population, Vol. I, Pt. 1 (U.S. Summary), Tables 12, 56, 106, 115 and 286; and Table 14 of Vol. I for each state. William H. Stewart and Maryland Pennell, Health Manpower Sourcebook, Section 10, Physicians' Age, Type of Practice and Location (Public Health Service, 1960), p. 8.

Table B.3. Death rates and independent variables for correlation analysis, white population, 48 states: United States, 1960

State	Age-adjusted death rates, 1959-61 (direct method, 1940 U.S. standard)						Infant mortality rate (white pop.)	Independent variables			
	White males			White females				Median years school, white pop. 25 & over	Median personal income, white males with income	Median family income, white families	% of white pop. in central cities of urb. areas
	All ages	65 & over	25-64 years	All ages	65 & over	25-64 years					
	X_A	X_B	X_C	X_A	X_B	X_C	X_D	X_1	X_2	X_3	X_5
UNITED STATES..	9.06	68.1	7.14	5.50	46.5	3.59	22.9	10.9	$4,319	$5,893	30.0
Alabama........	9.18	66.2	7.53	5.19	44.1	3.20	24.9	10.2	3,367	4,764	25.5
Arizona........	9.58	65.5	8.09	5.21	39.4	3.71	26.6	11.7	4,262	5,790	52.8
Arkansas.......	8.48	60.5	6.88	4.77	40.2	2.92	22.5	9.5	2,486	3,678	13.6
California.....	8.89	65.9	7.12	5.26	42.5	3.66	22.5	12.1	5,109	6,857	32.7
Colorado.......	8.60	62.2	6.76	5.26	42.5	3.49	26.9	12.1	4,228	5,816	36.1
Connecticut....	8.76	69.5	6.60	5.52	48.4	3.55	20.0	11.1	5,033	6,971	32.4
Delaware.......	9.23	71.9	7.13	5.73	50.1	3.79	17.8	11.6	4,879	6,570	18.4
Florida........	8.43	55.9	7.39	4.68	36.7	3.29	23.6	11.6	3,743	5,147	23.9
Georgia........	9.41	67.7	7.82	5.11	43.2	3.27	24.6	10.3	3,374	5,027	21.1
Idaho..........	8.47	62.9	6.42	5.01	41.0	3.25	22.7	11.8	3,866	5,275	0.0
Illinois.......	9.35	71.8	7.29	5.74	48.8	3.79	22.2	10.7	5,056	6,757	37.3
Indiana........	9.04	69.0	6.95	5.52	47.3	3.55	22.6	10.9	4,456	5,879	26.7
Iowa...........	8.33	64.0	6.28	4.97	42.8	3.09	21.7	11.3	3,708	5,077	21.5
Kansas.........	8.14	61.4	6.20	4.85	41.3	3.03	21.3	11.8	3,968	5,360	16.5
Kentucky.......	9.03	64.1	7.39	5.54	46.3	3.52	26.0	8.7	2,928	4,193	14.1
Louisiana......	9.61	69.6	7.97	5.34	45.7	3.37	22.6	10.5	4,001	5,288	31.0
Maine..........	9.51	71.9	7.29	5.79	48.4	3.81	25.7	11.0	3,275	4,882	14.2
Maryland.......	9.69	74.8	7.63	5.90	50.8	3.86	22.3	11.0	4,875	6,703	23.7
Massachusetts..	9.31	71.7	7.35	5.75	49.4	3.80	21.1	11.6	4,422	6,311	33.7
Michigan.......	9.08	70.9	6.84	5.63	48.2	3.65	22.1	11.0	4,984	6,442	28.0
Minnesota......	8.24	63.5	6.14	5.02	43.2	3.15	21.6	10.8	4,012	5,586	26.7
Mississippi....	8.95	63.9	7.33	5.11	43.6	3.09	26.6	11.0	2,757	4,209	7.4
Missouri.......	8.84	66.6	6.92	5.26	44.8	3.36	21.4	9.8	3,851	5,281	27.9
Montana........	9.47	67.9	7.55	5.44	44.6	3.68	24.2	11.7	3,993	5,453	16.4
Nebraska.......	8.12	62.6	6.02	4.84	41.7	2.99	21.3	11.7	3,497	4,883	29.2
Nevada.........	10.83	76.1	9.10	5.95	44.5	4.35	29.6	12.2	5,076	6,866	39.5
New Hampshire..	9.48	73.0	7.18	5.61	48.2	3.52	23.7	10.9	3,845	5,641	14.6
New Jersey.....	9.30	73.0	7.18	5.95	51.3	3.93	21.9	10.8	5,172	6,957	16.0
New Mexico.....	8.84	61.0	7.00	5.57	43.4	3.76	30.9	11.5	4,101	5,543	22.3
New York.......	9.40	73.1	7.28	6.03	52.2	3.94	21.5	10.8	4,798	6,542	52.9
North Carolina.	9.30	66.5	7.77	5.19	45.0	3.13	22.3	9.8	3,035	4,588	15.4
North Dakota...	7.96	61.2	5.84	4.95	43.1	2.96	24.1	9.3	3,134	4,558	7.5
Ohio...........	9.07	69.8	7.01	5.69	48.9	3.71	22.2	11.0	4,903	6,312	30.9
Oklahoma.......	8.69	63.4	7.00	4.84	39.5	3.18	22.7	10.7	3,446	4,824	27.1
Oregon.........	8.83	65.0	6.92	5.12	42.2	3.40	23.0	11.8	4,470	5,912	23.2
Pennsylvania...	9.64	74.3	7.57	6.12	52.8	4.04	22.6	10.3	4,348	5,824	27.2
Rhode Island...	9.15	71.8	7.14	5.82	50.7	3.76	22.4	10.0	3,848	5,624	32.9
South Carolina.	10.03	73.3	8.35	5.53	46.6	3.59	23.9	10.3	3,195	4,893	9.5
South Dakota...	8.38	62.2	6.36	4.87	41.8	3.01	24.2	10.5	3,043	4,300	9.9
Tennessee......	8.90	65.4	7.05	5.31	45.1	3.25	25.3	9.0	2,932	4,333	20.0
Texas..........	8.65	63.5	6.76	4.92	40.1	3.14	26.3	10.8	3,728	5,239	45.1
Utah...........	8.23	61.9	6.37	5.09	43.0	3.27	18.8	12.2	4,558	5,921	35.2
Vermont........	9.48	72.7	7.21	5.63	47.9	3.60	24.2	10.9	3,320	4,892	0.0
Virginia.......	9.25	68.8	7.42	5.40	46.7	3.35	24.6	10.8	3,734	5,522	22.2
Washington.....	8.82	66.3	6.96	5.18	43.5	3.39	22.7	12.1	4,689	6,265	30.1
West Virginia..	9.44	66.4	7.86	5.74	47.7	3.77	24.8	8.8	3,470	4,650	13.2
Wisconsin......	8.54	66.1	6.34	5.37	46.9	3.33	21.2	10.4	4,417	5,950	27.1
Wyoming........	9.11	64.9	6.91	5.24	43.2	3.38	27.5	12.1	4,435	5,917	0.0

Source: X_2 from Bureau of the Census, 1960 Census of Population, Vol. I, Pt. 1, Table 139. Other variables from sources cited in Table B.2.

Table B.4. Death rates and independent variables for correlation analysis, nonwhite population, 43 states: United States, 1960

State	Age-adjusted death rates, 1959-61 (direct method, 1940 U.S. standard)						Infant mor-tality rate (non-white pop.)	Independent variables					
	Nonwhite males			Nonwhite females				Median years school, nonwhites 25 & over	Median personal income, nonwhite males with income	Median family income, nonwhite families	Of nonwhite population		
											% in central cities of urb. areas	Percent Japa-nese	Percent non-Negro
	All ages	65 & over	25-64 years	All ages	65 & over	25-64 years							
	X_A	X_B	X_C	X_A	X_B	X_C	X_D	X_1	X_2	X_3	X_5	X_8	X_{16}
UNITED STATES.	11.85	66.4	11.78	8.79	49.5	8.76	43.2	8.2	$2,273	$3,161	50.5	2.3	...
Alabama.......	12.40	65.6	12.82	9.58	50.3	10.04	45.0	6.5	1,417	2,009	29.5	0.1	0.3
Arizona.......	11.18	46.2	11.83	7.91	41.7	7.31	60.8	7.0	1,845	2,457	26.3	1.1	67.3
Arkansas......	10.41	60.1	9.82	8.13	44.3	8.23	38.7	6.5	993	1,636	12.5	0.1	0.5
California....	9.00	58.4	7.96	6.44	42.2	5.64	29.7	10.5	3,515	4,971	62.9	12.5	30.0
Colorado......	9.88	62.6	8.49	6.52	40.4	5.74	44.0	11.2	3,163	4,531	77.2	12.9	24.9
Connecticut...	11.74	76.7	10.35	8.33	57.4	7.12	36.9	9.1	3,516	4,554	78.1	0.6	3.6
Delaware......	13.65	78.1	13.38	9.96	62.2	9.38	50.6	8.4	2,421	3,559	40.5	0.2	2.1
Florida.......	12.53	58.8	13.79	9.35	42.0	10.64	46.1	7.0	2,073	2,798	33.3	0.1	0.8
Georgia.......	13.66	63.8	15.43	9.85	44.4	11.43	48.1	6.1	1,489	2,188	31.5	0.1	0.3
Illinois......	12.27	73.0	11.93	9.17	54.7	8.95	39.6	9.0	3,613	4,590	82.3	1.3	3.1
Indiana.......	11.76	72.0	10.95	8.81	51.8	8.67	37.7	9.0	3,448	4,363	83.6	0.4	1.7
Iowa..........	10.51	76.6	8.29	9.03	62.2	7.37	35.2	9.5	3,141	4,301	71.6	2.1	12.1
Kansas........	10.24	67.1	8.85	8.08	51.4	7.72	33.4	9.6	2,636	3,801	31.0	1.4	8.5
Kentucky......	13.20	74.7	13.23	9.66	56.1	9.56	48.3	8.2	1,764	2,570	40.2	0.4	1.0
Louisiana.....	11.74	67.5	11.18	8.91	50.7	8.72	46.9	6.0	1,565	2,238	35.8	0.0	0.6
Maryland......	13.20	77.5	12.92	9.65	58.3	9.31	44.6	8.1	2,756	3,926	62.3	0.3	1.6
Massachusetts.	10.82	70.2	9.75	7.91	52.1	7.05	34.4	10.3	2,984	4,383	74.5	1.5	10.8
Michigan......	10.27	63.2	9.64	8.16	48.7	7.98	40.4	9.1	3,728	4,407	79.6	0.4	2.7
Minnesota.....	10.99	70.2	9.71	7.54	51.7	6.45	22.6	9.9	2,616	4,151	61.7	4.1	47.3
Mississippi...	11.48	67.0	10.44	8.81	51.5	8.14	54.3	6.0	890	1,444	5.6	0.0	0.5
Missouri......	12.66	71.6	12.77	9.24	52.0	9.31	45.4	8.7	2,570	3,426	76.9	0.4	1.5
Montana.......	12.77	68.5	12.23	11.00	55.3	11.20	34.5	8.7	1,461	3,011	6.4	2.5	93.9
Nebraska......	13.63	76.3	13.83	9.29	51.9	9.38	34.3	9.6	2,882	3,981	78.4	2.5	20.0
Nevada........	11.09	55.8	10.80	9.91	54.7	9.76	33.9	8.8	3,184	4,623	54.0	2.5	38.2
New Jersey....	12.11	69.8	11.81	8.91	53.4	8.43	41.7	8.8	3,341	4,571	47.5	0.7	2.4
New Mexico....	10.21	50.0	9.76	6.56	36.7	5.38	52.8	7.1	2,009	2,484	7.9	1.2	77.3
New York......	12.43	68.9	12.45	8.51	51.7	7.92	41.6	9.4	3,307	4,441	85.1	0.6	5.2
North Carolina	13.18	68.8	13.70	9.28	52.2	9.24	52.4	7.0	1,286	1,992	17.5	0.1	3.5
North Dakota..	13.52	81.8	11.47	10.74	65.5	10.13	43.3	8.4	1,416	2,553	1.8	1.0	94.0
Ohio..........	11.65	70.1	11.33	8.61	51.6	8.37	39.4	9.1	3,433	4,431	82.9	0.4	1.3
Oklahoma......	10.55	58.2	10.20	7.95	46.9	7.48	42.8	8.6	1,613	2,378	34.3	0.3	30.5
Oregon........	11.46	58.2	11.99	7.62	50.2	6.34	29.2	9.9	3,019	4,549	58.9	13.7	50.5
Pennsylvania..	12.16	72.4	11.81	8.94	52.8	8.71	40.6	8.9	3,216	4,142	78.3	0.3	1.5
Rhode Island..	12.48	90.1	10.76	8.32	55.4	7.14	44.4	9.5	2,503	3,483	60.2	0.9	11.8
South Carolina	14.42	59.3	17.51	10.30	42.1	12.54	48.5	5.9	1,135	1,699	10.0	0.1	0.3
South Dakota..	15.44	73.4	15.20	11.97	76.7	9.10	76.0	8.6	964	2,162	2.1	0.7	95.9
Tennessee.....	12.11	67.9	12.25	9.50	54.8	9.51	43.5	7.5	1,598	2,292	53.2	0.1	0.4
Texas.........	11.10	59.0	11.41	8.17	42.0	8.56	43.9	8.1	1,917	2,591	54.3	0.3	1.5
Utah..........	11.82	68.3	10.58	7.13	41.1	6.16	54.0	10.1	2,739	4,242	40.3	26.0	75.3
Virginia......	13.06	74.5	12.97	9.61	55.4	9.60	45.5	7.2	1,906	2,780	36.2	0.2	1.0
Washington....	10.57	63.7	9.52	6.89	42.4	6.29	36.7	10.5	2,989	4,705	58.0	16.4	52.0
West Virginia.	12.11	71.0	12.24	8.62	52.5	8.23	37.7	8.4	2,097	2,874	18.3	0.2	1.0
Wisconsin.....	10.26	64.3	9.14	8.03	53.6	6.81	35.3	9.0	3,631	4,653	80.4	1.5	19.7

Source: From sources cited in Tables B.2 and B.3. Five states with less than 10,000 nonwhite population in 1960 were excluded from the analysis.

Table B.5. Age-specific death rates (per 1,000 population) by marital status, color, sex and age: United States, 1959-61

Color, sex and age	Corrected for discrepancies in reporting of marital status				Uncorrected			
	Single	Married	Widowed	Divorced	Single	Married	Widowed	Divorced
WHITE MALES								
15-19 years.....	1.226	1.187	-- [a]	-- [a]	1.215	1.227	-- [a]	-- [a]
20-24 years.....	2.117	1.144	-- [a]	2.681	2.056	1.158	-- [a]	3.595
25-29 years.....	2.529	1.173	-- [a]	3.409	2.409	1.159	-- [a]	4.413
30-34 years.....	3.535	1.422	-- [a]	4.473	3.335	1.391	-- [a]	5.736
35-39 years.....	5.259	2.100	5.956	6.855	4.955	2.051	6.226 [b]	8.651
40-44 years.....	8.135	3.617	8.658	10.662	7.650	3.527	9.039	13.431
45-49 years.....	12.179	6.113	12.914	17.401	11.465	5.998	12.991	20.266
50-54 years.....	18.129	10.341	20.265	25.318	17.058	10.142	20.368	29.468
55-59 years.....	24.862	15.756	27.098	33.131	23.152	15.456	27.420	39.486
60-64 years.....	39.198	24.904	38.582	45.572	36.535	24.451	39.075	54.364
65-69 years.....	56.593	36.943	54.449	59.082	53.035	36.235	55.296	72.563
70-74 years.....	80.127	53.476	71.996	75.852	75.090	52.450	73.117	93.159
75-79 years.....	116.294	79.719	102.820	96.570	106.581	78.035	104.479	128.979
80-84 years.....	175.997	126.679	152.927	146.727	160.898	123.696	155.010	195.487
85 years & over.	259.169	206.692	251.388	248.297	237.663	198.082	256.610	267.089
WHITE FEMALES								
15-19 years.....	.484	.534	-- [a]	-- [a]	.480	.535	-- [a]	-- [a]
20-24 years.....	.792	.510	-- [a]	1.039 [b]	.774	.503	-- [a]	1.372 [b]
25-29 years.....	1.289	.620	-- [a]	1.608	1.277	.614	-- [a]	1.707
30-34 years.....	1.914	.867	1.908 [b]	2.036	1.891	.856	2.107 [b]	2.155
35-39 years.....	2.600	1.324	2.353	2.545	2.590	1.301	2.475	2.845
40-44 years.....	3.697	2.115	3.409	3.788	3.679	2.078	3.585	4.231
45-49 years.....	4.889	3.368	4.922	5.026	4.886	3.317	5.050	5.504
50-54 years.....	6.528	5.170	6.879	7.007	6.509	5.083	7.043	7.656
55-59 years.....	8.702	7.591	9.145	9.834	8.390	7.440	9.596	10.538
60-64 years.....	14.396	12.615	14.759	15.280	13.793	12.287	15.388	16.276
65-69 years.....	21.195	20.335	23.507	20.614	20.725	19.670	24.057	24.508
70-74 years.....	35.268	33.813	37.900	33.586	34.299	32.529	38.575	39.702
75-79 years.....	60.627	56.775	63.737	69.265	59.744	53.948	64.792	68.521
80-84 years.....	111.532	101.346	110.805	121.746	109.139	95.622	111.847	119.602
85 years & over.	223.948	173.320	207.667	172.046	213.446	139.273	211.133	199.934
NONWHITE MALES								
15-19 years.....	1.600	-- [a]	-- [a]	-- [a]	1.573	-- [a]	-- [a]	-- [a]
20-24 years.....	3.242	2.112	-- [a]	-- [a]	3.141	2.088	-- [a]	-- [a]
25-29 years.....	5.301	2.687	-- [a]	3.454 [b]	5.174	2.489	-- [a]	6.369 [b]
30-34 years.....	8.318	3.501	-- [a]	4.473 [b]	8.002	3.196	-- [a]	8.122 [b]
35-39 years.....	11.334	4.957	10.729 [b]	8.676	11.342	4.483	13.979 [b]	12.345
40-44 years.....	16.956	7.476	15.192	13.219	16.881	6.729	19.669	18.717
45-49 years.....	19.272	10.548	20.336	25.347	20.183	9.674	26.568	25.396
50-54 years.....	24.837	16.381	28.453	36.009	25.814	14.910	36.898	35.795
55-59 years.....	28.665	21.040	40.324	40.377	25.581	19.901	45.379	41.857
60-64 years.....	52.546	34.223	57.425	61.533	46.581	32.148	64.184	63.349
65-69 years.....	59.561	43.310	74.296	61.369	54.964	41.340	74.674	79.519
70-74 years.....	78.248	53.701	86.854	70.561	72.236	51.280	87.348	91.469
75-79 years.....	97.624	65.169	88.586	80.301	81.647	61.432	93.028	94.887
80-84 years.....	145.841	95.804	128.438	92.455	120.567	89.277	133.345	107.687
85 years & over.	196.022	128.045	186.817	101.487	154.714	125.617	184.533	187.227
NONWHITE FEMALES								
15-19 years.....	.798	1.018 [b]	-- [a]	-- [a]	.783	1.003 [b]	-- [a]	-- [a]
20-24 years.....	1.707	1.215	-- [a]	-- [a]	1.659	1.184	-- [a]	-- [a]
25-29 years.....	2.743	1.819	-- [a]	-- [a]	3.070	1.682	-- [a]	-- [a]
30-34 years.....	4.670	2.721	5.030 [b]	3.673 [b]	5.258	2.529	5.829 [b]	3.920 [b]
35-39 years.....	7.195	3.933	7.114	4.517	7.220	3.666	7.736	6.073
40-44 years.....	9.869	5.924	9.608	6.117	9.911	5.520	10.451	8.221
45-49 years.....	13.626	7.967	12.695	8.422	12.642	7.484	13.844	10.703
50-54 years.....	15.882	12.060	19.715	11.769	14.574	11.204	21.263	14.813
55-59 years.....	15.888	15.434	25.141	17.627	14.070	14.396	26.664	19.345
60-64 years.....	31.717	23.075	37.089	25.297	27.695	21.223	38.797	27.403
65-69 years.....	36.836	25.934	40.313	36.877	30.159	24.364	41.471	34.136
70-74 years.....	51.568	34.763	52.131	47.002	41.865	32.377	53.153	43.220
75-79 years.....	61.161	46.081	61.383	51.378	51.144	42.733	61.933	51.587
80-84 years.....	97.907	71.082	86.837	80.460	81.472	65.647	87.253	80.460
85 years & over.	153.597	94.375	137.994	151.275	124.417	83.900	139.435	86.192

Source: Uncorrected death rates and indexes based on tabulations of 1959-61 deaths and 1960 population as compiled by NCHS and Bureau of the Census from characteristics reported on each record. Corrected rates and indexes based on estimates of deaths corrected for discrepancies in the reporting of marital status on death certificates and census records (see text for details of correction procedure).

[a] Rate not shown because less than 200 deaths reported in this subgroup of the population.

[b] Only 200-499 deaths reported in this age-sex-color-marital status subgroup of the population.

NOTES

Chapter 2. Education and Income Differentials

1. Earlier studies have referred to restricted universes. For example, an inverse relationship between 1955 earnings and 1955-59 mortality was found among males 20-64 years of age insured under the Old Age and Survivors Insurance system (based on a one-percent sample of wage-earners covered by the Bureau of Old Age and Survivors Insurance in 1955 and followed for mortality through 1959).

2. The mortality differentials obtained from the 1960 Matched Records Study are limited to persons 25 years of age and over. Although death records for persons under 25 years of age were also matched with the 1960 census records—and their match rates were not substantially lower than other age groups—two problems complicate the estimation of differential mortality for persons under 25. First is the fact that most of these deaths refer to infants, and most of the infants who died between May and August 1960 were born after April 1, the census date; this greatly complicates the problem of computing "expected deaths" for the age group under one. Second, a socioeconomic index for persons under 25 would have to be something like family income or father's occupation, items that were not available for all persons under 25.

3. Although the mortality ratios derived from the Matched Records Study are based on age-adjusted ratios of actual to expected deaths—sometimes called indirectly standardized mortality ratios—they are not direct measures of conventional ratios in the sense that the subpopulations whose ratios are 1.00 did not provide the death rates for computing expected deaths for each of the more detailed subgroups into which the subpopulation is divided; for example, in Table 2.1 death rates for males 25-64 years old were not used to calculate expected deaths for each of the education subgroups into which these males are divided. Rather, age-specific death rates for the total population in the United States in 1960 were used to calculate expected deaths in each color-sex-education subgroup of the population, and each ratio in Table 2.1, for example, is a "relative" which expresses the ratio of actual to expected deaths for a particular education or income level as a proportion of the same ratio for the color-sex-age subtotal to which it belongs. In other words, the ratio of actual to expected deaths for each color-sex-age subgroup (for example, white males 25-64 years of age) was arbitrarily set equal to 1.00 to enable direct comparison of the size and pattern of education and income differentials in different subgroups of the population. The procedures used to calculate actual and expected deaths are described in Appendix A.

4. There were too few persons 65 and over with 4 years or more of college to permit computation of separate ratios for 1-3 years and 4 years of college. If, in order to be comparable with men 65 and over, the category "college 1 year or more" is used as the highest education level for men 25-64 years old, the education differential is reduced from 64 to 49 percent, still a much greater differential than for men 65 and over.

5. The education variable was selected for this calculation in the Matched

Records Study because after about age 25 education is completed and remains fixed for each individual. Consequently, the assumptions of the life table model apply more readily to education than to income, occupation, and other socioeconomic characteristics, which may change over the lifespan of an individual. The procedures used to derive abridged life tables for persons with different levels of education assume, essentially, that the pattern of education differentials derived from May-August deaths *within each sex-color-age subgroup* represents the pattern for the entire year. These procedures are elaborated in Appendix A.

6. The statistical significance of the difference between the income differentials of 64 and 50 percent for unrelated individuals and family members, respectively, has not been tested. All of the estimates from the Matched Records Study are subject to sampling and other errors (see the discussion of reliability in Appendix A). For this reason more emphasis should be placed on consistency of patterns—for example, continuous decreases in mortality as level of education or income increases or the repetition of stronger associations below age 65 than above age 65 among males and females, whites and nonwhites, etc.—than on precise measures of the difference in mortality ratios among adjacent income levels.

7. Income reported in the 1960 census included wages, salary, commissions or tips from all jobs; profits or fees from working in own business, professional practice, or farm; and income from Social Security or other pensions, veteran's payments, rent (minus expenses), interest and dividends, unemployment insurance, welfare payments, or other sources.

8. This fact was documented in a special tabulation of decedents by number of weeks worked during 1959, which showed, for example, that a much lower proportion of the male decedents 25-64 years of age had worked throughout 1959 than was the case for the total male population of the same age. (This tabulation was made by the Population Research Center, University of Chicago, from the sample of May-August deaths included in the NCHS Special Sample Survey [see Appendix A].)

9. Theoretically, if deaths from each cause were distributed uniformly throughout the year *and if* the Stage II census sample had included exactly 25 percent of the total population of the United States, then the indexes in column 7 of Table A.14 should be 8.3 percent (that is, one-twelfth, or one-third times one-fourth). Actually, slightly less than one-third—31 percent to be exact—of all deaths in the United States in 1960 occurred during the four-month period May through August, and slightly less than 25 percent of the May-August deaths were designated to be in the total Stage II census.

Chapter 4. Socioeconomic Differentials in a Metropolis

1. The Chicago SMSA includes Cook, DuPage, Kane, Lake, McHenry, and Will counties, Illinois; the ring is the portion of the SMSA outside the city of Chicago.

2. The death statistics by socioeconomic group for 1929-31 were compiled by Hauser for his Ph.D. dissertation (1938), from death certificates in the files of the city of Chicago Board of Health and the County Clerk of Cook County;

death statistics by socioeconomic group for 1940 were compiled by Mayer for his Ph.D. dissertation (1950) using punched cards provided by the Chicago Board of Health and original death certificates filed in the Cook County Recorder's office; 1950 death statistics by census tract for the city of Chicago were obtained from the Chicago Board of Health (which provided a duplicate deck of their mortality cards for deaths occurring in Chicago to Chicago residents) and the Illinois Department of Public Health (which provided a deck of cards for deaths occurring outside Chicago to Chicago residents); 1960 death statistics by census tract for the city of Chicago were provided by the Illinois Department of Public Health, in the form of census tract summary cards for 1960 deaths to Chicago residents. The 1950 and 1960 death statistics for the Chicago SMSA were provided by the Illinois Department of Public Health. Deaths for the Chicago SMSA and the city in 1950 and 1960 included deaths occurring anywhere in Illinois to Chicago residents, as well as some occurrences outside the state that were reported to the State Department of Public Health through reciprocal agreements with other states. Death statistics for the city of Chicago in 1930 and 1940 covered all deaths that occurred in Cook County to residents of the city. Both Hauser and Mayer cite evidence that the registration of deaths for Chicago was virtually complete, and that no corrections for underregistration were needed.

3. For example, if both the white and the nonwhite population in tracts with less than $3,250 median family income had been assigned to socioeconomic Group 1 in 1950, this group would have included 18 percent of the total population of Chicago and would, therefore, be in line with the proportion of the total population in Group 1 in earlier years. However, Group 1 would then have included 88 percent of the nonwhite population in 1950 as compared with 22 percent in 1930 and 1940, and only 6 percent of the white population in 1950 as compared with 17 percent in 1930 and 1940.

4. The 1950 median was calculated by subtracting the income distribution for Lake County, Indiana, and adding the distribution for McHenry County, Illinois, to the income distribution for the Chicago Standard Metropolitan Area as defined in 1950, in order to obtain 1950 data for the area as it was defined in 1960. (Sources of income data: *1950 Census of Population*, vol. 2, pt. 13, tables 37 and 45, and pt. 14, table 45; *1960 Census of Population, Census Tracts, Chicago, Illinois SMSA*, table P-1.)

5. A comparison with life expectancy in the United States is omitted in Table 4.8 because abridged life tables for the Chicago Study were calculated by a simpler method than that used for the official United States abridged life tables. The Chicago life tables for 1930 to 1960 were calculated as follows: (1) The infant mortality rate (deaths divided by births) was taken as equal to q_0. (2) The $_nq_x$ probabilities for whites were calculated from the Reed-Merrell tables, using age-specific death rates ($_nm_x$) for the age group 1-4, for 10-year age intervals between ages 5 and 45, and for 5-year age intervals thereafter up to ages 85 and over; $_nq_x$ probabilities for nonwhites were calculated using the Reed-Merrell tables and $_nm_x$ values for the age group 1-4 and for 10-year age intervals thereafter up to ages 75 and over. (3) The functions ℓ_x and $_nd_x$ were calculated from the formulas inherent in their definition. (4) The $_nL_x$ function for ages 1-4 was derived from the approximation,

$$_nL_x = 3400 + 1.184 \, \ell_1 + 2.782 \, \ell_5;$$

for age intervals up to the terminal open-ended interval; $_nL_x$ was calculated from the approximation, $_nL_x = _nd_x \div _nm_x$; $_\infty L_x$ for the last open-ended age interval was calculated from the same approximation, namely, $_\infty L_x = T_x = \ell_x \div _\infty m_x$. (5) T_x was then calculated Σ_nL_x, and $\overset{\circ}{e}_x$ as $T_x \div \ell_x$; both by definition. The one exception to this procedure was that 1930 life tables for the white population were calculated from the same 10-year age intervals used for nonwhites on all four dates.

Chapter 5. Socioeconomic Differentials by Cause of Death

1. Most of this analysis is taken from Kitagawa and Hauser, "Education Differentials in Mortality by Cause of Death, United States, 1960," *Demography*, 5, (1968), 333-53.

2. Deaths were classified (by the NCHS) in accordance with the Seventh Revision of the International Lists of Diseases and Causes of Death (see *Manual of the International Statistical Classification of Diseases, Injuries, and Causes of Death, Based on the Recommendation of the Seventh Revision Conference, 1955*, vol. 1, Geneva, Switzerland, World Health Organization, 1957).

3. Sex differentials could not be computed for all of the causes reported in Table 5.2 because the estimation procedures for males and females were independent, and larger numbers of deaths were required for reliable sex differentials by education and age than for education differentials within each sex-age group.

Chapter 6. Differential Mortality by Race, Nativity, Country of Origin, Marital Status, and Parity

1. Estimates of corrected deaths by age have been published by the National Center for Health Statistics in a report on the comparability of age on death certificates and census records (June 1968, table 8). The final estimates differ slightly from the preliminary estimates sent to us at the time computations were made for the present analysis. The revisions were so minor that recomputation of the corrected rates did not seem worthwhile, the only difference between the two estimates being a minor adjustment to retain the total number of reported deaths for each sex-color group. The preliminary estimates by age yielded totals that differed slightly from the reported numbers, as is evident in the small "percent differences" for three of the sex-color subtotals in rate no. 2 of Table 6.1.

2. The selection of "census age" as the basis for corrected rate no. 2 was determined by the nature of the data available for this correction and not by any evidence that age was reported more accurately on the census record than on the death record. That is, the sample of matched deaths for which a cross classification of census age by death certificate age was available provided a reasonable basis for estimating the census age of decedents from their reported death certificate age, but it did not necessarily provide a reasonable basis for correcting the reported census age of the total population.

3. Given the acknowledged roughness of the estimated net census under-counts (Siegel, 1968, p. 3), and the fact that the adjustments for discrepancies in age reporting were derived from deaths matched with census records, there is no direct way to determine inconsistencies in the two sets of corrections. However, one can rationalize as follows: (1) if it is assumed that age is reported correctly on the death certificate and that discrepancies between death certificate age and census age for matched decedents are representative of age misstatement in the census population, age misstatement in the census can be estimated as roughly equal to the "percent differences" for rate no. 2 in Table 6.1 *only with the signs reversed*; (2) next, differences between these estimates of census age misstatement and Siegel's estimates of net census undercounts—which are approximately by the "percent differences" for rate no. 3 in Table 6.1 and which include both age misstatement and census underenumeration—can be used to infer "net census underenumeration." In other words, if one adds the percent differences reported in Table 7.1 for rates no. 2 and no. 3 (which is equivalent to subtracting the negative of no. 2 from no. 3) one can infer net census underenumeration by age, sex, and color given the assumptions stated above. This procedure cannot be applied to the five-year intervals above age 65, of course, because of the assumption of constant net undercount above this age. However, the net undercount for age 65 and over (shown for each age above 65 in rate no. 3, Table 7.1) can be compared with the following corrections for age discrepancies (rate no. 2) for the age interval 65 and over: −0.8 and −0.9 percent for white males and females, respectively, and 6.8 and 13.7 for nonwhite males and females. The major inconsistencies in the two sets of corrections—following from these assumptions—are, first, an implied overenumeration of white males and females in several groups under age 45 and, second, an implied overenumeration of nonwhites over age 65 compensated for by high under-enumeration between ages 50 and 65. It is difficult to determine which assumption is at fault in the case of the first inconsistency, but the second inconsistency is probably due in large part to errors in estimates of the net census undercounts at the older ages.

4. The correction for discrepancies between the reporting of race on the two records was made by converting the reported distribution of 1959-61 deaths by "death certificate race" to an estimated distribution of deaths by "estimated census race," using a cross classification of race on the death certificate by race on the 1960 census record for all matched Stage I decedents included in the 1960 Matched Records Study (NCHS, May 1969). The estimates were made by allocating reported 1959-61 deaths for each race to an estimated census classification by race according to the cross classification of that death certificate racial group by census race in the tabulation of matched Stage I decedents mentioned above, and then summing the estimated census distributions over all the death certificate racial groups.

5. The same abridged method was used to construct life tables for each of the racial groups. The life expectancies obtained for whites and nonwhites are very close to the official United States life tables, 1959-61, for whites and nonwhites. The life expectancies for the Japanese females are slightly lower than those obtained by Hechter and Borhani (1965) for California, a somewhat

unexpected result because the regional differentials in Chapter 7 suggest that the West has slightly higher mortality than the total United States. However, the difference may well be within the range of the combined effect of sampling error, the area covered, and the method of constructing the abridged life tables. The life tables by race were calculated (using 10-year age intervals) as follows: (1) the infant mortality rate was taken as q_0; (2) $_nq_x$ was calculated from the Reed-Merrell tables of equivalent values for $_nm_x$ and $_nq_x$; (3) $_nL_x$ was calculated from the equations, $_1L_0 = 100,000 - (1 - f_0)d_0$; $_4L_1 = 3,400 + 1.184\ \ell_1 + 2.782\ \ell_5$; $_{10}L_5 = 5(\ell_5 + \ell_{15})$; for ages 15-64, $_{10}L_x = 5(\ell_x + \ell_{x+10}) + .41667\ (_nd_{x+10} - _nd_{x-10})$; $_{10}L_{65} = .83333\ (-\ell_{55} + 8\ell_{65} + 5\ell_{75})$; $_\infty L_{75} = \ell_{75} \div _\infty m_{75}$; (4) ℓ_x, $_nd_x$, T_x and $\overset{\circ}{e}_x$ calculated by definition.

6. Correction for discrepancies in the reporting of nativity on the two records was made by converting the reported distribution of 1959-61 deaths by "death certificate nativity" to an estimated distribution of deaths by "estimated census nativity" following a procedure similar to that described in note 4 for race. In this case, the conversion was based on a cross classification of nativity on the death certificate by nativity on the 1960 census records by 10-year age intervals for white matched Stage II decedents included in the 1960 Matched Records Study (see Appendix A and NCHS, May 1969).

7. Conversion of country of birth reported on the death certificate for the foreign born to estimated census country of birth was based on a cross classification of country of birth on the death certificates by country of birth on the census records for matched Stage II decedents included in the 1960 Matched Records Study who were reported as foreign-born white on *both* records (NCHS, May 1969). As stated in the text, it would have been preferable to have the cross classification include the native population as well so that the relative under-reporting of foreign born in the census could have been reflected in the corrections for deaths. The net result is that the correction procedure used adjusts only for discrepancies in the specification of countries for those who were foreign-born white on both records. The fact that the comparison of response classification referred to foreign-born whites rather than all foreign born probably did not affect the results significantly, however, since virtually all of the foreign born were white in the comparison of response tabulation by nativity and race simultaneously (of the total 13,800 reported as foreign born on the death certificates 13,554 were white, and of the total 12,772 reported as foreign born in the 1960 census records 12,554 were white).

8. The corrections for discrepant reporting of marital status were made by converting the reported marital status distribution of 1959-61 deaths, within ten-year age intervals of the four sex-color subgroups, to an estimated census marital status distribution using a cross classification of death certificate marital status by census marital status within each ten-year age interval of the four sex-color subgroups; this cross classification was tabulated from all matched Stage II deaths in the 1960 Matched Records Study (NCHS, May 1969). The corrections were made by allocating each reported marital status category of 1959-61 deaths according to its cross classification by census marital status for matched Stage II deaths, and then summing the results of the allocations for each marital category.

Chapter 7. Geographic Differentials and Socioeconomic Correlates

1. For procedures followed in the delineation of the economic subregions see Donald J. Bogue and Calvin L. Beale, *Economic Areas of the United States*, Glencoe, Ill.: the Free Press, 1961, pp. xxxix-xc.

2. In preparing the maps shown in Figures 7.1 to 7.6, three categories of subregions are differentiated: (*a*) those with death rates below Q_1, (*b*) those with death rates above Q_3, and (*c*) those with death rates between Q_1 and Q_3 or the middle half of the subregions. Thus, the boundaries of the class intervals for death rates on the maps conform to the quartiles reported in Table 7.5.

3. Similar correlations between death rates for whites and Negroes (indirectly standardized for age) are substantially higher, 0.60 for all males and 0.30 for all females, indicating that the almost complete lack of association between white and nonwhite rates may be due in large part to the varying proportions, in the nonwhite group, of other races (especially Japanese) with much lower mortality than the Negroes.

4. The correlation analysis for 1950 was made as part of an intensive analysis of 1950 materials supported by a research grant (R 4397) from the National Institutes of Health to the Population Research Center, University of Chicago. Similar analyses were not carried out for other years during the 30-year period for which data are reported in Chapter 4.

5. Initially, the following classes of census tracts were excluded from the correlation analysis: (*a*) 38 tracts with less than 50 families reporting income (that is, with income data based on less than 10 families because income data were collected in the 20 percent sample of the 1950 census), (*b*) 12 tracts with less than 50 percent of their population in dwelling units (excluded because the income and housing indexes covered less than one-half the population of the tract); (*c*) 7 tracts with more than 10 percent of their population in institutions or more than 5 percent residing in homes for the aged (excluded because the institutional population might unduly influence death rates); (*d*) tracts with less than 1,500 total population (excluded because of small numbers); and (*e*) tracts containing a public housing project (excluded because of the "abnormal" relation between housing and income for residents of public housing projects). In all, these excluded tracts had 8 percent of the city's total population, and 14 percent of the city's Negro population. The selection of tracts for the correlation analyses was made from the remaining tracts as follows: (*a*) *Tracts with 90 percent or more Negro population*. All remaining census tracts with 90 percent or more Negroes were included in the correlation analysis for this group (55 tracts); in the correlation analysis for Negro males and females, an additional 11 tracts were discarded because they had less than 10 (actual or expected) male or female deaths. (*b*) *Tracts with 90 percent or more white population*. A random sample of 84 tracts was selected from the tracts with 90 percent or more white population which were not excluded from the analysis for one of the reasons cited above; in the correlation analysis for males and females an additional 15 tracts were discarded because they had less than 10 (actual or expected) male or female deaths. (*c*) *Random sample of all tracts*. A random sample of 115 census tracts from all the tracts not excluded for one of the reasons cited above was selected by supplementing the sample of "tracts with 90 percent or more white

population," with a similar proportion of tracts from the universe of tracts with less than 90 percent of the population white and which were not excluded for reasons cited above.

6. Of course, the variations in death rates and socioeconomic indexes were much less among the large, heterogeneous populations of states and economic subregions than among the small, more homogeneous populations of census tracts. In other words, much more of the variation in mortality and socioeconomic level among individuals is buried within the large state and subregion areas than is buried within the small census tract subdivisions of a large metropolitan area. Consequently, the correlations obtained with census tracts as geographic units more closely approximate relationships among individuals than do correlations based on states and economic subregions.

Chapter 8. Summary and Implications

1. Problems relating to the delivery of medical services in the United States are under increasing scrutiny and are now receiving unprecedented attention. Medicare and Medicaid are but intial steps in the improvement of medical care and will undoubtedly be followed by more comprehensive programs, public and private, to provide the nation and especially lower socioeconomic classes with better medical attention.

2. The differentials reported here are based on age-adjusted death rates corrected for discrepancies in the reporting of marital status on death certificates and census schedules. As was pointed out in Chapter 6, differences in mortality by marital status based on death and census statistics as reported on their respective records are exaggerated by an overstatement of mortality for divorced and widowed persons and an understatement of mortality for single and married persons.

3. Age-adjusted death rates standardized by the direct method were used for the analyses based on tabulations of U.S. death statistics for 1959-61, and for Chicago area death statistics for the entire period 1930-1960, whereas age-adjusted mortality ratios standardized by the indirect method were of necessity used for most of the analyses based on the United States 1960 Matched Records Study.

4. Direct calculations of excess deaths from each cause—comparable to the calculations made for all causes of death summarized in Table 8.1—would have required that age-specific death rates for college-educated males and females be applied to the age composition of the three less educated groups. The necessary age-specific death rates for each cause were not available, however. Instead, indirect approximations were made by calculating the number and percentage of the estimated "total Stage II Census deaths" (see column 4, Table A.14) from each cause that would *not* have occurred if the mortality indexes for each education group had been the same as that obtained in Table 5.2 for white persons of the same sex who had completed one or more years of college. These estimated percentages for each cause were then applied to the total number of 1960 deaths from that cause, separately for white males and females in the two age groups, to obtain estimates of excess deaths in the white population in 1960. Net excess deaths for all causes combined (in Tables 8.2 and 8.3) and for the

three general cause groups—malignant neoplasms, major cardiovascular-renal diseases, and all accidents—were estimated by summing excess deaths, negative as well as positive, for their component specific causes. Specific causes of death with negative "excess deaths" are positively associated with education, and there would have been a larger number of deaths from these causes if the less educated groups had the same mortality as the college educated.

5. The indirect calculations estimate that 9 percent of the white male deaths and 29 percent of the white female deaths, 25 and over, were excess, as compared with estimates of 10 and 27 percent, respectively, by the direct calculation. The largest difference between the two calculations of excess deaths pertain to white males 25-64, for whom 21 percent of the deaths were excess by the direct calculation as compared with 25 percent by the indirect calculation.

6. The countereffect of causes positively related to education was much greater among men than women, "net excess" mortality for males being a net balance of 94,000 deaths that would not have occurred (from causes inversely associated with education) and 21,000 additional deaths that would have occurred (from causes positively associated with education), as compared with a net balance for females of 179,000 deaths that would not have occurred and 5,000 additional deaths that would have occurred.

Appendix A

1. For example, see *Vital Statistics—Special Reports*, vol. 53, no. 1 (June 1961), *The Comparability of Reports on Occupation from Vital Records and the 1950 Census.*

2. The decision to limit the study to deaths occurring during the four-month period was made after several discussions with Census Bureau personnel and examination of the match rates by month in the 1950 matching of death and census records for the report on comparability of occupational responses. April deaths were excluded because of potentially high "nonmatch" rates due to the fact that the census enumeration period—especially for the 25-percent sample schedules—was spread over a significant part of the month, and a significant proportion of the April decedents may have died before their households were enumerated. In the 1950 matching operation, the "nonmatch" rate for August was 23 percent compared with 20 percent for June and July, and 22 percent for May. This encouraged the inclusion of deaths for August, but left uncertain how quickly "nonmatch" rates might increase for later months. Because of this uncertainty—and the real, though unknown, risks involved in extending the period to a year to avoid potential seasonal bias—it was decided to confine the study period to May-August deaths.

3. The weighted count of 533,742 deaths covered by the study (see Table A.3), based on tabulations of punched cards for the 340,033 deaths selected for the match operation, differs from the total number of 534,623 deaths for May through August 1960, reported in *Vital Statistics of the United States, 1960*, vol. 2, part A, table 5-3, for a variety of reasons, including processing errors in selection of the sample and handling of the cards through the census match operation and tabulation procedures.

4. Monroe G. Sirken, James W. Pifer, and Morton L. Brown, *Design of*

Surveys Linked to the Death Record, National Center for Health Statistics, September 1962.

5. The Census match operation itself had to await the completion of the regular processing of the 1960 census records by the Census Bureau, as well as the preparation of duplicate copies of the death certificates and punched mortality cards by NCHS, who then forwarded them to the Census Bureau for the match operation. It was clear from the beginning that it would take at least two to three years to identify unmatched decedents, and it was judged too risky, in terms of potentially high nonresponse rates and poor quality of information, to wait this long to attempt a Survey follow-up of unmatched decedents.

6. The procedures followed in the match operation are relevant to these alternative explanations for unmatched decedents. Matching was done manually, first by allocating the residence address reported on each death certificate to its enumeration district (ED) in the 1960 census, and then searching the Stage I census records for the ED until the record for the decedent was located. If the decedent was not listed in any of the possible ED's assigned to his residence address *and* if he had died in an institution, the institution's address was then allocated to an ED and this ED's file of census records was searched for the decedent. Decedents whose Stage I census records were located and were designated for inclusion in the Stage II (25-percent) sample were then searched in the Stage II files in the locations indicated on their Stage I records. Special procedures for decedents under one year of age—most of whom were born after April 1, 1960, the official census date—included a search for the mother of the decedent (whose name was listed on the infant's death certificate) in the ED file of Stage I Census records. The fact that the nonmatch rates for infants under one were no higher than the rates for young women 15-34 years (their mothers' ages, in most cases) indicates the success of this procedure for locating infants who had not been born at the time of the census.

7. See Jacob S. Siegel, "Completeness of Coverage of the Nonwhite Population in the 1960 Census and Current Estimates, and Some Implications," in David Heer, ed., *Social Statistics and the City* (Cambridge, Mass.: Harvard University Press, 1968).

8. The NCHS Sample Survey is the only source of information on match bias by social and economic characteristics which are not reported on the death certificate. Consequently, the rates in Tables A.5 to A.8 are based on relatively small numbers and subject to larger sampling errors than the rates in Tables A.2 and A.3.

9. This procedure for estimating the "Stage II Census equivalent" of unmatched deaths was necessary because the match operation was made in two steps. First, the 340,033 death records were matched with Stage I (100-percent enumeration) census records and separated into two groups, matched Stage I deaths and unmatched Stage I deaths. Second, only the matched Stage I decedents who were identified as in the Stage II (25-percent) census sample were searched in the Stage II census records. The net result was that the following sets of basic tabulations of deaths were possible after the match operation was completed: (1) tabulations of matched (Stage I) deaths by either Stage I census or death certificate characteristics, (2) tabulations of unmatched Stage I deaths by death certificate characteristics, (3) tabulations of matched Stage II deaths by either Stage II census or death certificate characteristics.

10. Exact values of unweighted numbers were not known because Stage II deaths were tabulated by census age and color in weighted numbers only, whereas the sample was selected on the basis of death certificate age and color. Consequently, unweighted numbers were estimated by applying sampling proportions (one for white decedents 25-64 years of age and for all nonwhites, one-half for white decedents 65-74, and one-fifth for white decedents 75 years and over) to the weighted tabulation of matched Stage II deaths.

11. This choice was made not because of any evidence that the census characteristics are more accurate than the characteristics reported in the NCHS survey or on the death certificate, but because this was the best alternative for consistent numerators and denominators for our mortality indexes given the basic data available from the study.

12. Tabulations of matched Stage II deaths in the Matched Records Study were made for 41 causes of death, based on recommendations by authors of eight of the monographs in the APHA series of monographs on Vital and Health Statistics (each monograph covering a general cause of death); the 23 causes for which education differentials in mortality were estimated include those recommended causes which had sufficiently large number of deaths, and combinations of more detailed causes when numbers were small and the combined cause group was thought to be meaningful. The nonmatch rates in Table A.8 do not cover exactly the same 23 causes of death because the tabulations of matched and unmatched Stage I deaths from which they were computed identified 29 causes of death which could not be collapsed to the same 23 categories.

13. In several cases it was necessary to compute ratios of matched Stage II deaths from a given cause to matched Stage I deaths from a more general cause, but these ratios could then be applied to unmatched Stage I deaths from the same more general cause of death to obtain the unmatched Stage II control totals for the given cause. This was done for seven of the causes of death listed in the stub of Table A.14 as follows: (1) Cause 2a, because matched and unmatched Stage I deaths referred to ISC codes 150-156A and 157-159 combined instead of code 151 only; in 1960, deaths coded 151 comprised 25 percent of the white male deaths and 18 percent of the white female deaths from causes assigned codes 150-156A and 157-159 combined. (2) Cause 2b, because matched and unmatched Stage I deaths referred to ISC codes 150-156A and 157-159 combined instead of codes 152-154 only; in 1960, deaths coded 152-154 comprised 41 percent of the white male deaths and 51 percent of the white female deaths from causes assigned codes 150-156A and 157-159 combined. (3) Cause 2c, because matched and unmatched Stage I deaths referred to ISC codes 160-164 instead of codes 162-163; in 1960, deaths coded 162-163 comprised 92 percent of the white male deaths and 91 percent of the white female deaths from causes assigned codes 160-164. (4) Cause 2e, because matched and unmatched Stage I deaths referred to ISC codes 171-179 instead of codes 171-175; in 1960, deaths coded 171-175 comprised 96 percent of the white female deaths assigned codes 171-179. (5) Cause 2f, because matched and unmatched Stage I deaths referred to ISC codes 171-179 instead of code 177 only; in 1960, deaths coded 177 comprised 94 percent of the white male deaths assigned codes 171-179. (6) Cause 4c, because matched and unmatched Stage I deaths referred to ISC codes 420-422 instead of codes 420 and 422; in 1960, deaths coded 420 and 422 comprised 99 percent of both the white male and

white female deaths assigned codes 420-422. (7) Cause 4d, because matched and unmatched Stage I deaths referred to ISC codes 440-447 and 451-468 combined instead of codes 440-447 only; in 1960, deaths coded 440-447 comprised 71 percent of the white male deaths and 84 percent of the white female deaths assigned codes 440-447, 451-468.

14. The education distribution within each cause of death is not reported in Table A.14, as it is for all causes combined in Table A.12.

15. The unweighted counts in Table A.1 indicate that although 24.6 percent (64,675) of the 262,966 matched Stage I decedents were assigned to the Stage II sample, only 23.7 percent (62,405) were included on the final matched Stage II tape file from which the tabulations of deaths for this study were run.

16. Occupation information (current or last) was reported on 88 percent of the NCHS survey questionnaires returned for white male decedents 25 years and older who had worked at some time during or since 1950. The percentages with occupation reported were higher in the younger ages and for decedents matched with census records, but it did not go below 80 percent in any of the age groups used in the analysis, as is indicated in the figures below:

	25 Years & Over	25-44 Years	45-64 Years	65-74 Years
White males	88	92	91	87
Matched with census	89	94	92	89
Not matched with census	82	87	84	81

These percentages are based on NCHS survey decedents for whom questionnaires were returned, including those for whom the question on "year last worked" was not answered (6.0 percent of the white males with questionnaires returned did not have information on date last worked); this allocation of "unknown work experience" is in accord with 1960 census procedures.

17. The decisive factor in selecting marital status as reported on the death certificate rather than as reported on the survey questionnaire as the preliminary estimate for unmatched NCHS survey decedents (column 2, Table A.19), was the availability of the cross classification shown in Table A.20 which permitted conversion of death certificate marital status to estimated census marital status on a more reliable basis than would have been possible if survey marital status had to be converted to estimated census marital status using a cross classification of survey by census marital status for the much smaller number matched decedents who were included in the NCHS Sample Survey. The very small proportions of widowed and divorced at some ages made the larger numbers especially desirable for the marital status adjustment by the three age groups shown.

18. Nathan Keyfitz, "Sampling Variance of Demographic Characteristics," *Human Biology*, 38, no. 1 (February 1966), 22-41, and "Sampling Variance of Standardized Mortality Rates," *Human Biology*, 38, no. 3 (September 1966), 309-317.

19. See National Center for Health Statistics, *Vital Statistics–Special Reports*,

vol. 9, no. 54, *A Short Method for Constructing an Abridged Life Table*, by Lowell J. Reed and Margaret Merrell (June 1949).

20. See National Center for Health Statistics, *Vital Statistics of the United States, 1960*, vol. 2, pt. A, table 2.2.

21. The formulas are taken from T.N.E. Greville, "Short Methods of Constructing Abridged Life Tables," *The Record of the American Institute of Actuaries*, vol. 32, pt. 1, no. 65, June 1943.

REFERENCES

Altenderfer, Marion E. (1947). "Relationship between Per Capita Income and Mortality, in the Cities of 100,000 or More Population," *Public Health Reports*, 62 (no. 48), 1681-1691.

Antonovsky, Aaron (1967). "Social Class, Life Expectancy and Overall Mortality," *The Milbank Memorial Fund Quarterly*, 45 (April 1967, part 1), 31-73.

Benjamin, B. (1965). *Social and Economic Factors Affecting Mortality*. The Hague and Paris: Mouton.

Berkson, Joseph (1962). "Mortality and Marital Status," *American Journal of Public Health*, 52 (no. 8), 1318-1329.

Bourgeois-Pichat, Jean (1971). *Present State of Demographic Research with Regard to Economic and Social Development*. United Nations, Economic and Social Council, Expert Working Group on Population Research in National Institutions, Lyon, France, 3-11 June 1971 (E/CN.9/AC.13/R.2).

Dollar, Melvin L. (1942). *Vital Statistics for Cook County and Chicago*. Chicago: Works Projects Administration Publications in Research and Records.

Dublin, Louis I., Alfred J. Lotka, and Mortimer Spiegelman (1949). *Length of Life*, rev. ed. New York: Ronald Press.

Duncan, Otis Dudley (1961). "Occupational Components of Educational Differences in Income," *Journal of the American Statistical Association*, 56 (December 1961), 783-792.

Duncan, Otis Dudley (1964). "Residential Areas and Differential Fertility," *Eugenics Quarterly*, 2 (June 1964), 82-89.

Edwards, Alba W. (1943). *Comparative Occupation Statistics for the United States, 1870 to 1940*, Sixteenth Census of the United States: 1940. Washington, D.C.

Farr, William (1885). *Vital Statistics: A Memorial Volume of Selections from the Reports and Writings of William Farr* (edited by Noel A. Humphreys). London: Offices of the Sanitary Institute and Edward Stanford.

General Register Office (1958). *1951 Census of England and Wales, General Report*. London: H.M. Stationery Office.

Gordon, Tavia (1957). "Mortality Experience among the Japanese in the United States, Hawaii, and Japan," *Public Health Reports*, vol. 72, pp. 543ff.

Gordon, Tavia (1967). "Further Mortality Experience among Japanese Americans," *Public Health Reports*, 82 (no. 11), 973-984.

Grove, Robert D., and Alice M. Hetzel (1968). *Vital Statistics Rates in the United States, 1940-1960*, National Center for Health Statistics. Washington, D.C.

Guralnick, Lillian, and Charles B. Nam (1959). "Census-NOVS Study of Death Certificates Matched to Census Records," *The Milbank Memorial Fund Quarterly*, 36 (April 1959), 144-153.

Hamilton, C. Horace (1955). "Ecological and Social Factors in Mortality Variation," *Eugenics Quarterly*, 2 (September 1955), 212-223.

Hauser, Philip M. (1938). "Differential Fertility, Mortality and Net Reproduction in Chicago, 1930," unpublished Ph.D. dissertation, Department of Sociology, University of Chicago, 1938.

Hechter, H.H., and N.O. Borhani (1965). "Longevity in Racial Groups Differs," *California's Health*, 22 (no. 15, February 1), 121-122.

Hodge, Robert W., and Paul M. Siegel (1968). "The Measurement of Social Class," *International Encyclopedia of the Social Sciences,* vol. 15, pp. 316-325.

Keyfitz, Nathan (1968). *Introduction to the Mathematics of Population.* Reading, Mass.: Addison-Wesley Publishing Co.

Kitagawa, Evelyn M. (1964). "Standardized Comparisons in Population Research," *Demography*, 1 (1964), 296-315.

Kitagawa, Evelyn M. (1966). "Theoretical Considerations in the Selection of a Mortality Index, and Some Empirical Comparisons," *Human Biology*, 38 (September 1966), 293-308.

Kitagawa, Evelyn M. (1971). "Social and Economic Differentials in Mortality in the United States, 1960," in *International Population Conference, London, 1969*, vol. 2, pp. 980-995. Liège, Belgium: the International Union for the Scientific Study of Population.

Kitagawa, Evelyn M., and Philip M. Hauser (1964). "Trends in Differential Fertility and Mortality in a Metropolis—Chicago," in E.W. Burgess and Donald Bogue (eds.), *Contributions in Urban Sociology*, pp. 59-85. Chicago: the University of Chicago Press.

Kitagawa, Evelyn M., and Philip M. Hauser (1971). "Education and Income Differentials in Mortality, United States, 1960," in Minoru Tachi and Minoru Muramatsu (eds.), *Population Problems in the Pacific: New Dimensions in Pacific Demography*, pp. 157-166. Tokyo, Conveners of Congress Symposium no. 1, the Eleventh Pacific Science Congress, Tokyo, 1966.

Linder, Forrest E., and Robert D. Grove (1943). *Vital Statistics Rates in the United States, 1900-1940*, U.S. Bureau of the Census. Washington, D.C.

MacMahon, B. (1970). "Infant Mortality Rates by Socioeconomic Characteristics, United States, 1964-66." Paper presented at meetings of American Public Health Association, Houston, Texas, October 1970.

Mayer, Albert J., and Richard V. Marks (1954). "Differentials in Infant Mortality, by Race, Economic Level and Cause of Death, for Detroit: 1940 and 1950," *Human Biology*, 26 (May 1954), 143-155.

Moriyama, Iwao M., and Lillian Guralnick (1956). "Occupational and Social Class Differences in Mortality," in *Trends and Differentials in Mortality.* New York: Milbank Memorial Fund.

National Center for Health Statistics (September 1951). *Vital Statistics—Special Reports*, Selected Studies, vol. 33, no. 10, *Mortality, Occupation and Socioeconomic Status* (by Jean Daric). Washington, D.C.

(May 1956). *Vital Statistics—Special Reports*, vol. 39, no. 7, *Mortality from Selected Causes by Marital Status.* Washington, D.C.

(June 1961). *Vital Statistics—Special Reports*, vol. 53, no. 1, *The Comparability of Reports on Occupation from Vital Records and the 1950 Census* (by David L. Kaplan, Elizabeth Parkhurst, and Pascal K. Whelpton). Washington, D.C.

(1963). *Vital Statistics of the United States, 1960*, vol. 2, pt. A. Washington, D.C.

(1964). *United States Life Tables, 1959-61.* Washington, D.C.

(June 1966). *Vital and Health Statistics*, series 20, no. 2, *Mortality Trends in the United States, 1954-63.* Washington, D.C.

(1968). *Vital and Health Statistics*, series 4, no. 8, *The 1968 Revision of the Standard Certificates.* Washington, D.C.

(June 1968). *Vital and Health Statistics*, series 2, no. 29, *Comparability of Age on the Death Certificate and Matching Census Record, United States, May-August 1960.* Washington, D.C.

(January 1969). *Vital and Health Statistics*, series 2, no. 30, *Comparison of the Classification of Place of Residence on Death Certificates and Matching Census Records, United States, May-August 1960.* Washington, D.C.

(May 1969). *Vital and Health Statistics*, series 2, no. 34, *Comparability of Marital Status, Race, Nativity, and Country of Origin on the Death Certificate and Matching Census Record, United States, May-August 1960.* Washington, D.C.

(December 1970). *Vital and Health Statistics*, series 20, nos. 8A and 8B, *Mortality from Selected Causes by Marital Status.* Washington, D.C.

Reiss, Albert J., et al. (1961). *Occupations and Social Status.* New York: Free Press of Glencoe.

Sauer, Herbert I. (1962). "Epidemiology of Cardiovascular Mortality—Geographic and Ethnic," *The American Journal of Public Health*, 52 (no. 1), 94-105.

(1970). "Geographic Differences in the Risk of Premature Death," *Business and Government Review*, University of Missouri (May-June 1970), pp. 19-26.

and Frank R. Brand (1971). "Geographic Patterns in the Risk of Dying," in Helen L. Cannon and Howard C. Hopps (eds.), *Environmental Geochemistry in Health and Disease*, pp. 131-150. Boulder, Colo.: Geological Society of America.

Seidman, Herbert, Lawrence Garfinkel, and Leonard Craig (1962). "Death Rates in New York City by Socio-Economic Class and Religious Group and by Country of Birth, 1949-51," *Jewish Journal of Sociology*, 4 (December 1962), 254-273.

Shapiro, Sam, Edward R. Schlesinger, and Robert E.L. Nesbitt, Jr. (1968). *Infant, Perinatal, Maternal, and Childhood Mortality in the United States.* Cambridge, Mass.: Harvard University Press.

Sheps, Cecil, and J.H. Watkins (1947). "Mortality in the Socio-Economic Districts of New Haven," *The Yale Journal of Biology and Medicine*, 20 (October 1947), 51-80.

Sheps, Mendel C. (1961). "Marriage and Mortality," *American Journal of Public Health*, 51 (no. 4), 547-555.

Shurtleff, D. (1956). "Mortality among the Married," *Journal of American Geriatrics Society*, 4 (July 1956), 654-666.

Siegel, Jacob S. (1968). "Completeness of Coverage of the Nonwhite Population in the 1960 Census and Current Estimates, and Some Implications," in David

M. Heer (ed.), *Social Statistics and the City*, pp. 13-54. Cambridge, Mass.: Harvard University Press.

Spiegelman, Mortimer (1966). *Significant Mortality and Morbidity Trends in the United States since 1900*, rev. ed. Bryn Mawr, Pa.: The American College of Life Underwriters.

Stockwell, Edward (1961). "Socioeconomic Status and Mortality in the United States," *Public Health Reports*, 76 (no. 12), 1081-1086.

     (1963). "A Critical Examination of the Relationship between Socioeconomic Status and Mortality," *American Journal of Public Health*, 53 (no. 6), 956-964.

United Nations (1967). *Demographic Yearbook, 1966*. New York: United Nations.

U.S. Bureau of the Census (1945). *Vital Statistics—Special Reports*, vol. 23, no. 2, *Mortality by Marital Status by Age, Race, and Sex, Urban and Rural, United States, 1940*. Washington, D.C.

     (1963). *U.S. Census of Population: 1960, Educational Attainment*, Final Report PC(2)-5B. Washington, D.C.

U.S. Department of Health, Education and Welfare (1969). *Toward a Social Report*. Washington, D.C.

deVise, Pierre (1967). *Chicago's Widening Color Gap*. Chicago: Community and Family Study Center, University of Chicago.

Wiehl, Dorothy G. (1948). "Mortality and Socio-Environmental Factors," *The Milbank Memorial Fund Quarterly*, 26 (October 1948), 336-365.

Yeracaris, Constantine A. (1955). "Differential Mortality, General and Cause-Specific in Buffalo, 1939-41," *Journal of the American Statistical Association*, 50 (December 1955), 1235-1247.

INDEX

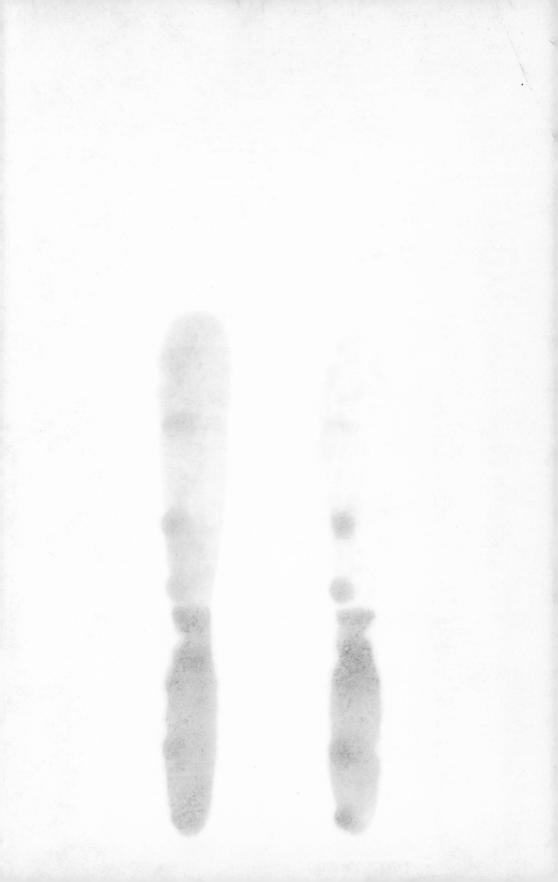

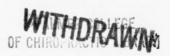